Are Your Health ~~Problems~~ Yeast Connected?

If your answer is "yes" to any question, circle the number in the right hand column. When you've completed the questionnaire, add up the points you've circled. Your score will help you determine the possibility (or probability) that your health problems are yeast connected.

	YES	NO	SCORE
1. Have you taken repeated or prolonged courses of antibacterial drugs?	☐	☐	4
2. Have you been bothered by recurrent vaginal, prostate or urinary infections?	☐	☐	3
3. Do you feel "sick all over," yet the cause hasn't been found?	☐	☐	2
4. Are you bothered by hormone disturbances, including PMS, menstrual irregularities, sexual dysfunction, sugar craving, low body temperature or fatigue?	☐	☐	2
5. Are you unusually sensitive to tobacco smoke, perfumes, colognes and other chemical odors?	☐	☐	2
6. Are you bothered by memory or concentration problems? Do you sometimes feel "spaced out"?	☐	☐	2
7. Have you taken prolonged courses of prednisone or other steroids; or have you taken "the pill" for more than 3 years?	☐	☐	2
8. Do some foods disagree with you or trigger your symptoms?	☐	☐	1
9. Do you suffer with constipation, diarrhea, bloating or abdominal pain?	☐	☐	1
10. Does your skin itch, tingle or burn; or is it unusually dry; or are you bothered by rashes?	☐	☐	1

Scoring for women: If your score is 9 or more, your health problems are probably yeast connected. If your score is 12 or more, your health problems are almost certainly yeast connected.

Scoring for men: If your score is 7 or more, your health problems are probably yeast connected. If your score is 10 or more, your health problems are almost certainly yeast connected.

"An outstanding book! It will help physicians provide cost-effective treatment for many patients."

George C. Miller II, M.D., Fellow, American College of Obstetrics and Gynecology, Lewisburg, Pennsylvania

"Like the late Linus Pauling, Orian Truss and William Crook have given us food for thought. We will need to pursue their ideas for generations to come. They are a stimulus to students and scholars. They help tie together practical medicine with research . . ."

Milan L. Brandon, M.D., Diplomate, American Board of Allergy and Immunology, San Diego, California

"Recommendations in this book may be the key to wellness for many people plagued with chronic health disorders."

Harold Hedges, M.D., Fellow, American Academy of Family Practice, Little Rock, Arkansas

"Without question, Dr. Crook has opened a window on women's medical care. This book should be read by every woman who has ever taken antibiotics without proof of an infection."

Larrian Gillespie, M.D., Urologist and Urogynecologist, Beverly Hills, California

"*The Yeast Connection and the Woman* informs readers of the latest findings and workable approaches to many disorders which affect women. My patients and I are eternally grateful."

C. Richard Mabray, M.D., Fellow, American College of Obstetrics, and Gynecology, Victoria, Texas

"Children with allergies, recurrent ear infections, and developmental problems frequently respond to the medical approaches recommended by Dr. Crook in his new book."

Richard E. Layton, M.D., Fellow, American Academy of Pediatrics, Towson, Maryland

"Dr. Crook provides real answers rather than simply masking the symptoms or creating new problems. His book is an absolute must for anyone who desires to achieve lifelong health."

Michael T. Murray, N.D., President, VITAL Communications, Bellevue, Washington

"Dr. Crook's best book yet—a fine and comprehensive look at yeast and the insidious role it plays in many illnesses."

Marguerite Kelly, Author and Syndicated Columnist, Washington, D.C.

The
Yeast.
Connection
and the
Woman

WILLIAM G. CROOK, M.D.

PROFESSIONAL BOOKS, INC.
Jackson, Tennessee

DISCLAIMER

This book describes relationships which have been observed between the common yeast germ *Candida albicans* and health problems which affect people of all ages and both sexes—especially premenopausal women. *I have written it to serve only as a general informational guide and reference source for both professionals and nonprofessionals.*

For obvious reasons I cannot assume the medical or legal responsibility of having the contents of this book considered as a prescription for anyone.

Treatment of health disorders, including those which appear to be yeast connected, must be supervised by a physician or other licensed health professional. Accordingly, you and the professional who examines and treats you must take the responsibility for the uses made of this book.

Published by Professional Books, Inc., Box 3246, Jackson, Tennessee 38303.

Cover art, book design and typography by ProtoType Graphics, Inc., Nashville, Tennessee.

Library of Congress Catalog Card Number: 95–067424

ISBN: 0-933478-22-4

Manufactured in the United States of America
1 2 3 4 5 6 7 8 9 10 — 00 99 98 97 96 95

To my daughters

Elizabeth
Nancy
Cynthia

What You'll Find
in This Book

◆

In *The Yeast Connection and the Woman,* you'll find

- notes about the common yeast, *Candida albicans,* and how and why superficial yeast infections often cause symptoms in many parts of the body.
- a special message to physicians which includes a discussion of the yeast connection controversy. Included also will be information about new and old studies which provide scientific support for the yeast/human interaction.
- a discussion of health problems which affect *only* women, including recurrent vaginal yeast infections, vulvodynia (burning vulva), PMS and endometriosis.
- answers to the question, "Why do yeast-related problems affect women 8 to 10 times more often than men?"
- information about common health problems which affect women much more often than men, including cystitis and interstitial cystitis, sexual dysfunction and infertility.
- a discussion of still other problems which affect women more often than men, including chronic fatigue syndrome (CFS), fibromyalgia syndrome (FMS), multiple chemical sensitivity syndrome (MCSS), headache, depression and manic depression, multiple sclerosis and other autoimmune diseases.
- yeast-related disorders which affect both sexes, including psoriasis and asthma.
- an easy-to-follow discussion of the steps you'll need to take to regain your health.
- a comprehensive discussion of diets which contain more vegetables and fewer animal products, less protein and fat, but which contain the essential fatty acids.

- new scientific studies to show how and why sugar in the diet promotes yeast overgrowth in the intestinal tract, with answers to the question, "If I can't use sugar, what can I use?"
- a detailed discussion of vitamins and other nutritional supplements.
- *brand new information about nonprescription antiyeast natural remedies, including citrus seed extracts and mathake.* Also, an up-to-date discussion of *Lactobacillus acidophilus* (and other probiotics), Kyolic (and other garlic products), caprylic acid and Tanalbit, a tannic acid medication.
- updated information about nystatin, Nizoral (ketoconazole) and a discussion of the new and highly effective prescription yeast-control medications, Diflucan (fluconazole) and Sporanox (itraconazole).
- a comprehensive discussion of food allergies. Included is information about the "leaky gut" and why food allergies are common in patients with yeast-related disorders.
- detailed instructions for tracking down hidden food allergies.
- a discussion of psychological support and the mind/body connection.
- information about exercise and immunotherapy.
- a discussion of thyroid and other hormones.
- a discussion of laboratory studies. *Yet, I'll emphasize that the diagnosis of a yeast-connected health problem continues to be based mainly on your clinical history and your response to a sugar-free special diet and prescription or nonprescription antiyeast medication.*
- stories and letters from men with yeast-related health problems.
- information about yeast-related health problems in children, including recurrent ear infections, hyperactivity, attention deficits and autism.
- information on many other subjects, including intestinal parasites, dental fillings, yeast-related drunkenness, AIDS, free radicals and health care costs.
- and much, much more.

Acknowledgments

◆

If I listed all the people who have helped me and all the sources which have contributed to this book, the bibliography would be massive and the names legion. Many colleagues and friends will come across their ideas on these pages. As they do, they will know how grateful I am to them for having shared their knowledge and experience with me.

I want to acknowledge my special indebtedness to C. Orian Truss, M.D., of Birmingham, Alabama. This brilliant and courageous internist and allergist first noted the relationship of superficial yeast infections to health problems which affect countless people—especially women.

In the very first chapters of his informative book, *The Missing Diagnosis,* Truss emphasized health problems which affect women. These included not only frequent cystitis and vaginitis, but also multiple other problems which caused countless women to feel "sick all over." Common symptoms included fatigue, depression, headache, PMS and sexual dysfunction—symptoms which had often been attributed to psychological causes.

In discussing yeast-related health problems, Truss said:

> "*This condition is devastating to a woman's ability to function, whether in a career, as wife and mother, or outside the home; its unpredictability often makes it impossible to plan activities requiring more than minimal responsibility. To be shown a physical alternative to psychological factors as the cause of this disability is to be given reason for renewed hope* [emphasis added].
>
> "It is the first small step in the restoration of self-esteem that, first shattered by illness itself, has been further eroded by the feelings of guilt and inadequacy engendered by the endless psychological explanations of this illness.
>
> "It enables an understanding of the principles that underlie the various components of the treatment program, and prepares them

for the inevitable setbacks that occur periodically along the way to recovery. Once understood, women with this condition can show great fortitude, and can accept the fact that patience and time will be required for full recovery."

Truss also noted that,

"Men and boys show the same problems and manifestations except for the severe symptoms related to interference with the hormone cycle in women—the symptoms resulting from yeast infections of the vagina and vulva—and the frequent attacks of urethritis and cystitis.

"Chronic candidiasis is a very real problem in infants and children, interfering in many ways with normal growth and development and performance in school, predisposing them to allergic membranes and a vicious cycle of infections and antibiotics."

During the past 15 years Dr. Truss has shared his knowledge and information with me on countless occasions.

Special thanks are also due to Drs. Sidney Baker, Leo Galland and Elmer Cranton. Their astute observations about yeast-related health problems and the nutritional, allergic, environmental, psychologic and biochemical factors that contribute to health have influenced me for over a decade.

As with my other publications, I'm grateful to John Adams and the entire staff at ProtoType Graphics, Inc., Nashville, Tennessee, for their skillful production services.

Special words of appreciation are due my daughter, Elizabeth, who helped me organize and complete this book and to my daughter, Cynthia, for her delightful illustrations. I'm also grateful to Gregg Bender for his superb illustration of the "antibiotic cascade" and to Jere Perry and the staff of Tennessee Industrial Printers for their graphics.

I'm grateful to Janet Gregory, who typed and re-typed the entire manuscript, and to my Professional Books staff, Georgia Deaton, Kaye Tankersley-Flowers, Karen Glover, Brenda Harris, Nell Sellers and Jan Torre, who helped me in various ways in putting this book together.

Table of Contents

◆

Foreword

◆

Since *The Yeast Connection* was first published in 1983, many new ideas have appeared relative to the role of yeast in human illness. During the past decade, the number of patients who have been diagnosed and successfully treated have been legion. Patient testimonies, many of which are cited in this text, are compelling. They have encouraged those of us who treat this and related disorders to continue our efforts.

The Yeast Connection and the Woman brings the public and interested professionals important and timely new information. While the title suggests this is a book for women with yeast-related disorders, it will interest any man, woman, or child with a chronic illness. This is especially true of the sections relating to lifestyle, exercise, and mind/body connection.

New information on certain vitamins and nutrients such as co-enzyme Q_{10}, pycnogenol, and acidophilus is exciting to anyone studying preventive health. There is considerable information presented relating to hormones such as thyroid, adrenal, estrogen, progesterone, and DHEA. The relationship between hormonal problems, yeast-related illness, and other chronic illness is thoughtfully reviewed.

The book cites countless references for those who wish to read further about how the yeast theory evolved, what evidence supports it, and what treatments appear to be effective.

During the past decade, we have learned a great deal about chronic fatigue and the importance of listening to and not dismissing patients who complain of it. Many individuals with chronic fatigue immune dysfunction syndrome (CFIDS) have responded well to treatment for yeast, suggesting there may be a relationship between yeast and this illness. Cognitive impairment, sometimes described as spaciness, poor memory, or loss of concentration, is an all too common complaint. After other causes of this have been systematically excluded, a trial of yeast-reduction therapy is suggested and is often remarkably effective.

Other common problems such as allergy, irritable bowel syndrome, PMS, depression, and fibromyalgia may also have a relationship to yeast. It has been suggested that certain autoimmune disorders and less common problems such as interstitial cystitis and vulvodynia may be related to yeast since they frequently respond to yeast-reduction therapy. If there is a relationship between these common and not so common disorders and yeast, then this must be better defined and acknowledged. The health of many depend on it.

James H. Brodsky, M.D.
Chevy Chase, Maryland
Diplomate, American Board of Internal Medicine
American College of Physicians
American Society of Internal Medicine
Clinical Instructor, Georgetown University Medical Center

Introduction

◆───────────◆

The Yeast Connection and the Woman is superb! I'm so impressed by:

- The author's willingness and ability to tackle such a comprehensive project.
- His fair approach in presenting all sides of controversial topics.
- His scholarship and research, including literature citations for those who wish to pursue a particular topic.
- His ability to utilize a vast network of health professionals who may be expert in fields where he is not and his careful use of quotes and attributions.
- His care in not making exaggerated health claims.

As with his previous publications, this book is well organized and written—immensely readable. In the areas of my expertise (gynecology, hormone therapy, chronic fatigue syndrome) I found the material to be up-to-the-minute, factual and practical.

I was intrigued by the sections on diet, alternative therapies, prescription and nonprescription medications, the environment, vitamins and mind/body connection.

In short, this is a book that will be useful to any reader. The suggestions are practical, affordable and scientifically based. Sick and well alike would benefit if each one were to adopt the healthy lifestyle proposed.

My only criticism is that the title is much too restricted. Yes, it is a book about women's issues, but *so much more*. It is for every member of the family. It is like a health encyclopedia.

Philip K. Nelson, M.D.
Fellow, American College of Obstetrics and Gynecology
Medical Advisor, Manasota, Florida, CFIDS Support Group
Sarasota, Florida

Preface

---◆---

As you may know, the first hardback edition of *The Yeast Connection* was published over a decade ago (December 1983). Then, almost before the ink was dry, I learned a lot of things that I hadn't known. To bring readers more and better information, I added 60 pages to the second edition which was published in the summer of 1984. Then, as the months went by, I learned still more.

In early 1985, I began working on an extensive revision of *The Yeast Connection*. In October 1986, a third edition was published. It contained an entirely new 100-page addition, *The Yeast Connection Update*. I also revised my diet recommendations. I began to feature more vegetables and other complex carbohydrates and I no longer asked readers to count grams of carbohydrates.

Early in 1987, I began working on a new book which was published in 1989. Its title, *The Yeast Connection Cookbook—A Guide To Good Nutrition And Better Living*. Since I wasn't a cook, I enlisted the help and collaboration of Marjorie Hurt Jones, R.N., author of the *Food Allergy Cookbook* (published by Rodale Press).

In carrying out research for the cookbook, I wrote to several dozen physicians who were knowledgeable and experienced in treating patients with yeast-connected health problems. I asked a number of questions, including: "How many of your patients with yeast-related health problems are bothered by food allergies." Each of the 25 physicians who responded said, "All of them."

My survey of the physicians, plus the feedback I received from my patients (and others who wrote or called me), showed that yeasty foods triggered reactions in most people. Yet, some individuals were able to tolerate these foods, especially after they had avoided them for several weeks.

During succeeding printings of *The Yeast Connection* (now in its 22nd printing), I made further modifications in my diet recommendations and a few minor additions and corrections.

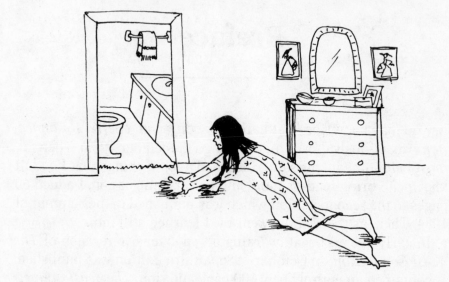

In April 1989, I attended a conference on Chronic Fatigue Syndrome (CFS) sponsored by the University of California, San Francisco, and other organizations. One of the featured speakers, Carol Jessop, an assistant clinical professor of medicine, UCSF, and an internist in private practice, described her findings in 1100 CFS patients—the majority of whom were women. In her report, Dr. Jessop said, "In many instances, CFS patients became so ill that they had to crawl to the bathroom."

At this conference and at a subsequent CFS conference in Charlotte, North Carolina, Dr. Jessop reported that 84% of her CFS patients responded to a sugar-free, alcohol-free diet and antiyeast medications, including Nizoral and Diflucan.

Dr. Jessop's reports and those of others, including Drs. Orian Truss and Jorge Flechas, led me to write and publish an illustrated book entitled, *Chronic Fatigue Syndrome and the Yeast Connection* in 1992.

During the past decade, I have developed an even stronger interest in women's health problems—especially those affecting females between 12 and 55.

Included have been women with chronic fatigue, headache, muscle aches, memory loss and other symptoms which made them feel "sick all over." In addition, I've received new information about

PMS, interstitial cystitis, vulvodynia (burning vulva), endometriosis, digestive problems, skin problems, infertility, loss of libido, loss of orgasm and other types of sexual dysfunction.

Although some women with these symptoms give a history of repeated (or persistent) vaginal yeast infections, other women develop their symptoms because of yeast overgrowth in the gut. Yet, they give a history of relatively few vaginal infections.

Increasing numbers of physicians, including especially gynecologists, have found that many of these health problems are yeast connected. They've also observed that a simple, but comprehensive, treatment program which features a sugar-free special diet and antiyeast medications has helped countless numbers of their patients regain their health and get their lives back on track.

In gathering material for this book, I consulted a number of board certified obstetricians and gynecologists, including Philip K. Nelson, Sarasota, Florida, George C. Miller, Lewisburg, Pennsylvania and Donald R. Lewis, Jackson, Tennessee.

Dr. Nelson: "I must admit for years I was a complete skeptic. Several things have changed my mind. I've had the opportunity of working with chronic fatigue syndrome patients over the past two years and seeing their response to both diet and antifungals has been impressive . . .

> ### I must admit for years I was a complete skeptic. Several things have changed my mind.

"The same regimen has helped many of my patients who have recurrent vaginal candidiasis. I think most experts agree that vaginal candidiasis has a bowel reservoir . . . I've been amazed at the number of patients who report an improved sense of well being by restricting sugar."

Dr. Miller: "I became interested in problems relating to the environment in 1981 when I became familiar with the pioneer work of

C. Orian Truss on the relationship of *Candida albicans* to a diverse group of health problems. Then in 1984 I read *The Yeast Connection* by Dr. William Crook.

"In the office on a day-to-day basis I began to see patients who had symptoms consistent with those described by Dr. Truss and Dr. Crook. *Nowhere in my medical training or background had anyone put these pieces of information together before . . .*"

Dr. Lewis: "After the initial skepticism, I decided to try the diet/nystatin approach . . . as much out of desperation as for other reasons . . . I was initially amazed and subsequently quite gratified to know that I did have an approach that promised success to a fairly large subset of my patients.

"If I might add, that it has also been interesting to talk with the patients, one or two months into the program. When I inquire about their vaginitis symptoms, they frequently say, 'Oh yes, that's better. But the greatest thing is my sinuses have opened up for the first time in several years.'

"So there are obviously other side benefits than can be gained from this approach that are far afield from the initial reason for treatment."

A Word About Men and Children

As I gathered material for this book, I planned originally to focus *only* on the health problems which affected women. Then, during recent months I received a number of letters from women concerned about the men in their lives. And many more who were concerned about their children. One of my consultants commented:

> *Don't forget the men! They get yeast problems too—especially those who have taken long term antibiotics.*

"Don't forget the men! They get yeast problems too—especially those who have taken long term antibiotics for skin problems, sinusitis or prostatitis. So do men who have taken inhaled, oral or injectible steroids for asthma or other disorders."

Several other consultants emphasized the "yeast connection" to recurrent ear infections, hyperactivity, attention deficits and autism—problems which are affecting growing numbers of children. Because I'm a pediatrician with a long-time interest in these disorders, and because women are the main caretakers of children, I'm including information about children in this book.

To summarize: This book is written for women, men and children—and those who care for them, including physicians and other professionals.

A Special Message to the Physician

◆

Like most physicians, you've heard about "the yeast connection." And, if you've read the 1985 Position Statement of the American Academy of Allergy and Immunology, you may feel that the relationship of superficial *Candida albicans* infections to a number of chronic health disorders is "speculative and unproven."

You may ask (as have many physicians), "Why haven't scientific studies been carried out to prove the yeast/human interaction which you so enthusiastically describe in your books? . . . Why haven't you published your observations in peer-reviewed journals?"

You may also say, "I read the report by Dismukes[1] and associates published in the *New England Journal of Medicine*. These investigators described women with recurrent vaginitis, fatigue, headache and other symptoms. And they stated that *the women in a control group responded just as well as those treated with oral and vaginal nystatin.* So it seems to me that the relationship of yeast infections to chronic illness is unproven."

I can understand your point of view and your criticisms. They obviously have merit. *Yet, there are always two (or more) sides to any controversial issue.* Here are several of them.

Flaws in the Dismukes Study
Comments by John E. Bennett, M.D.

In an editorial which accompanied the Dismukes article, Bennett, a mycologist at the National Institute of Allergy and Infectious Diseases, said:

> "Few illnesses have sparked as much hostility between the medical community and a segment of the lay public as the chronic can-

didiasis syndrome. Those who argue for the existence of this complex of symptoms . . . have leveled a serious charge against the medical community, claiming it is not fulfilling one of its most important obligations to its patients. The charge is simply put: *You physicians are not listening to your patients* [emphasis added]."

> ## *Few illnesses have sparked as much hostility between the medical community and . . . the lay public as the chronic candidiasis syndrome.*

In his continuing discussion, Dr. Bennett pointed out that physicians tend to pay more attention to laboratory tests than to what their patients are saying. They also seem . . .

"unwilling to learn from their patients when they claim to have been helped or cured by regimens not considered acceptable by the medical community.

"These charges are difficult to refute for a profession that appears to be spending too much time ordering and interpreting tests and not enough time talking to patients. Even more damaging is the profession's apparent refusal to study chronic candidiasis. How can science reject an idea that has not been tested, when science is purportedly open to new ideas? . . .

> ## *None of the proponents of this syndrome have recommended the use of nystatin alone.*

"Those who argue for the existence of the chronic candidiasis syndrome will complain that diet was not controlled and that it is an important aspect of treatment. In addition, candida allergy shots, injunctions to avoid moldy environments and other therapeutic approaches are often included in treatment regimens.

*"In fact, none of the proponents of the syndrome have recom-
mended the use of nystatin alone, and they are not likely to consider
the Dismukes study an adequate test of their hypothesis* [emphasis
added]."

In the concluding sentence of his editorial, Bennett said:

"Additional scientifically sound studies will be needed to determine whether this syndrome does or does not exist, and if it does,
what the optimal treatment is for patients."[2]

I'm happy to report that the first of these studies has been
funded to provide the scientific support for the candida/human
interaction which the skeptics have been demanding.*

Other Comments on the Dismukes Study

A number of professionals took exception to the Dismukes observation and wrote letters to the editor of the *New England Journal of Medicine* and to other publications. Some were published
and some were not. Here are excerpts of several letters which were
published in the May 30, 1991, issue of *NEJM*. C. Orian Truss, M.D.,
and associates, in analyzing the study by Dismukes and associates
made a different interpretation. And they said:

"We see in these data strong support for the proposal that generalized symptoms caused by toxins or other mechanisms may accompany mucosal yeast infections."

Marjorie Crandall, Ph.D., also disagreed with the conclusions by
Dismukes, et al, and said:

"I challenge the conclusion by Dismukes, et al, that the candidia-
sis/hypersensitivity syndrome 'is not a verifiable condition.' This
negative conclusion is not substantiated by the results of their clinical study, which show a strikingly positive effect of the all nystatin
regimen in women with the presumed syndrome."

*See Chapter 20.

In my own *NEJM* letter to the editor, I expressed agreement with the comments of Bennett, and I said:

"Additional scientifically sound studies are desperately needed. I hope that pharmaceutical companies or the National Institute of Health will provide funds for carrying out such studies . . . I would especially urge the investigators to look at the important role (and intricacies) of diet. A diet low in sugar (and other simple carbohydrates) was an essential part of the treatment program first outlined by Truss."[3]

I also received copies of letters which were sent to *NEJM* by a number of other candida clinicians which were not published, or were published in other periodicals. Here are several of them:

"Candida-related illness is never an illness unto itself . . . Patients who suffer from almost any dysfunction related to candida . . . always have food intolerances and these may be severe. Generally sugar in virtually any form is the most consequential offender . . . Candida-related illness must always be treated, at least initially, with *stringent* dietary control in addition to any antifungal therapy . . . *There is practically no hope of successful treatment of this problem without dietary restrictions."* W. A. Shrader, Jr., M.D.

> **There's no hope of successful treatment of this problem without dietary restrictions.**

"I would like to report that I have now treated over 5000 patients using Truss' protocol. I have seen the dramatic multisystem improvement in the majority of these people, just as described by Truss, Crook and others—Not one of Truss' critics referenced by Dismukes and Bennett has ever reported treating a single patient using Truss' complete protocol. I would like to recommend that any researcher who evaluates Truss' protocol, *use* Truss' protocol." Dennis W. Remington, M.D.

"It is very difficult to treat a yeast problem with a one-pronged approach. The startling aspects of their paper, however, is that they ignored the diet. Some women need only to eat a bar of candy and they develop an immediate vaginal discharge. The study is sort of analogous to designing a study on diabetes and insulin while letting the patients eat sugar . . ." Doris J. Rapp, M.D.

Observations of Carol Jessop, M.D.

At the April 1989 conference on chronic fatigue syndrome sponsored by the San Francisco Department of Public Health, the San Francisco Medical Society, the University of California (SF) Department of Medicine and the University of California (SF) School of Nursing, Carol Jessop, M.D., Diplomate, American Board of Internal Medicine, and assistant Clinical Professor of Medicine at UCSF, described her experiences. Here's a summary of Dr. Jessop's presentation as described in *American Medical News*:

"Beginning last year, Dr. Jessop treated 900 of her CFS patients with ketoconazole, a drug used to treat candidiasis, and placed them on a sugar-free diet. Since then 529 have returned to their previous health and another 232 have shown improvement.

> *Often patients with chronic fatigue feel abandoned by the traditional medical community.*

"Dr. Jessop said that her patients have taught her about CFS. She said, 'I didn't learn it in medical school.' She urged more physicians to listen to complaints from fatigued patients . . . Often such patients 'feel abandoned' by the traditional medical community."[4]

In a subsequent presentation at a November 1990 conference sponsored by the CFIDS Association, Inc., in conjunction with the Charlotte Area Health Education Center and other organizations, Jessop discussed her findings in working with 1324 patients with chronic fatigue syndrome seen between 1984 and 1990. Jessop said:

"Bacterial, viral, fungal and parasitic agents need to be examined as possible contributors to this disease ... If they have a yeast overgrowth, my treatment of choice is three weeks of fluconazole (Diflucan), 100 mgs. daily [emphasis added]."

In her foreword to my recent book which focused on the relationship of repeated antibiotics and yeast overgrowth to the chronic fatigue syndrome, Jessop said:

"Ten years ago I was very frustrated working with CFS patients because of deeply ingrained skepticism about theories such as the 'yeast connection.' However, following further research and a trial of some of these therapeutic interventions with my patients, my work has become both intellectually rewarding and fun."[5]

Comments by Other Physicians

In a statement discussing candida-related illness in September 1989, Douglas H. Sandberg, M.D., Professor of Pediatrics, Division of Gastroenterology and Nutrition at the University of Miami, said:

"Confirmation of the diagnosis remains difficult, evaluation of efficacy of therapeutic measures incomplete; and tools for monitoring a therapeutic response are below the standards we've come to expect in modern medical practice.

"In spite of these shortcomings, *I'm convinced that this disorder exists and that it is important. It must be considered in differential diagnosis of patients with a variety of chronic complaints. Since diagnosis at times can be made only through determining response to a therapeutic trial, some patients would have to be treated without a firm diagnosis prior to institution of therapy* [emphasis added]."[6]

In an October 14, 1993, statement, James H. Brodsky, M.D., a diplomate of the American Board of Internal Medicine, and a member of the American College of Physicians, commented:

"Since my introduction to the relationship between yeast and human illness in the early 1980s, I've seen well over 1000 patients with some form of yeast-related illness ... I maintain a general internal medicine practice and make hospital rounds daily. *While I find all aspects of my practice fulfilling, nothing has been so rewarding as helping patients with yeast-related illnesses who have been unable to find help elsewhere.'*[7]

Nothing has been so rewarding as helping patients with yeast-related illnesses who have been unable to find help elsewhere.

Clinical Reports of the Effectiveness of a Therapy Often Precede Scientific Studies

Clinical reports that describe the effectiveness of a particular method of therapy may precede by decades (or even centuries) the scientific studies which provide support for the therapy.

Many therapies used in medicine today continue to be used because physicians (and nonphysicians) have found that they work. Moreover, many such therapies are safe and inexpensive. Yet, information about how and why a therapy works may not be known.

Over ten years ago, two physicians from the University of New Mexico School of Medicine published a fascinating article entitled, "The Tomato Effect." In the article they told about the rejection of tomatoes by North Americans for over 300 years because people thought they were poisonous. And they said:

> "Not until 1820 when Robert Gibbon Johnson ate a tomato on the steps of the courthouse in Salem, New Jersey, and survived, did the people of America begin—grudgingly—to consume tomatoes. The tomato effect in medicine occurs when an efficacious treatment for a certain disease is ignored or rejected because it does not 'make sense' . . ."

If you review medical history, you'll find many examples of the "tomato effect." And in their continuing discussion, Drs. Goodwin and Goodwin said:

"Modern medicine is particularly vulnerable to the tomato effect. Pharmaceutical companies have . . . turned to theoretical over practical arguments for using their drugs . . . *the only three issues that matter in picking a therapy are: Does it help? How toxic is it? How much does it cost?*"[8]

> ### *The only three issues that matter in picking a therapy: Does it help? How toxic is it? How much does it cost?*

In an editorial published the following year entitled, "The Gold Standard," Gene H. Stollerman, M.D., Professor of Medicine, Boston University School of Medicine, seemed to me to express a somewhat similar conclusion when he said:

"As the insights of medical bioscience and technology increase our medical powers, I find renewed strength in my clinical skills . . . *Clinical experience is the gold standard on which patient care should be based.*"[9]

Several thousand physicians in practice and a handful of academicians have found that a sugar-free special diet and nystatin, ketoconazole (Nizoral), fluconazole (Diflucan) or itraconazole (Sporanox) are effective in treating patients with a diverse group of health problems. These range from PMS, chronic fatigue syndrome, interstitial cystitis and psoriasis in adults to recurrent ear infections and other respiratory infections and the subsequent development of hyperactivity, attention deficits and autism in children.

I hope you'll take a careful look at the relationship of superficial yeast infections to chronic health disorders which affect people of all ages and both sexes. Included especially are premenopausal women who feel "sick all over" and other family members who give a history of repeated courses of broad spectrum antibiotic drugs. I feel that in so doing you'll be able to help many of your difficult patients and at the same time make your own practice more interesting and rewarding.

REFERENCES

1. Dismukes, W.E., Way, J.S., Lee, J.Y., Dockery, B.K., Hain, J.D., "A randomized double-blind trial of nystatin therapy for the candidiasis hypersensitivity syndrome." *N. Engl. J. Med.*, 1990; 323:1717–23.
2. Bennett, J.E., "Searching for the Yeast Connection," *N. Engl. J. Med.*, 1990; 323:1766–67.
3. Letters to the Editor, *N. Engl. J. Med.*, 1991; 324:1592–93.
4. Jessop, C., as quoted by Staver, S., *American Medical News*, April 1989.
5. Jessop, C., Foreword in Crook, W.G., *Chronic Fatigue Syndrome and the Yeast Connection*, Professional Books, Jackson, TN, 1992.
6. Sandberg, D.H., Statement, "Candida-Related Illness," September 22, 1989.
7. Brodsky, J.H., Statement, "The Importance of Candida-Related Health Problems," October 14, 1993.
8. Goodwin, J.S. and Goodwin, J.M., "The Tomato Effect," *JAMA*, 1984, 251:2287–90.
9. Stollerman, G.H., "The Gold Standard," *Hospital Practice*, January 30, 1985, Vol. 20 No. 1A, p. 9.

PART

ONE

An Overview

1

Are Your Health Problems Yeast Connected?

IF YOU . . .

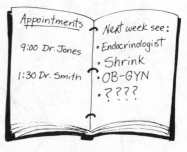

✱ feel "sick all over"

✱ have taken a lot of antibiotic drugs

✱ have sought help from many different specialists

Appointments
9:00 Dr. Jones
1:30 Dr. Smith

Next week see:
• Endocrinologist
• Shrink
• OB-GYN
• ????

have taken birth control pills and/or steroids ✱

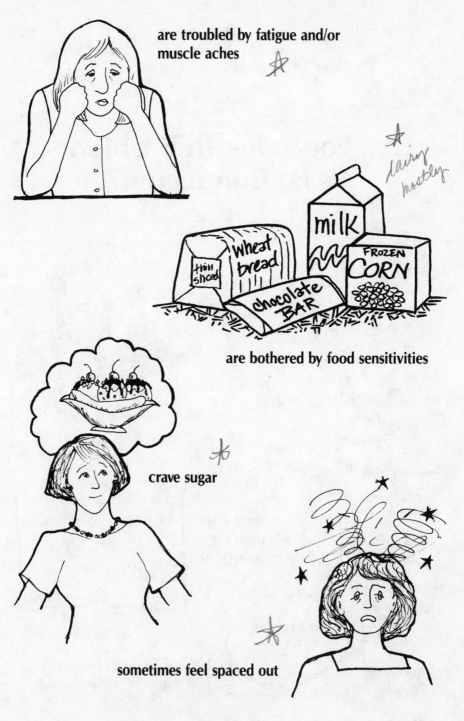

are troubled by fatigue and/or muscle aches

are bothered by food sensitivities

crave sugar

sometimes feel spaced out

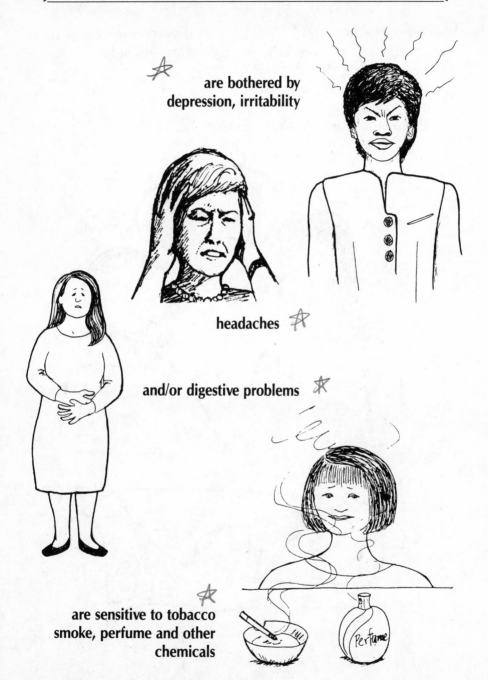

are bothered by
depression, irritability

headaches

and/or digestive problems

are sensitive to tobacco
smoke, perfume and other
chemicals

your health problems may be yeast connected.

Women between 20 and 55 are especially apt to develop yeast-related health problems. Common symptoms include:

- **Recurrent vaginal yeast infections**

- **Recurrent urinary tract infections**

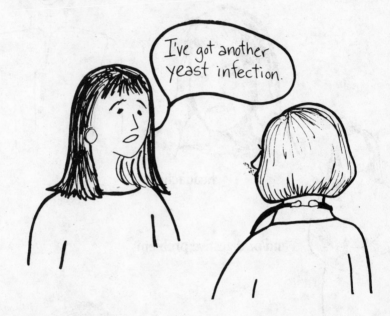

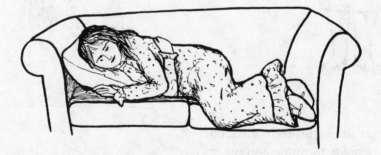

- **PMS**

- **Vulvodynia (burning vulva)**

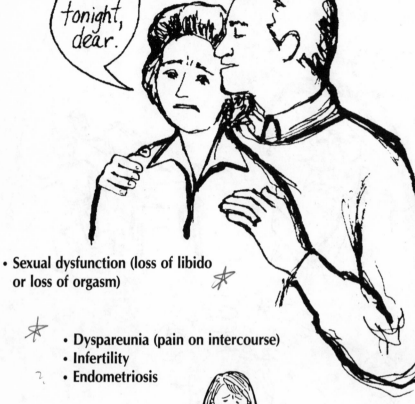

- Sexual dysfunction (loss of libido or loss of orgasm)

    - Dyspareunia (pain on intercourse)
    - Infertility
    - Endometriosis

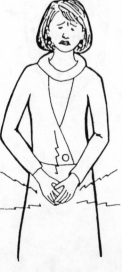

- Interstitial cystitis

MEN AND CHILDREN also develop yeast-related health problems, especially those who take many antibiotic drugs.

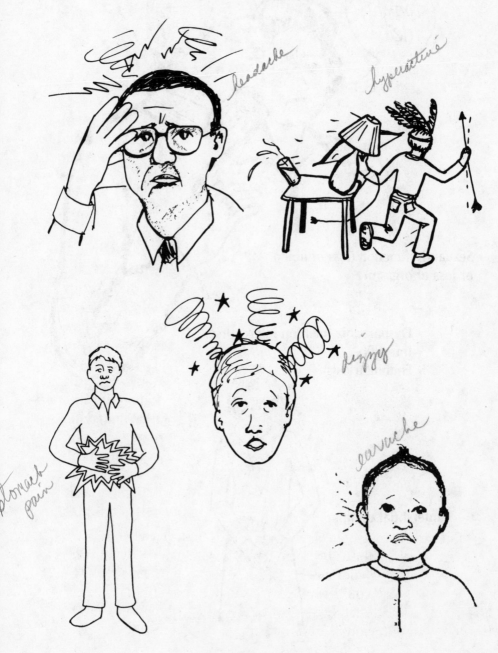

Other complaints and illnesses which may sometimes be related to the common yeast, *Candida albicans,* include:

- Numbness
- Multiple sclerosis
- Crohn's disease
- Sinusitis
- Scleroderma
- Rheumatoid arthritis
- Myasthenia gravis

- Tingling
- Eczema
- Acne
- Lupus erythematosus
- Asthma
- Psoriasis
- Chronic hives

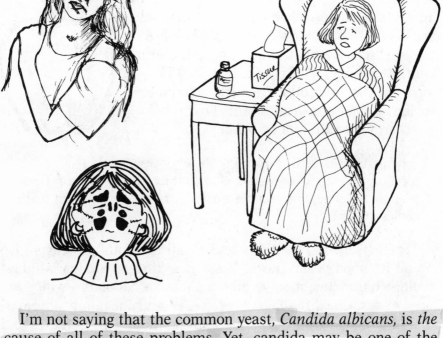

I'm not saying that the common yeast, *Candida albicans,* is *the* cause of all of these problems. Yet, candida may be one of the causes—even a major cause—of these and other health problems.

In this book you'll find easy-to-read-and-understand explanations of yeast-related health problems and a step-by-step program which will help you overcome them.

2

---◆---

Yeasts—What They Are and How They Make You Sick

---◆---

What Are Yeasts?

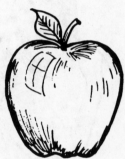

Yeasts are single cell living organisms which are neither animal nor vegetable. They live on the surfaces of all living things, including fruits, vegetables, grains and your skin. They're a part of the "microflora" which contribute in various ways to the health of its host.

According to Dr. Sidney Baker:

> "Polishing a fresh picked apple removes some of the coating of yeasts that inhabit its healthy surface. These friendly fungi help protect the apple from other germs that make apples moldy."

Yeast, itself, is nutritious and small amounts of yeasts give bread its good yeasty taste. Yeast is a kind of fungus. Mildew, mold, mushrooms, monilia and candida are all names which are used to describe different types of yeast. And one family of yeasts, *Candida albicans*, normally lives on the inner warm creases and crevices of your digestive tract and vagina. Quoting Dr. Baker again:

> "Yeasts have some very animal-like behavior and they must consume other substances such as sugar and fats in order to survive."[1]

In addition, *Candida albicans* has been referred to as a "Dr. Jekyll and Mr. Hyde" sort of critter. Here's why: It can branch from a single cell yeast form into a branching fungal form. And these branches can burrow beneath the surfaces of your mucous membranes.

Factors That Predispose to Yeast Infections*
Prescription Medications

Yeast infections are especially apt to trouble you if you have taken repeated or prolonged courses of amoxicillin, ampicillin, Ceclor, Keflex, tetracycline and/or other broad-spectrum antibiotics during infancy, childhood, adolescence, or since you've become an adult.

What do I mean by a "broad-spectrum" antibiotic? These antiotics are so powerful they destroy bacteria of many types. They include both "enemies" and "friends." And some of the important "friends" live normally in your digestive tract.

Candida yeasts aren't affected by antibiotics. Accordingly, if you took these products for acne (or for urinary, sinus, ear, chest or other infections), candida multiplied in your intestinal tract—and also in your vagina.

Medications that your doctor prescribes play an important part in causing yeast infections. In discussing the iatrogenic (doctor-induced) factors that predispose to candida infections, Dr. F.C. Odds, a world famous candida authority, commented:

> "All antibacterial antibiotics possess the ability in theory to eliminate from human microbial habitats bacteria that normally compete with yeast for nutrients. Such alterations in the microflora may lead to yeast overgrowth and consequent yeast infection because yeasts themselves are unaffected by antibacterial antibiotics.
>
> "In practice, only treatment with broad-spectrum antibiotics, or multiple narrow-spectrum antibiotics, appears to produce this effect to any significant extent. The relationship between antibiotic therapy and candidosis is far from unequivocally proven . . ."

*See Chapter 9.

Odds then cites large numbers of studies which indicate that yeast carriage is increased in individuals who have been treated with broad-spectrum antibiotics, as well as other studies which are less inclusive. Yet, he said:

"There is clearly a strong consensus view in favor of antibiotic enhancement of yeast carriage . . ."[2]

In his continuing discussion of doctor-induced causes of candida infections, Odds noted that contraceptives, steroids (oral or inhaled) and metronidazole (Flagyl) encourage the proliferation of candida.

Sugar and Other Simple Carbohydrates

Many clinicians have noted the role of sugar (and other simple carbohydrates) in promoting yeast overgrowth. Moreover, their clinical observations have been confirmed by several research studies. (See Chapter 9.)

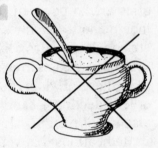

Other Factors

As every woman knows, nylon underwear and tights may make you more apt to develop genital yeast infections. And such infections are especially apt to occur if your skin or mucous membranes are mechanically irritated or macerated. Similarly, they may occur in the mouth of people with dentures.

Hormonal changes in pregnancy also encourage yeast overgrowth, especially during the last trimester. Sexual transmission is also an important factor with many women. And in their book, *A Woman's Guide to Yeast Infections*, gynecologist Naomi Baumslag and D.L. Michels said:

"Leading researchers agree that the sexual partner(s) should always be treated in any situation where a sexually active woman is suffering from recurrent yeast vaginitis. One standard medical text, *Harrison's Principle of Internal Medicine* states, 'Unless the sexual partner is treated when candidiasis is present there will be a constant retransfer of the infection.'

"By treating a partner harboring yeast, you remove a predisposing factor of vaginitis and are that much closer to breaking the cycle of infection, especially for sexually active women with recurrent infection."[3]

A Yeast Infection Is More Than a Vaginal Infection

If you're like most people, when you read or hear about a "yeast infection" you immediately think of a vaginal infection. And such infections do cause millions of women to experience itching, irritation, burning, and/or other types of discomfort involving their genitalia.

> *Every woman with a vaginal yeast infection has an accompanying overgrowth of yeast in her digestive tract.*
> **Mary Miles, M.D., JAMA, Oct. 28, 1977**

Yet, every woman with a vaginal yeast infection has an accompanying overgrowth of yeasts in her digestive tract as noted by researchers at Michigan State University.[4] Symptoms which may result include diarrhea, constipation, bloating and abdominal pain. Yet, remarkably enough, many women may experience few, if any, digestive symptoms.

What Is "The Yeast Connection"?

It is a term to indicate the relationship of superficial yeast infections in your vagina and digestive tract to fatigue, headache, depression, PMS, irritability and other symptoms which can make you feel "sick all over."

Other causes must also be considered. If you're like most people with a candida-related health problem, you resemble an overburdened camel. To regain your health, to look good, feel good and enjoy life, you'll need to unload many "bundles of straw." This may take months—even a year or two—but then your camel will be off and running.

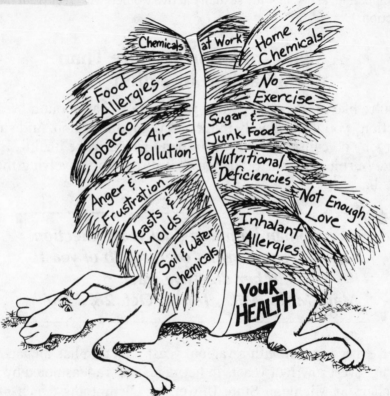

How Superficial Yeast Infections Cause Symptoms in Distant Parts of Your Body

There are several possible mechanisms:

Immune System Disturbances Studies by Japanese researchers Iwata and Yamamoto (Department of Microbiology, Faculty of Medicine, University of Tokyo) show that *Candida albicans* puts out high and low molecular weight toxins that can weaken your immune system.[5]

In one of these studies carried out in mice the researchers stated:

"Upon *Candida albicans* infection the toxin produced in the invaded tissues may act as an immunosuppressant to impair host defenses involving cellular immunity."[6]

In case of infection with a virulent strain of *Candida albicans*, a selective decrease in the number of T cells was characteristically noted.

Symposium *Medical Mycology*
Flims, January 1977

mykosen, Suppl. 1, 72 – 81 (1978)
© Grosse Verlag 1978

Department of Microbiology, Faculty of Medicine, University of Tokyo, Japan
(Director: Prof. Dr. K. Iwata)

Cellular Immunity in Experimental Fungus Infections in Mice: The Influence of Infections and Treatment with a Candida Toxin on Spleen Lymphoid Cells

K. Iwata and K. Uchida

Summary

Mice whose cellular immunity was congenitally deficient (athymic nude mice) or artificially lowered by treatment with anti-thymocyte serum or cyclophosphamide were much more susceptible to lethal infections with Candida albicans, Histoplasma capsulatum and Fonsecae (Phialophora) pedrosoi than were untreated normal mice. Germfree mice were susceptible to lethal infection with Histoplasma capsulatum, but rather resistant to that with Candida albicans or Fonsecaea pedrosoi.

When normal specific pathogen-free mice were infected with each of these pathogenic fu there occured a marked change in the fractions of certain subpopulations of spleen lymp cells during the course of infection; in the case of infection with a virulent strain of Can albicans, a selective decrease in the number of T cells was characteristical. . . . In vit sponsiveness to mitogens of spleen lymphoid cells isolated fro— . . . s varia extent, depending on species of mitogens tested and . . . m m fected with the virulent Candida albi— . . . . ive canavalin A than comparable — . . . ga also caused decrease—

When injected phoid cells simila This indicates the invaded tissues ma ing cellular immuni tion with such toxi

"...Upon *Candida albicans* infection the toxin produced in the invaded tissues may act as an immunosuppressant to impair host defense mechanisms involving cellular immunity..."

Résumé

Chez les souris aya chez celles présentant antithymocyte ou cyclo toplasma capsulatum et . normales, non traitées. L tions léthales à Histoplas. Candida albicans ou à Fonsecaea pedrosoi.

Lorsqu'on a inoculé un changement notable dans une fraction de certai tions spécifiques, il y a eu au cours de l'évolution de l'infe tions des cellules lymphoides de la rate; ceci au cours de Candida albicans on a re inoculation d'une souche virulente de cellules T. Les cellules lym . . . . sélective du nombre de . . . une sensibilité variable aux . . . . . . souris inf

Further evidence of the adverse effect of *Candida albicans* on the immune system was noted in 1985 by Steven S. Witkin, Ph.D. (Cornell University Medical College), who said:

> "*Candida albicans* infection, often associated with antibiotic in-duced alterations in microbial flora, may cause defects in cellular immunity . . .
>
> "In addition to creating an increased susceptibility to *Candida* re-infection, the immunological alterations may also be related to sub-sequent endocrinopathies [hormone dysfunction] and autoantibody formation . . .
>
> "Reports that immunological or endocrine abnormalities have been reversed following successful antifungal antibiotic therapy for *Candida* infection lend credence to the idea that these abnormalities can arise as secondary consequences of fungal infection."[7]*

Michigan State University researchers also noted the possible relationship of intestinal and vaginal yeast infections to immuno-logical problems. And they commented:

> "*Extending the gut reservoir concept may explain other forms of candidiasis and the immunological phenomena found in some peo-ple* [emphasis added]."[4]

Recently, researchers in Finland carried out studies on the rela-tionship of *Candida albicans* to atopic dermatitis, and they com-mented:

> "Although the immunological factors involving *C. albicans* . . . are still not thoroughly understood, the observed linkage between high anti-*C. albicans*, IgE and *C. albicans* colonization and severity of AD (Atopic dermatitis) may provide a model for the understanding of the pathogenesis and immunoregulation of the disease."[8]

Absorption of Food Antigens—and Toxins   Based on clinical and research studies by many different observers, candida overgrowth

---

*You'll find more recent references to Witkin's research studies on women with vaginitis in Chapter 9.

in the intestinal tract may create what has been called a "leaky gut." As a result, food antigens and toxins may be absorbed which play a part in making you feel "sick all over."

Allergies to Candida   According to James H. Brodsky, M.D.:

"There is much evidence to suggest that *C. albicans* is one of the most allergenic microbes. Both immediate and delayed hypersensitivity reactions to Candida are very common in the adult population. The relationship between yeast and urticaria has been established in a well designed double-blind trial.

> ### There's much evidence to suggest that C. albicans is one of the most allergenic microbes.

"The investigators estimate that in about 26% of patients with chronic urticaria, *C. albicans* sensitivity is an important factor. Significant clinical improvement was seen with anti-candida therapy and a low yeast diet."[9]

A number of other physicians have also noted that candida allergies may play an important role in causing symptoms.[10]

REFERENCES

1. Baker, S., Notes on the yeast problem, Gesell Institute, New Haven, CT, 1985.
2. Odds, F.C., *Candida and Candidosis,* University Park Press, Baltimore, 1979; pp 82–83.
3. Baumslag, N. and Michels, D.L., *A Woman's Guide to Yeast Infections,* Pocket Books, New York, 1992; p 56.
4. Miles, M.R., Olsen, L. and Rogers, A., "Recurrent Vaginal Candidiasis: Importance of an Intestinal Reservoir," *JAMA,* 238:1836–1837, October 28, 1977.
5. Iwata, K. and Yamamoto, Y., "Glycoprotein Toxins Produced by *Candida*

albicans," Proceedings of the 4th International Conference on the Mycoses, June 1977, PAHO Scientific Publication No. 356.

6. Iwata, K. and Uchida, K., "Cellular Immunity in Experimental Fungus Infections in Mice: The influence of infections in treatment with a candida toxin on spleen lymphoid cells," *Mykosen, Suppl.* 1, 72–81 (1978), Symposium Medical Mycology, Flims, January 1977.

7. Witkin, S.S., "Defective Immune Responses in Patients with Recurrent Candidiasis," *Infections in Medicine,* May/June 1985, pp 129–131.

8. Savolainen, J., Lammintausta, K., Kalimo, K. and Viander, M., *Clinical and Experimental Allergy,* Vol. 23, 1993, pp 332–339.

9. Brodsky, J.H., as quoted in the Foreword of *The Yeast Connection,* Third Edition, paperback, by W.G. Crook, M.D., Professional Books, Jackson, TN and Vintage Books, New York, 1986.

10. Liebeskind, A., *Annals of Allergy,* 1962; 20:394–396; Hosen, H., *Texas Medicine,* 1971; 67:58; Kudelko, N.M., *Annals of Allergy,* 1971; 29:266; Palacios, H.J., *Annals of Allergy,* 1976; 37:110–113; and Truss, C.O., *J. of Ortho. Psych.,* 1980; 9:287–301.

3

Why You May Develop
Yeast-Related Health
Problems

The common yeast, *Candida albicans,* normally lives in your body—

especially in your intestines and vagina.

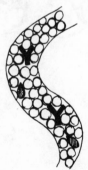 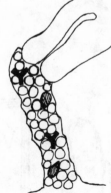 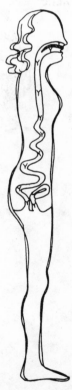

Y- yeasts   **O** - friendly germs

◖ - enemies

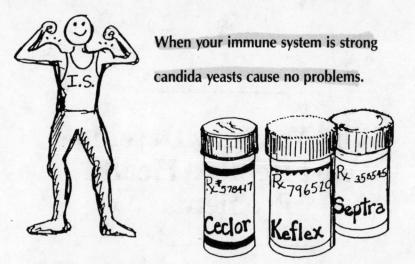

When your immune system is strong candida yeasts cause no problems.

BUT, when you take broad-spectrum antibiotics for

acne   respiratory infections

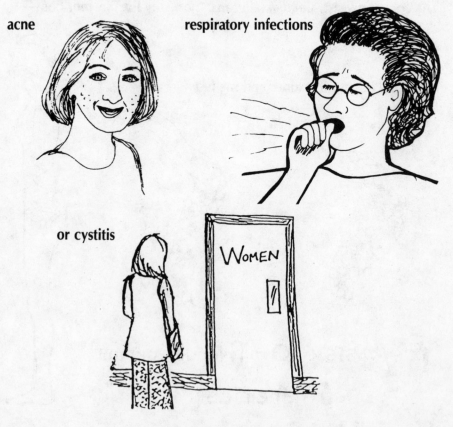

or cystitis

these drugs knock out friendly germs while they're knocking out enemies.

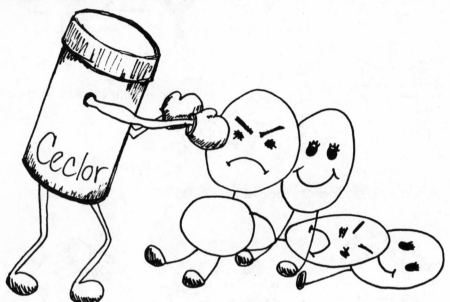

Candida yeasts aren't
affected by antibiotics.

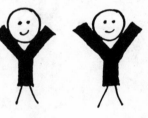

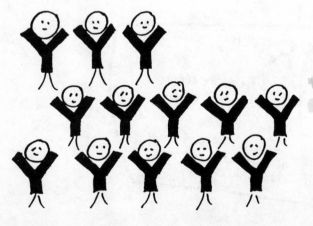

So they multiply and
raise large families.

These candida yeasts put out toxins

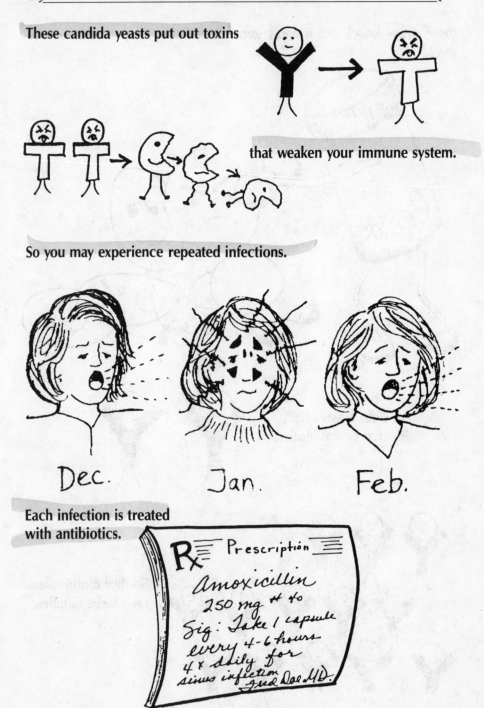

that weaken your immune system.

So you may experience repeated infections.

Dec. Jan. Feb.

Each infection is treated
with antibiotics.

R℞ ═══ Prescription ═══
Amoxicillin
250 mg # 40
Sig: Take 1 capsule
every 4-6 hours
4 × daily for
sinus infection
Fred Doe M.D.

So a vicious cycle develops.

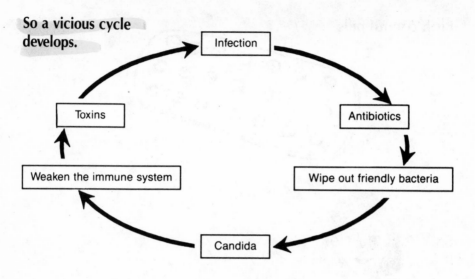

Other Causes of Yeast Overgrowth Include

Hormonal changes associated with the normal menstrual cycle

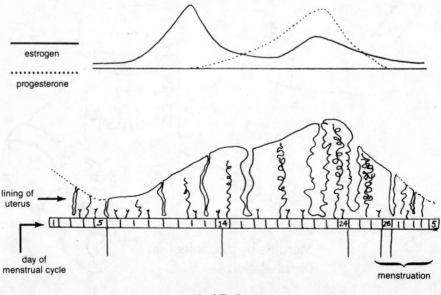

Birth control pills

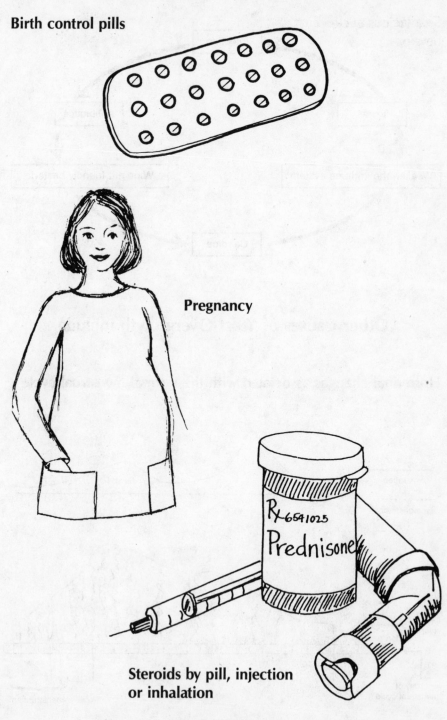

Pregnancy

Steroids by pill, injection or inhalation

Genital irritations and abrasions

Re-infection from your sexual partner

Diabetes

Sugar rich diets

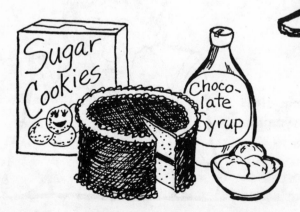

Candida overgrowth in your intestine may cause a leaky gut. Toxins and food allergens may then pass through this membrane and go to other parts of your body.

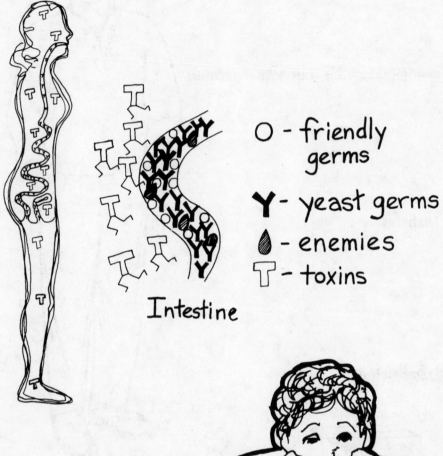

O - friendly germs

Y - yeast germs

♦ - enemies

T - toxins

Intestine

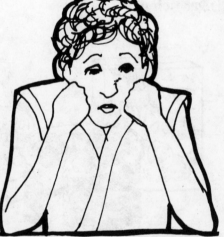

Candida allergies may also contribute to your symptoms.

Still Other Factors Often Play a Role in Making You Sick

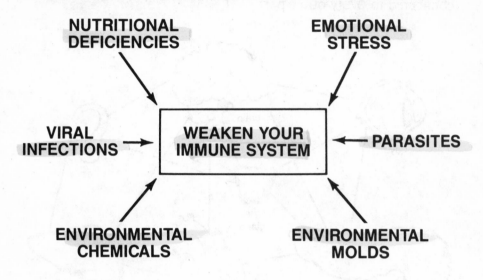

Many of your yeast-related symptoms, including PMS, sexual dysfunction, headache and depression, develop because your immune system, your endocrine system and your brain are intimately related —

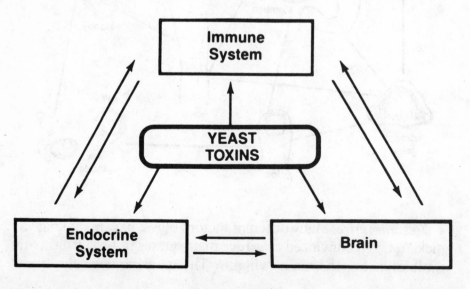

—and (although we sometimes forget it) every part of your body is connected to every other part.

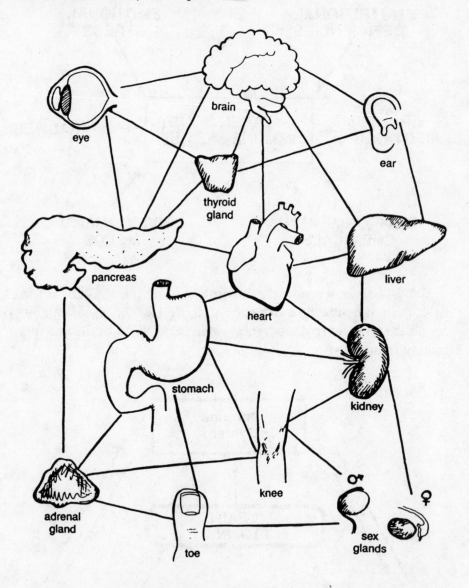

To summarize: Many different factors play a part in making you sick. Yet, I'm convinced that repeated courses of broad spectrum antibiotics are the main "villain." These antibiotics cause yeast overgrowth in your intestinal tract and vaginal yeast infections. And these infections, like a stream cascading down a mountain set off disturbances which can make you feel "sick all over."

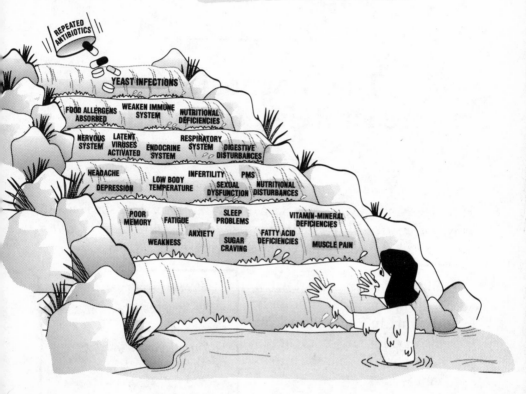

4

The Diagnosis of a
Yeast-Related Disorder

How does your physician make a diagnosis? How does she find out **why** *you're troubled by fatigue, headache, depression or other symptoms?* She bases her conclusions on—

- *Your history or story.* Such a history includes not only your main complaints, but also symptoms or events in your past that may be important.
- *Your physical examination.* It should include not only your skin, eyes, heart, lungs and other parts of your body, but also an overall look at you.
- *Laboratory examinations,* other tests and x-rays.

> MEDICAL HISTORY
> * Repeated antibiotics during childhood
> * Acne during teen years
> * Recurrent urinary infections
> * Frequent vaginitis
> * Menstrual problems
> * PMS
> * Fatigue, depression, headache
> * Visits to many different physicians
> * Digestive symptoms
> * Crave sweets
> * Sick all over, etc., etc.

With some health disorders, a diagnosis can be made easily. Here are examples: You develop a slight sore throat, a cough and other mild respiratory symptoms. Then you sit through an entire football game on a cold, windy day. That night your cough worsens. And early the next morning your teeth begin to chatter and you shiver and shake. You're having a chill.

Then your fever jumps up to 104 and you experience a sharp pain in your chest. You go to a hospital emergency room. The physician there listens to your story and examines you. Then she orders a chest x-ray and lab tests of various sorts, including a white blood count and a urinalysis.

After reviewing these findings, she says, "You have lobar pneumonia. With a shot of penicillin today, you'll be a lot better by tomorrow. Then, with a few days of rest and a little more penicillin, you'll be well in a week."

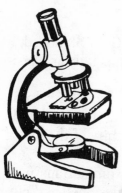

Another example might be: You develop urinary frequency and burning and you note blood in your urine. Microscopic examination shows that your urine is loaded with blood cells, pus cells and bacteria. You have an acute urinary tract infection. The doctor says, "Drink lots of fluid and take this antibiotic for a few days and the problem will soon go away."

With a yeast-related problem, the situation is entirely different. Here's why: a physical examination and tests do not provide an answer. They do not enable your physician to make a diagnosis. Nevertheless, if you feel "sick all over," you should go to a physician for a checkup. You'll need to make sure your symptoms aren't caused by some other disorder.

If your physical examination and "routine" laboratory tests are normal and your history suggests a yeast-related problem, the diagnosis is made by noting your response to a simple, but comprehensive, treatment program. Such a program features a sugar-free special diet and prescription or nonprescription antiyeast medications.

You'll find a discussion of diagnostic studies which a number of physicians have found helpful in Chapter 38.

5

Candida Questionnaire and Score Sheet

Gene H. Stollerman, M.D., in an editorial "The Gold Standard,"[1] stressed the importance of the medical history, especially as physicians "learn better questions to ask."

As I learned about yeast-related illnesses over a decade ago from Orian Truss, Sidney Baker and other physicians, and from my patients, I was impressed by the remarkable uniformity of the histories found in these patients.

Because the usual physical and laboratory examinations provided little or no help in making the diagnosis, I designed and put together a long questionnaire and score sheet which was published originally in the first edition of *The Yeast Connection*.[2]

During the past decade, minor changes have been made in this questionnaire. It has also been copied and published elsewhere many, many times. It was, and is, designed for adults and the scoring system is *not* appropriate for children. And because your spouse, companion, friend or male relative may also be troubled by yeast-related problems, this questionnaire is designed for people of both sexes.

Questions in Section A focus especially on factors in your medical history which promote the growth of *Candida albicans* along with items in the history which are frequently found in people with yeast-related health problems.

In Section B you'll find a list of 23 symptoms which are often present in patients with yeast-related health problems. Section C consists of 33 other symptoms which are sometimes seen in people with yeast-related problems—yet they may also be found in people with other disorders.

Filling out and scoring this questionnaire should help you and your physician evaluate the possible role Candida albicans contributes to your health problems. Yet, it will not provide an automatic yes or no answer.

Section A: History

	Point Score
1. Have you taken tetracyclines or other antibiotics for acne for 1 month (or longer)?	35
2. Have you at any time in your life taken broad-spectrum antibiotics or other antibacterial medication for respiratory, urinary or other infections for 2 months or longer, or in shorter courses 4 or more times in a 1-year period?	35
3. Have you taken a broad-spectrum antibiotic drug— even in a single dose?	6
4. Have you, at any time in your life, been bothered by persistent prostatitis, vaginitis or other problems affecting your reproductive organs?	25
5. Are you bothered by memory or concentration problems—do you sometimes feel spaced out?	20
6. Do you feel "sick all over" yet, in spite of visits to many different physicians, the causes haven't been found?	20
7. Have you been pregnant . . .	
2 or more times?	5
1 time?	3
8. Have you taken birth control pills. . .	
For more than 2 years?	15
For 6 months to 2 years?	8

9. Have you taken steroids orally, by injection
   or inhalation?

   For more than 2 weeks?   15

   For 2 weeks or less?   6

10. Does exposure to perfumes, insecticides, fabric
    shop odors and other chemicals provoke . . .
    Moderate to severe symptoms?   20 ✓

    Mild symptoms?   5

11. Does tobacco smoke *really* bother you?   10 ✓

12. Are your symptoms worse on damp, muggy days
    or in moldy places?   20 ✓

13. Have you had athlete's foot, ring worm, "jock itch"
    or other chronic fungous infections of the skin or
    nails? Have such infections been . . .
    Severe or persistent?   20

    Mild to moderate?   10 ✓

14. Do you crave sugar?   10 ✓

Total Score, Section A ___204___

Section B: Major Symptoms

For each of your symptoms, enter the appropriate figure in the
Point Score column:

If a symptom is *occasional or mild*. . . . . 3 points
If a symptom is *frequent and/or moderately severe*. . . . 6 points
If a symptom is *severe and/or disabling* . . . . 9 points
Add total score and record it at the end of this section.

Point
Score

1. Fatigue or lethargy   6

2. Feeling of being "drained"   9

3. Depression or manic depression   9

4. Numbness, burning or tingling   _9_

5. Headache   _9_

6. Muscle aches   _9_

7. Muscle weakness or paralysis   _9_

8. Pain and/or swelling in joints   _9_

9. Abdominal pain   _6_

10. Constipation and/or diarrhea   _3_

11. Bloating, belching or intestinal gas   _9_

12. Troublesome vaginal burning, itching or discharge   _6_

13. Prostatitis   _____

14. Impotence   _____

15. Loss of sexual desire or feeling   _9_

16. Endometriosis or infertility   _____

17. Cramps and/or other menstrual irregularities   _9_

18. Premenstrual tension   _6_

19. Attacks of anxiety or crying   _3_

20. Cold hands or feet, low body temperature   _9_

21. Hypothyroidism   _____

22. Shaking or irritable when hungry   _6_

23. Cystitis or interstitial cystitis   _3_   ?

Total Score, Section B   _138_

Section C: Other Symptoms

For each of your symptoms, enter the appropriate figure in the
Point Score column:

If a symptom is *occasional or mild*.................. 1 point
If a symptom is *frequent and/or moderately severe*.... 2 points
If a symptom is *severe and/or disabling*............. 3 points
Add total score and record it at the end of this section.

	Point Score
1. Drowsiness, including inappropriate drowsiness	2
2. Irritability	2
3. Incoordination	2
4. Frequent mood swings	2
5. Insomnia	2
6. Dizziness/loss of balance	3
7. Pressure above ears . . . feeling of head swelling	3
8. Sinus problems . . . tenderness of cheekbones or forehead	2
9. Tendency to bruise easily	3
10. Eczema, itching eyes	3
11. Psoriasis	1
12. Chronic hives (urticaria)	
13. Indigestion or heartburn	2
14. Sensitivity to milk, wheat, corn or other common foods	3
15. Mucus in stools	
16. Rectal itching	1

17. Dry mouth or throat ___1___

18. Mouth rashes, including "white" tongue _____

19. Bad breath ___2___

20. Foot, hair or body odor not relieved by washing ___1___

21. Nasal congestion or postnasal drip ___2___

22. Nasal itching ___2___

23. Sore throat ___1___

24. Laryngitis, loss of voice ___1___

25. Cough or recurrent bronchitis ___3___

26. Pain or tightness in chest ___3___

27. Wheezing or shortness of breath ___2___

28. Urinary frequency or urgency ___3___

29. Burning on urination ___2___

30. Spots in front of eyes or erratic vision ___3___

31. Burning or tearing eyes ___3___

32. Recurrent infections or fluid in ears ___1___

33. Ear pain or deafness ___3___

Total Score, Section C ___64___

Total Score, Section A ___204___

Total Score, Section B ___138___

GRAND TOTAL SCORE ___406___

The Grand Total Score will help you and your physician decide if your health problems are yeast connected. Scores in women will run higher, as 7 items in the questionnaire apply exclusively to women, while only 2 apply exclusively to men.

403-406

Yeast-connected health problems are almost certainly present in women with scores *over 180,* and in men with scores *over 140.*

Yeast-connected health problems are probably present in women with scores *over 120,* and in men with scores *over 90.*

Yeast-connected health problems are possibly present in women with scores *over 60,* and in men with scores over 40.

With scores of less than 60 in women and 40 in men, yeasts are less apt to cause health problems.

REFERENCES

1. Stollerman, G.H., "The Gold Standard," *Hospital Practice,* 1985; 20: January 30, p 9.
2. Crook, W.G., Candida Questionnaire and Score Sheet, *The Yeast Connection,* First Edition, Professional Books, Jackson, TN, 1983; pp 29–33.

6

---◆---

Women with Yeast-Related Problems Are Often "Sick All Over"

---◆---

During the past 15 years I've received thousands of letters and phone calls from women with complaints which focused on a specific problem or "disease" on a particular part of the body. Examples include endometriosis, PMS, migraine, interstitial cystitis, multiple sclerosis, psoriasis and infertility. Yet, I've received an even greater number of calls and letters from women who, when asked about their medical history, say, "It's hard to know where to begin . . . I feel 'sick all over.'"

If you are such a person, it *is* important for you to seek out and find a physician who is not only competent, but also caring and compassionate. And, during the course of an examination or evaluation, he/she will usually be able to rule out many diseases and disorders. Yet, even a careful and comprehensive examination may fail to come up with a "diagnosis."

In discussing this situation, Martin H. Zwerling, M.D., Kenneth N. Owens, M.D., and Nancy H. Ruth, RN, BS, commented:

> "Consider the following 'incurable' patient who is being treated by several specialists. Her gynecologist is treating her recurrent vaginitis and irregular menstrual periods while an otolaryngologist is trying to control her external otitis and chronic rhinitis.

"At the same time, an internist is unsuccessfully attempting to manage symptoms of bloating, indigestion and abdominal pain and a dermatologist is struggling with bizarre skin rashes, hives and psoriasis.

"Lastly, psychiatrists have been unable to convince the patient that her nerves are the cause of her extreme irritability, inability to concentrate and depression. We've all been guilty of labeling such patients as 'psychosomatic' and since there is 'nothing physically wrong,' conclude that we cannot cure them.

"Incurable? Not if you think yeast. This patient and thousands like her are suffering from chronic candidiasis."[1]

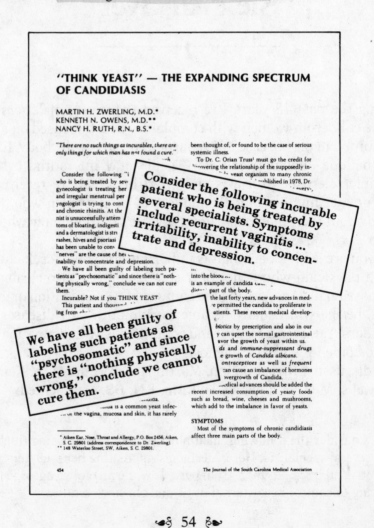

"THINK YEAST" — THE EXPANDING SPECTRUM OF CANDIDIASIS

MARTIN H. ZWERLING, M.D.*
KENNETH N. OWENS, M.D.**
NANCY H. RUTH, R.N., B.S.*

"There are no such things as incurables, there are only things for which man has not found a cure."

Consider the following "i... who is being treated by sev... gynecologist is treating her... and irregular menstrual per... yngologist is trying to cont... and chronic rhinitis. At the... nist is unsuccessfully attem... toms of bloating, indigesti... and a dermatologist is str... rashes, hives and psoriasi... has been unable to con... "nerves" are the cause of her... inability to concentrate and depression.

We have all been guilty of labeling such patients as "psychosomatic" and since there is "nothing physically wrong," conclude we can not cure them.

Incurable? Not if you THINK YEAST This patient and thousan... ing from ch...

> Consider the following incurable patient who is being treated by several specialists. Symptoms include recurrent vaginitis ... irritability, inability to concentrate and depression.

> We have all been guilty of labeling such patients as "psychosomatic" and since there is "nothing physically wrong," conclude we cannot cure them.

...ua is a common yeast infec-
... of the vagina, mucosa and skin, it has rarely

been thought of, or found to be the case of serious systemic illness.

To Dr. C. Orian Truss[1] must go the credit for ...covering the relationship of the supposedly in... ... yeast organism to many chronic ... ...blished in 1978, Dr. ... ...very-,

into the blood ...
is an example of candida ca... ...
diet... part of the body.

the last forty years, new advances in med- ...e permitted the candida to proliferate in atients. These recent medical develop- ...

biotics by prescription and also in our ...y can upset the normal gastrointestinal ...avor the growth of yeast within us. ...ds and *immune-suppressant drugs* ...e growth of *Candida albicans*. ...ontraceptives as well as *frequent* ...can cause an imbalance of hormones ...vergrowth of Candida. ...dical advances should be added the recent increased consumption of yeasty foods such as bread, wine, cheeses and mushrooms, which add to the imbalance in favor of yeasts.

SYMPTOMS
Most of the symptoms of chronic candidiasis affect three main parts of the body.

* Aiken Ear, Nose, Throat and Allergy, P.O. Box 2456, Aiken, S. C. 29801 (address correspondence to Dr. Zwerling).
** 148 Waterloo Street, SW, Aiken, S. C. 29801.

454   The Journal of the South Carolina Medical Association

Observations of Dr. C. Orian Truss

On the cover of his classic book, *The Missing Diagnosis*, Dr. C. Orian Truss said:

> "You may seem neurotic . . . but do you experience . . . depression, anxiety, irrational irritability, bloating, diarrhea, constipation, heartburn, indigestion, loss of self-confidence, inability to cope, lethargy, symptoms from contact with food and chemical odors, acne, migraine headaches . . . urethritis, cystitis, repeated vaginal yeast infections, premenstrual tension and menstrual problems? . . . These may be symptoms of a correctable illness."

And in a chapter entitled, "The Woman," Dr. Truss commented:

> "Repeatedly disappointed by the failure of past medical and psychiatric therapeutic approaches faithfully tried, disillusioned patients become increasingly skeptical of each new suggestion."

And in his continuing discussion, Dr. Truss described how yeast overgrowth could upset a woman's immune system, her hormones and affect many different organs of her body. He said:

> "Each woman with this problem will have experienced during the course of the illness perhaps 80% or more of the many manifestations that characterize this chronic yeast problem . . .

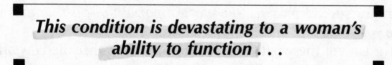

> ## *This condition is devastating to a woman's ability to function . . .*

> "This condition is devastating to a woman's ability to function, whether in a career as wife and mother or outside the home; its unpredictability often makes it impossible to plan activities requiring more than minimal responsibility.
> "To be shown a physical alternative to psychological factors as a cause of this disability is to be given reason for renewed hope. It is the first small step in the restoration of self-esteem, that, first shat-

tered by the illness itself, has been further eroded by the feelings of guilt and inadequacy engendered by the endless psychological explanations of this illness."

He also pointed out that when a woman understands the things she needs to do to overcome her problems, she must realize also that setbacks may occur. He said:

"Women with this condition can show great fortitude, and can accept the fact that patience and time will be required for a full recovery."[2]

Observations On My Own Patients

After learning about the relationship of superficial yeast infections to chronic illness from Dr. Truss in 1979, I began to see and help many patients with candida-related health problems. The great majority of these patients were women and over three-quarters were in their thirties. And I was gratified—even excited—when most of them responded favorably.

Their complaints included fatigue, irritability, PMS, headache and depression. Most gave a history of recurrent vaginal infections, loss of libido, painful intercourse and recurrent urinary tract infections.

The four patients whose stories I'm including in this section were all seen for the first time in the early '80s. And I'm featuring them for several reasons; *the most important one is that they will give you hope and optimism for the future.*

The first of these patients, 38-year-old Deborah, called my office for an appointment in October 1984. Here are excerpts from a six-page letter she sent me prior to her first visit.

Deborah's Story

"For over 15 years I've been bothered by recurrent urinary tract infections and persistent vaginal yeast infections. For at least 10 years I've had to make myself get out of bed every morning. I couldn't hear an alarm clock so my husband would literally have to drag me out. Many days I would feel tired and dazed, like a rag doll or a wet washrag.

> ### *For at least 10 years I've had to make myself get out of bed every morning.*

"Over the years I've been to all sorts of doctors because of my many complaints, including aching in my neck, joints and legs, noises in my ears, constipation, bloating, poor memory and a feeling of being 'spaced out.' As a result of all of these symptoms I've had absolutely no interest in sex.

"I've been hospitalized several times but the tests never showed anything. Chemicals of all sorts bothered me, including several brands of perfume. My symptoms also get worse when I eat sweetened foods or drink milk."

Because of her typical history, I put Deborah on a sugar-free, milk-free special diet, the antiyeast medication nystatin and nutritional supplements. She also got rid of the odorous chemicals in her home.

Two weeks after beginning treatment, Deborah reported:

"I'm much better. Less vaginal itching and burning, and less frequent urination. My energy level has improved significantly. I no longer feel bloated."

In the ensuing months, she steadily improved. However, she would notice a flare-up of symptoms when she ate foods containing sugar, or when she was exposed to chemicals. At a follow up visit six months after starting her treatment program, she reported:

"I've had an excellent winter. I'm symptom free and well except when I cheat on my diet."

In a Christmas card Deborah sent me several years ago she said:

"Just wanted you to know I'm really doing well. Thanks so much for your help."

Then in March 1993, I received a letter from her in which she said:

"I'm doing great. I'm happy and healthy. I rarely ever experience symptoms unless I'm exposed to chemicals or cheat too much on my diet."

Sara's Story

As readers of *The Yeast Connection* may recall, I looked after Sara as a newborn and on through childhood.[3] Like many youngsters during my early years of practice, Sara received many courses of antibiotic drugs for bacterial respiratory infections. Although my pediatric partners and I did our best to use antibiotics sparingly, if I'd been aware of the yeast-related health problems which might follow, I would have prescribed them less frequently.

During her teen years Sara developed occasional vaginal yeast infections, menstrual cramps, PMS and inappropriate drowsiness. In her early and mid-twenties, she developed additional problems, including urinary tract infections and more vaginal yeast infections.

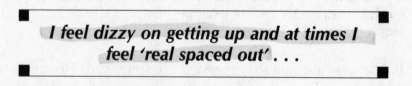

I feel dizzy on getting up and at times I feel 'real spaced out' . . .

Sara came back to see me as a patient at the age of 27. Here are excerpts from her medical record.

"I fall asleep anywhere and if I don't eat at frequent intervals I become weak. I feel dizzy on getting up and at times I feel 'real spaced out' like I'm not on this planet. My memory has been poor during recent years and at times I can't remember the names of people I know well. I feel uncoordinated, I stumble and drop things. My arms and legs ache. I'm also bothered by mood swings, frequent frontal headaches and severe menstrual cramps."

Because of the complexity of Sara's problems, I referred her to an endocrinologist for further study and workup. And on a treatment program which included a high protein diet and supplemental vitamins, Sara improved to a degree. Yet, she continued to be bothered by severe vaginal yeast infections and bouts of fatigue and lethargy.

Sara came back to see me again some months later and as I reviewed her history, I said:

"Sara, since you last came to see me, I've learned of the work of Dr. Orian Truss of Birmingham who feels that *Candida albicans*, the common yeast which causes vaginitis, plays an important role in causing health problems similar to those you've experienced over the years."

I prescribed nystatin, a yeast-free diet and nutritional supplements. Although Sara experienced a few ups and downs, she improved remarkably. When I saw her again in January 1983, she said:

"I feel great. No headaches, no spaced out feelings, lots of energy, only occasional mild premenstrual cramps. Life is full and exciting."

I felt her story would give other women with yeast-related health problems hope.

Because Sara's parents are close friends and across-the-street neighbors, I kept up with her over the years. And her health was so good I never again saw her as a patient. Yet, because I felt her story would give other women with yeast-related health problems hope, I'm including excerpts of my July 1993 conversation with Sara.

Crook: Sara, I know you've been doing well because I keep up with some of your many activities. Tell me a little bit more about what you've been doing.

Sara: Sure. I've had the busiest couple of weeks I can remember— because of all of my new business. It sort of exploded. People all over the country have been calling me. It's exciting.

Crook: That's great. I knew you were doing well because your parents brag on you from time to time. But let me ask you this. On a scale of one to ten, ten would be a state of health that no person achieves and one would be barely crawling out of bed. How do you rank?

Sara: Dr. Crook, I feel pretty fortunate. I'm far up on the scale. During the past decade I have, of course, experienced periods when I didn't feel good, along with periods when I felt okay and other periods when I felt really good. Right now, I'm close to the top of the scale. And to repeat, I feel fortunate, especially in comparing how I feel with other people I know.

Crook: How long did you have to take the nystatin? Your father told me you took it off and on for some years.

Sara: I'm still taking it—on occasion. I don't take it every day. I take it during the periods when I may feel a bit lethargic or get a trace of a yeast infection. Not like I used to, but it's sort of automatic. If I don't feel up to snuff, I tighten up on my diet and take nystatin.

Crook: How much do you take and how long do you take it?

Sara: I might take it for two or three months every day. Then when I get things under control I leave it off. When I first start taking it, I get some of those die-off symptoms. I feel like it's kind of working me over—if you know what I mean.

I don't really have a yeast problem any more because I know what to do about it.

Crook: Well, that's good evidence that you have some yeast in your intestinal tract that you're killing off. That proves it's doing you some good.

Sara: I don't really have a yeast problem any more because I know what to do about it. It's more of a nuisance now. I sure don't have the troubles I had ten years ago. I also take my nutritional supplements, including multivitamins, minerals, and primrose oil, especially the week before my period.

Crook: Any thing else you feel is important?

Sara: I don't drink alcohol. I haven't for the past four years. It seems like some of my friends were having problems with it so I stopped.

Crook: That's good because alcohol really triggers the yeast. Do you now have any headaches, muscle aches, constipation, bloating, skin rashes—any of those things?

Sara: None of the above.

Crook: How about exercise?

Sara: I've got an exercise bike in my bedroom. I also have weights. Every day I exercise with the weights and every other day I get on the bike.

Crook: Have you had to take any antibiotics in the last ten years?

Sara: No, I don't take antibiotics.

Crook: There could be an occasion when you need them. Especially for strep throat, pneumonia, sinusitis or a severe urinary tract infection. And if your doctor puts you on antibiotics, you'd need to take nystatin and, if that isn't helping promptly, I'd suggest Diflucan or Sporanox.

Sara: Thanks, Dr. Crook, for calling. I'll let you know if I have any problems.

Janet's Story

In 1982, Janet, a physician's daughter, came to see me searching for help. Here are excerpts from a letter she sent me prior to our first visit:

"I'm ready to find out if it's 'all in my head' and my symptoms are due to 'just getting older' or whether there's something that's really making me sick."

Janet then told me about many of the symptoms which had bothered her for years, including abdominal pain, aching in her fingers, headache, dizziness, nausea, persistent night cough, chest pain and chemical sensitivities, and she said:

"This spring I developed bladder problems; two infections and frequent urination. I've also been unable to empty my bladder without hard pushing. These symptoms took me to a urologist who diagnosed it as 'a small urethra and spasm.' He dilated me and gave medicine. Incidentally, frequent urination had been a part of my life, but not the pressure. (I have even wet the bed since I've been married.) I also am bothered by nervousness, fatigue, puffiness in my fingers, bloating, excessive weight gain and breast soreness during the week before my period."

On a simple but comprehensive treatment program which featured nystatin, dietary changes and nutritional supplements, Janet steadily improved. She moved to an adjoining state in 1985 and although I haven't seen her as a patient since that time, I've kept in touch with her through occasional letters and phone calls. And I knew she was doing well. To get an update I wrote her in March 1993 and asked her to send me a progress report. Here are excerpts from her letter:

"Thanks for your letter. I'm doing quite well and enjoying my forties healthwise much more than my thirties. I'm 43 now and am quite busy with three children. One almost 17, one 14 and one 5. I operate with my energy level much higher today than when we first began the 'yeast journey' together.

> *I'm doing quite well and enjoying my forties healthwise much more than my thirties.*

"I still don't eat bread, but I do have yeast in my diet, some sugar and other junk. But overall my eating is much healthier than ten years ago."[4]

Karen's Story

This registered nurse and mother of four first came to see me on October 1, 1981. Because her story illustrated so many important points, I reproduced in full a six-page letter she wrote me November 19, 1982, 13 months after she started on a comprehensive treatment program which included anticandida medication.[5]

Karen's story should give people with yeast-connected health problems hope that they can get well. Yet, it isn't always easy. And no physician can provide a quick fix. In Karen's case it took a lot of hard work, including home detective work. Karen gradually improved during the mid-1980s on a comprehensive program which included antifungal medications, immunotherapy for allergies, avoidance of environmental chemicals and oral antifungal therapy. Yet, at times there were setbacks.

To get an update on how she's getting along, I called her in June of 1993. Here are excerpts from our conversation.

"My severe vaginal problems which tormented me for so many years have gone away—almost as though the problem never existed. And I haven't had to take nystatin, amphotericin B, Nizoral or other oral antifungal therapy for over four years. Yet, I do notice some itching and burning during the spring and fall pollen seasons. I believe you told me it was a form of 'vaginal hay fever.'

My severe vaginal problems . . . have gone away.

"Several years ago I was tormented by urinary frequency and I had to urinate up to 60 times a day. Comprehensive examinations by a urologist, plus my home diet detective work, showed that the cause was an allergic cystitis. And the medication I was taking had a corn base and I am clearly sensitive to corn in any form.

"I was also sensitive to ordinary wheat bread. Through networking I found that I can tolerate whole living wheat, which is organically grown, and this enables me to have bread which I normally could not tolerate. I also take big doses of vitamin C and calcium and magnesium and take supplemental vitamins at times when I can afford them.

"But compared to my health ten years ago, my problems are literally nonexistent. I do have a sensitive bladder and have to urinate frequently, but I drink lots of fluid."

In a conversation with me in August 1994, she said in effect:

"My health is superb. And except for mild seasonal hay fever, I have no complaints. I'm delighted to know that you'll be including my story in your next book. It should give other women hope."

Comments of Dr. John Curlin

In the early '80s, John Curlin, a Jackson, Tennessee gynecologist, developed an interest in yeast-connected health problems. Here are comments he made at that time:

"Since entering practice, I've seen thousands of patients with various gynecological dysfunctions. Their complaints have included pelvic pain, menstrual irregularities, PMS, infertility, endometriosis, vaginitis, painful intercourse and absence of normal sexual interest and response.

"Two years ago I learned about yeast-related illness and began to use diet, nystatin and candida extracts in treating many of my patients. Although this program did not relieve all of their symptoms, the response in many of my patients has been gratifying. In addition to the typical gynecological problems that have responded, many patients with other health problems, including arthritis, colitis and other autoimmune disorders, have also improved."

In the spring of 1993, I was invited to give a presentation to a group of gynecologists at the University of Tennessee. In gathering information, I again asked Dr. Curlin for his observations and comments. Here's an excerpt from a letter he sent me:

"Since you stimulated my interest over 15 years ago, I've treated literally hundreds of patients with oral nystatin, sugar-free diet and emphasis on good health measures such as exercise . . .

"If a patient is willing to abide by the diet and take the nystatin, recurrent vaginal candidiasis can be successfully treated almost 100% of the time. And many patients with chronic fatigue and multiple other immune dysfunction symptoms can also be greatly helped.

> ## *Many patients with chronic fatigue and multiple other symptoms can also be greatly helped.*

"In talking to my patients I tell them of the controversy regarding the causes of the symptoms and the treatment. Yet, I've had no adverse effect from the therapy and many patients who found no relief in the orthodox medical community have been greatly helped by this simple therapy."

Patients of Dr. George E. Shambaugh, Jr.

Every person needs heroes—people who inspire them—people in whose footsteps they'd like to follow. Over the years, I've acquired a number of heroes, including Dr. Shambaugh. This 91-year-old practicing physician sees and helps many patients each week, gives lectures at international medical meetings and writes a newsletter. In the early 1990s, as I was gathering information for this book, I asked Dr. Shambaugh if he would tell me about some of his most exciting and gratifying patients. Here are some of their stories.

Paige Grant Pell: "I enjoyed generally good health except for headaches, which plagued me since I was a child. I also had frequent vaginal and urinary tract infections. Yet, I was able to control them with antibiotics. Before I was married I was a full time model and commercial actress and I never missed a day's work for illness.

"Then in my mid-30's I began to subtly slide into various problems. By 1990 I had very little energy, felt generally awful, slept a lot and was seeking medical help frequently. I started to feel like I was crazy because the doctors couldn't find out exactly what was wrong with me. They would usually give me antibiotics and I would get better, then I would get worse.

> ### Since 1984 I estimate that I saw about 50 different doctors for various ailments.

"Since 1984 I estimate that I saw about 50 different doctors for various ailments, including a psychotherapist, because I was beginning to think it might be 'all in my head.' My husband and I estimate my cost for this period at about $100,000.

"Finally I saw Dr. Alan McDaniel, a New Albany, Indiana ear, nose and throat specialist and an allergist. I think he saved my life. On a comprehensive program which included anticandida therapy and treatment for my allergies, I began to feel like a new person. Later I moved to Chicago and continued under the good care of Dr. George Shambaugh.

"I've been involved in many personal and community projects, which I never would have been able to do until now. I no longer have the irritability and mood swings. I only have headaches now when I eat the wrong food.

"I've had such a dramatic recovery that I would like to see other women reached by your work. Please let me know how I can help."

Nora: "I began developing health problems in 1984. My symptoms included PMS, severe fatigue, joint pain, irregular heart beat and low grade sore throat. I was so tired and sick that I had to quit my teaching job. I was incapacitated. I was also weak and emaciated and had lost 27 lbs.

"In 1987 I went to Dr. Shambaugh who put me on a comprehensive treatment program which included a sugar-free special diet, nystatin and acidophilus. This treatment helped me regain my health and get my life back on track. I'd been on birth control pills for about 5 years which probably contributed in part to my yeast infections and other problems. Yet, I didn't want to get pregnant because my health was too poor.

"Then, after my health improved, I stopped the birth control pills and I'm happy to say that I now have a year old, healthy child.

"I also read your book *The Yeast Connection* many times and it has helped me a lot in regaining my health. I'm also a born again Christian and I feel that prayer and faith all played an important part in helping me regain my health and important parts of my life."

Jeri: "During my twenties I craved sweets and had constant sore throats and didn't feel well. I experienced many illnesses and I had repeated headaches. In my efforts to find help I saw five different allergists. Nothing they did was effective. Then I was referred to Dr. Shambaugh and in two weeks after starting on a comprehensive program which included nystatin and a sugar-free diet, I began to improve.

"I also have two boys, ages 11 and 7, who in the past have experienced allergies of various sorts. Now, on a good diet and environmental control measures, they're healthy.

> ### I feel so good now that I'm sorry I didn't feel this way when I was in my twenties.

"I feel so good now that I'm sorry I didn't feel this way when I was in my twenties. At one point Dr. Shambaugh said to me, 'I hope that after you follow my treatment program, you'll feel as good as I do!'"*

Mary: "All of my adult life I have been bothered by fatigue and many other symptoms which came and went with no regularity or predictability. No doctor (and there were many) was able to find a cause or to provide me with help. The final condition which completely incapacitated me was extreme exhaustion and a 'fuzzy brain.' I just could not 'put things together.'

"Then I read the book *The Yeast Syndrome* and I found 'the story of my life.' It was a marvelous revelation which finally brought me to Dr. Shambaugh. On a comprehensive program including nystatin, a sugar free special diet, nutritional supplements, avoidance of food allergens and allergy vaccines, 90% of my symptoms have gone away."

---

*In an October 1994 message I received from Jeri, she said that she had only been "sick" once in the past six years and that was a slight cold.

Letters I've Received

During the past decade, I've received tens of thousands of letters in my office and in the office of the International Health Foundation and the great majority have come from women. *Some make me feel wonderful—excited, happy and gratified. Yet others make me feel frustrated, depressed and even angry.* First, I'll tell a story that has a happy ending.

Alexandria On a Saturday morning in November 1993, I went to my office to pick up a book and some papers. As I was leaving, the Federal Express man pulled up. He said:

> "Dr. Crook, I didn't really expect to find you here. Here's an overnight letter addressed to your office. I also have what seems to be a letter from the same person directed to your home address."

I opened the packets and the contents of each were identical three-page letters from 27-year-old Alexandria (not her name). Here are excerpts:

> ## *I cannot tell you enough the pain I'm in.*
> ## *. . . I feel I'm running out of time*

> "I cannot tell you enough the pain I'm in. I urge you to respond a.s.a.p. to this letter. I feel I'm running out of time . . . My problems began in 1981. I've had tons and tons of yeast infections. I've taken over 4000 pills and antibiotics for urinary tract infections, pelvic inflammatory disease and other infections. The yeast medications like Terazol, Monistat, Betadine, douche, yogurt, Gyne-Lotrimin and many others—you name it—haven't worked. I'm now very ill.
> "I never realized that yeast could be the reason for all of my problems. No one explained this to me and it's been going on for ten years. I've been hospitalized and they've done endoscopic examina-

tions on me. I've taken IV antibiotics which made me worse than ever. And surgery didn't help.

"I continued to have all sorts of symptoms, including urinary frequency, abnormal spotting, dizziness, headache and weird out feelings. I was so depressed. Also abdominal pain and weakness—I've almost fainted.

"The bleeding is worse now than it was over a year ago. I've seen three gynecologists who said they find no bladder infection, no chlamydia and no gonorrhea. Nevertheless, they gave me more antibiotics and Bactrim. Symptoms again became worse. Now they feel I need another laparoscopy/hysteroscopy.

"I read your book for the first time yesterday and after reading the stories of others I believe in my heart my problems are yeast-related. I've taken birth control pills, had an abortion, have a little endometriosis and eat sugary foods—crave them. I can't get rid of the yeast infections. My bladder feels like it's pressing down to make me urinate. *It's really bad!* I can't get anyone to care enough to help me or to listen, or to look deep enough.

"I don't want a hysterectomy. I don't want to keep taking antibiotics. They don't work. I'll fly to Tennessee to see you. I'm really scared I'm dying. I can't believe this is happening to me. I almost didn't get this letter out fast enough. My typewriter ribbon stopped just as I was typing so I'm writing you long hand. I need you desperately. I don't want to show up on your doorstep, but I'm scared and I'm lost."

Alexandria's letter really got my attention. And I responded at once. Fortunately, she lived only about 50 miles from a kind and caring physician, who was also knowledgeable in treating yeast-related health problems.

In March 1994 I received a letter from Alexandria telling me that she was improving, and, to check on her, I called her in August 1994. Here's an excerpt of what she had to say:

"Before starting on treatment my worst symptoms were constant abdominal pain, vaginal itching and more especially the feeling of being 'sick all over.' I'm now at least 90% along the road to being completely well. I'm working every day as a supervisor of a marketing research firm and have a wonderful relationship.

> ## *I'm now at least 90% along the road to being completely well.*

"I cut out all sugar and most of the red meat. I eat lots of vegetables. I also stopped fruits for two months, but then I was able to start them again and they don't bother me.

"I took the Diflucan prescribed by my doctor, but I didn't have to take it very long. I also took vitamin/mineral supplements and acidophilus. I'm taking no prescription medicine now and sex causes no problems. I'll send you a further report, in a few months, as I get even healthier."

Other Letters That Make Me Feel Good

Nan: "I'm a 41-year old female enthusiastically starting on your candida control diet.

"A persistent vaginal infection is what finally caused me to seek out your book. Perhaps my history would be of interest to you. At least it must be very gratifying to know how helpful your book has been to me—as it has to so many others.

"I've been tired all of my life. Damp days are the worst. I've had joint aches, itchy patches of skin, vaginal infections, painful intercourse, asthma and allergies and depression. I tried to commit suicide when I was 20.

"My slumber is deep and I awake in a stupor. Mental confusion, dizziness and feeling spacy and anxious are all part of my daily routine. These in turn have caused feelings of inadequacy because I can't cope with daily life. Trying to keep up with three children, plus all the necessary household chores. And as you might guess, my interest in sex has become nonexistent. . . .

"I've always craved sugar and wheat. I could go on with more problems, but those I've mentioned are the major ones and seem so similar to various patients you described. After reading your book I knew beyond a shadow of a doubt that the anticandida diet is what I need."

In her continuing discussion, Nan said that after starting on the diet and taking caprylic acid and garlic she's improving. And she said:

"Already I'm not as bloated. My fingers aren't as fat and stiff in the morning. Fatigue and spaciness are improving."

She also told of some ups and downs and she said:

"Yesterday was rainy and damp and I felt terrible. My drowsiness was nearly narcoleptic. Today I awoke feeling just as bad and very depressed and discouraged about the diet. However, I improved immediately after a bowel movement. I continued to 'stay the course' and got through the day without lying down . . .

"While it is somewhat frustrating there isn't treatment to zap the candida and free me instantly from all of my symptoms, I'm resigned to work very hard to achieve good health. I realize it may be a lengthy process. I intend to seek the help of Dr. Harold Walmer who treats candidiasis . . .

"Truly I'm not writing you to obtain a response. I only wanted to let you know how grateful I am to you for the prospect of changing my life."

Susan: "I believe I can trace my yeast-related symptoms back to my childhood as I was plagued with constant ear and throat infections. I've never taken birth control pills, but have consistently ingested a diet high in sugar and yeasty foods.

> ## I would have bouts of tremendous bloating, constipation and overall lethargy.

"Dating back to high school I would have bouts of tremendous bloating, constipation and overall lethargy which was to me disturbing, but unexplainable.

"The episodic bloating/constipation/lethargy continued through my twenties and into my thirties. Eventually I realized that my symptoms appeared the worst immediately after eating. Following some detective work of my own, I presumed I was allergic to wheat. Yet, when my symptoms returned immediately after eating wheat-free yeast bread, I decided to look at the yeast connection more closely.

"As I have eliminated sugar, fruits and white flour and rice from my diet, I have felt like I never dreamed was possible. I never realized all the systemic effects that the yeast was having on me. I thought the spaciness, insomnia, constipation, bloating, lethargy, funny feeling in my extremities and terrible headaches were a normal part of life.

"I now see that this is not the case; my sinuses have cleared completely (I didn't realize how stuffed my nose was); my PMS has nearly subsided; I can fit into my clothing more easily and the list goes on. Suffice to say that I'm grateful and hooked. Curiously, however, all the symptoms return if I inadvertently happen upon some yeast in food."

Linda: "Thank you so much for sending me information about candida. I greatly appreciated it. I'm writing to give you a report. First, for the good news. I started the whole family on the diet beginning two weeks ago. I noted a strange thing. We're urinating a lot without drinking much. I assumed it was our own bodies excreting extra fluids. By the third or fourth day I noted that the little "fat pooch" below my umbilicus was gone. I always thought it was a normal female thing to have a little fat pooch there. I guess not. It was just extra fluid.

"Even without medication I began feeling better. My symptoms have been depression, insomnia, gas, vaginal infection, migraines (onset one and a half years ago), memory and concentration loss and extreme fatigue.

"We all started getting better. My husband's symptoms, including allergies, muscle and joint aches and pains, low endurance, constipation/diarrhea cycles of 2 to 3 weeks/2 to 3 days, respectively, improved also. He only sneezed six times in one week—could breathe. His soreness after activity was minimal, BM's more normal and increased energy.

"Now for more really good news. Yesterday, I went to see Dr. R. Gapal Mallad in Holyoke, Massachusetts. He gets 5 stars in my book and so does his staff. *He was willing to see the whole family.* He listened and also did a brief exam of the kids. He stated that he suspected candida in all of us.

"He addressed all my concerns and wanted me to feel comfortable and knowledgeable about the medication and diet plan. His personality was warm and kind and his knowledge of the disorder was extensive. He then referred me to a staff of nurses who all helped me with diet questions, food and vitamin sources, etc.

"They have an excellent and comprehensive compilation of diet information and sources to get food products locally, as well as menus and recipes. They were all extremely nice and helpful. An answer to prayer! They were also willing for me to call anytime with questions and concerns. His fee was also very reasonable.

"Lastly, I would like to know how I can personally help expose the reality of this disorder to the public and physicians, and/or help the foundation.

"I plan to send the information you sent me to our family doctor who does not believe in this diagnosis. I would also like to send some more to the OBGYN clinic in our town. I'm personally distressed at how hard help is to find. I've had symptoms for ten years; initially treated, but not comprehensively, and thus not completely. I then tabled any thoughts of candida until recently when symptoms got so bad I knew it was candida again.

"I'll look forward to hearing from you. God Bless."

Some Disheartening Letters

These are the letters which make me feel sad, yet, which make me work harder to bring the relationship of yeast to chronic illness into the medical mainstream:

Eleanor: "I'm very sick and need help. *The doctors around here refuse to believe anything about yeast-related illness.* I've read books and have been treating myself with some things from a health food store. I get better, then I get bad again. I feel like I'm slowly being poisoned.

"I've been in many doctors' offices and hospitals and they don't find anything wrong. Yet, I don't get well and all I've been given are more nerve pills and antidepressants, which make me sicker.

> *If there's anyone in the country who can help me I'll travel there.*

"I have so many doctor and hospital bills piled up that if I could find a doctor to help me I really don't know how I would pay him. Very slowly I guess. If there's anyone in the country who can help me I'll travel there. I'm sick, I'm desperate, I'm broke and I'm scared—real scared. If there's research going on anywhere, I would volunteer to be a part of it.

"Here's a list of my symptoms I've had for the last 10 years, and the last 6 months these symptoms have been worse:

vaginal infections	pain in jaw	PMS
depression	dizziness	thrush
muscle and joint pain	always tired	headache
pain down back	tightness in chest	nausea
sinusitis	shortness of breath	bloating
constipation	no feeling in vagina	colitis

If you could help me in any way I would be grateful. I want to stop this before it goes into something more serious. I have a lot to live for and I just want to get well."

> **The past year my life has been a living hell. I've seen eight different doctors, none could help.**

Amy: "I'm a white 25-year-old female. The past year my life has been a living *hell*. I've seen eight different doctors, none of whom could help. Most decided my many symptoms must be 'all in my mind.'

"The medications the doctors have tried me on include Tagamet, Zantac, Valium, vaginal cream, Keflex and steroids for sinus trouble. The tests I've gone through include endoscopies (upper GI and small intestine), ultra sound and hundreds of blood tests.

"The doctors I've gone to have tested me for ulcers, mono, leukemia, Hodgkin's disease, Epstein Barr Virus and cancer. I continue to be ill and my symptoms during the past year include: nausea, unbelievable chest and stomach pains, gas, dizziness and feeling spaciness, fatigue, insomnia, depression (crying every day and became suicidal when no one was helping me).

"Also unbelievable postnasal drip, black circles under my eyes, shortness of breath (I'm a dance instructor and could not even teach), heart spells, muscle weakness, ear fluid and pain, skin rashes on my elbows, constipation alternating with diarrhea, anxiety and irritability and trouble breathing.

"I crave sugar and bread and if I don't eat at frequent intervals I feel weak with fatigue, irritability, headache, stomachache and belching.

"I'm also bothered by exposure to perfume, colognes, paints, hair spray, beauty parlors and grocery store detergent isles.

"I'm supposed to be married soon but I don't want to make his life a living hell. I'm afraid to have children because I'm afraid whatever I have will kill them.

> ## My only wish is to get better and to get on with my life.

"I've come close to losing my business over this and I've been a total burden on my family for the past year. My only wish is to get better and to get on with my life. Whatever this illness is, it has destroyed an entire year of my life and of my family's life.

"I came upon your book, *The Yeast Connection,* and it gave me hope. I scored 245 on the test. My biggest problem, I've been to every doctor in my area and none of them have the slightest idea about the yeast connection. I'm at the end of my rope and I don't know where to turn. I'll go anywhere for help. I'm too young to give up on life so soon.

"PLEASE HELP!"

Sophia: "I'm writing you this letter with great hope. I read your book *The Yeast Connection* and it was as though a light bulb went off in my head. So many of the female case histories you cited in your book sounded like me.

"For all of my adult life (I am now 51, and my symptoms began in my teens) I've suffered from a painful, persistent vaginitis which has defied diagnosis by medical experts. I've seen literally dozens of specialists over the years ranging from gynecologists young and old, dermatologists, various clinics and even a psychiatrist. I know my problem is not in my head, and yet on every test nothing conclusive appears.

"This vaginitis has made my life miserable with its periodic outbreaks and I can readily identify with the woman in your book who said that at times she even considered 'ending it all.' It is wrenching to suffer from a physical ailment only to be told 'there's nothing wrong.'

"The problem has now reached the crisis state. My husband of 30 years is a loving, understanding and supportive man. But after so many years of patience he is reaching his limit. I have absolutely no interest in sex (we've not had sexual relations in over a year). Even if I am 'symptom free' at the moment, the fear of having sex and a subsequent flare up it causes for me, I am totally afraid to try.

"I'm also totally fatigued all the time, even after a week of 9 to 10 hours of sleep and I'm bothered by a constantly red, cracked tongue covered with a coat.

"I had to write to you as your book is the first glimmer of hope I've had. Since you cared enough to write this book to help yeast sufferers, I have to think you might have time to help me as well. Please recommend a doctor in the Los Angeles area who understands yeast. I could even come to Tennessee, that's how willing I am to be helped."

Judy: "I'm sure you've heard this before, but one more time can't hurt:

"I'M D-E-S-P-E-R-A-T-E !!!!!

"After finally tracking down a logical cause for what has been ailing me for the past two years, *I discovered that the waiting list to see sympathetic physicians ranges from 6 months to a year!* I'm at the wrist-slitter's stage . . . The thought of postponing knowledgeable help is unbearable!

"Hysteria is not my style . . . forgive me. I would appreciate any help you can give . . . to find a doctor in my area (Gulfcoast area of Alabama, Mississippi, Florida, or a recommended specialist in the Southeast) who might see me sooner than next February.

"Thanks in advance for your support. As soon as I learn more about this syndrome and how to conquer it, I want to form a self-help group for other would-be wrist-slitters. It's nice to know we're not crazy or alone."

> # *I've gone to six different doctors and they all tell me I'll have to live with it.*

Cora: "I need to find a physician who is well versed in treating yeast infections, as I've had one for almost three years now. I've gone to six different doctors and they all end up telling me, 'You'll have to live with it. We do not know what else to try.'

"I need someone to take an active interest in my case and not just treat me as one of the 'herd.' I need a physician who will be willing to try different combinations of drug therapy and work with me to solve my problem.

"Since March 1991, I've had the following symptoms: vaginal burning, itching and discharge. My entire bottom, including my vulva and my rectum, is bright red. Any rubbing or friction makes the area more painful, burning and red. (This includes wiping and wearing pantyhose.) I've also had repeated urinary tract infections.

"I hope you can help me as I am desperate."

My Comments

How have I responded to these desperate pleas for help? I've tried a number of different approaches. Ten years ago, with the help of friends and relatives, I established the International Health Foundation (IHF). It obtained its charter from the State of Tennessee in 1985 and received approval by the Internal Revenue Service as a non-profit organization in 1986.

The goals of the foundation included:

- Providing people who wrote and called IHF with information and help.
- Establishing a roster of physicians interested in yeast-related disorders.
- Working to obtain credibility for the yeast/human interaction.
- Providing information to physicians and other professionals.

In certain ways, IHF has succeeded. We were able to help many people find physicians. We also organized and carried out two conferences on the candida/human interaction. Participants included prominent physicians from North America and Europe. Then, in 1994, IHF received a grant from a major pharmaceutical company, which, along with donations from friends, is being used to fund scientific studies on the relationship of superficial yeast infections to multiple sclerosis and other chronic illnesses.

Yet, in certain ways, we failed. The number of physicians on our IHF referral list never grew as much as we hoped that it would. Although we had 90 physicians on our California list, in some states (even populous ones) there were fewer than ten and in other states there were none!

Another problem: A number of physicians on our list had so many requests for their services that persons seeking help had to wait six months or longer for an appointment.

Where Can You Find Help?

If your physician is kind and caring, even if she is skeptical of the yeast connection, write her a letter. First, thank her for her kindness and for her interest in your health problems. Next, say "I feel that my health problems are yeast-related and I would appreciate your help."

> *If your physician is kind and caring, even if she is skeptical of the yeast connection, write her a letter.*

Then, copy and enclose selected pages from this book, including "A Special Message to the Physician" and the Preface, which cites the comments of three board certified obstetricians and gynecologists. If she shows interest, lend her the whole book. Or, if she'll write or call me, I'll send her several articles from the medical literature.

If you do not have a physician who fits into the above category, call your local hospital or medical society and obtain a list of gynecologists and/or family physicians in your community. Select the names of several and write a one to two-page letter summarizing your symptoms and medical history. Then say, "I feel that my health problems may be yeast-related. Will you help me?" Also ask for an estimate of charges.

If you're unable to find a physician (M.D. or D.O.), you may find help from other licensed professionals, including nutritional doctors (NDs), chiropractors (DCs), registered nurses (RNs) and other knowledgeable counselors.

In some communities, there are support groups for people with the candida related complex (CRC), multiple chemical sensitivity syndrome (MCSS), chronic fatigue syndrome (CFS/CFIDS) and many others. By getting in touch with these groups, you may be able to obtain the names of knowledgeable and interested professionals who can help you. See Part Nine for further information.

REFERENCES

1. Zwerling, M.H., Owens, K.N. and Ruth, N.H., "Think Yeast—The Expanding Spectrum of Candidiasis," *South Carolina Med. Assoc.*, 1984; 80:454–456.
2. Truss, C.O., *The Missing Diagnosis*, P.O. Box 26508, Birmingham, AL 35226, 1983 and 1986; pp 19–21.
3. Crook, W.G., *The Yeast Connection*, Third Edition, Professional Books, Jackson, TN and Vintage Books, New York, 1986; pp 175–177.
4. Crook, W.G., *The Yeast Connection*, Third Edition, Professional Books, Jackson, TN and Vintage Books, New York, 1986; pp 5–8.
5. Crook, W.G., *The Yeast Connection*, Third Edition, Professional Books, Jackson, TN and Vintage Books, New York, 1986; pp 224–228.

7

---◆---

Why Women Develop
Yeast-Related Health
Disorders More Often
Than Men

---◆---

During the early and mid-1980s, I reviewed the records of 100 consecutive adult patients with yeast-related problems. There were 86 females and 14 males. Three women were older than 55 and two were younger than 21. The peak age of women who were affected was 33–37. Yet, there were many women in their late 20s and early 30s or in their late 30s and early to mid-40s.

Why did I see many more women in their mid-30s than in other age groups? I'm not certain that I know the answer, but here's one possible explanation.

Women in their 30s that I saw during the early and mid-1980s were born in the late 1940s and early 1950s. Those were the years when the broad-spectrum antibiotics were first introduced and began to be widely used in treating children with respiratory and other infections. As pointed out by Dr. Carol Jessop in her presentations on the chronic fatigue syndrome, most of her patients were women and almost all gave a history of repeated courses of antibiotic drugs in infancy, childhood and adolescence.

Based on the calls and letters I've received during the 1990s, the ages of women during the last several years have changed. Now, women in their 40s seem to be troubled by yeast-related health problems as much as women in their 30s.

Why do women develop yeast-related problems more often than men? And why do pre-menopausal women appear to be especially susceptible?

Although I don't claim to possess a scientific answer for these questions, here are my thoughts:

Anatomical differences   Women are more apt to develop yeast-related health problems because of the differences in their anatomy.

They frequently develop urinary infections because the urethra (the tube leading from the urinary bladder to the outside) is short. Accordingly, bacteria are much more apt to enter the woman's bladder and set up an infection.

Urinary tract infections are especially apt to occur in women following frequent or prolonged sexual intercourse ("honeymoon cystitis"). When these infections occur, they're usually treated with antibiotic drugs.

The candida yeasts which live normally in the intestinal tract, multiply when a woman takes antibiotics. The proximity of the anal opening to the vulva and vagina increases a woman's chances of developing a genital infection.

> ### Since yeasts thrive on the warm, dark, interior membranes of the body, the vagina furnishes a hospitable home.

Since yeasts thrive on the warm, dark, interior membranes of the body, the vagina furnishes a hospitable home. By contrast, males are much less apt to develop a genital yeast infection.

The Pill   In his classic book, *The Missing Diagnosis,* Dr. C. Orian Truss listed the various factors which cause candida-related health problems and their prevention. Included were antibiotics, dietary factors, immunosuppressive drugs and birth control pills. Here are excerpts:

"The advent of the contraceptive hormones commonly known as the 'birth control pill' or simply 'the pill' had a further impact on the yeast problem in the female population . . . Approximately 35% of women using 'the pill' were having severe chronic yeast vaginitis . . . Alternate methods of contraception are available and should replace the use of these hormones in women susceptible to their impact on yeast growth."[1]

Ellen Grant, a British obstetrician/gynecologist has, for many years, expressed concern about possible adverse effects of the pill. I met Dr. Grant at a medical conference in Florida over ten years ago and in 1985 my wife, Betsy, and I had dinner at her home in Surrey. During our visit, she gave me a copy of her 270-page book, *The Bitter Pill*, which discussed the adverse effects of the pill on young women who take it. And in commenting on yeast problems, she said:

"Candidiasis is caused by the yeast *Candida albicans*, a normal habitant of our digestive tract . . . It can overgrow and cause irritating white plaques in the vagina when a woman's resistance is lowered by taking the pill . . . taking antibiotics . . . or eating too much sugar. Candidiasis is at least doubled among pill users . . ."[2]

Hormonal changes associated with the normal menstrual cycle encourage yeast colonization So do hormonal changes during pregnancy. Quoting Dr. Truss again:

"Estrogen is produced throughout the monthly cycle. Progesterone is produced in very small quantities prior to ovulation, but thereafter in large quantity until the onset of the next period. This high level of progesterone persists throughout pregnancy when conception occurs . . . By unknown mechanisms, progesterone greatly aggravates yeast growth in women . . . Also, women with chronic yeast vaginitis usually are aware that their symptoms are worse from ovulation to the next period, coinciding with the interval of increased progesterone production and the monthly cycle."[3]

Pre-menopausal women go to physicians more often than men
Some of these visits are for routine check-ups and Pap smears.
Others are for pregnancy—or for vaginal yeast infections. By contrast, men between the ages of 15 and 45 rarely go to a physician
unless they experience an athletic injury or go for an insurance
exam.

So, a young woman is apt to develop a personal relationship
with a physician. Accordingly, when she develops a fever, cough or
cold, she's apt to call her physician and say, "We're beginning our
family vacation this week and I don't want to be sick . . . *Please*
send me an antibiotic."

Many times the obliging physician answers her request and antibiotics promote the growth of yeasts.

Prolonged antibiotics for teenagers with acne Teenagers, especially girls, are concerned about their complexions. So they're
more apt to consult a phy-
sician and to be put on
long-term antibiotics. These
drugs, including minocy-
cline (Minocin), doxycycline
(Vibramycin) and/or other
tetracyclines are apt to be
prescribed for teenage girls

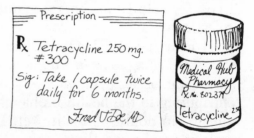

more often than for teenage boys. Although these drugs seem to
help some youngsters with acne, they wipe out normal bacteria in
the intestinal tract. As a result, yeasts multiply and a "cascade" of
other health problems often develop.

REFERENCES

1. Truss, C.O., *The Missing Diagnosis,* P.O. Box 26508, Birmingham, AL,
   35226, 1993.
2. Grant, E., *The Bitter Pill,* Corgi, Elm Tree/Hamish Hamilton Edition,
   London, 1986; p 174.
3. Truss, C.O., *The Missing Diagnosis,* P.O. Box 26508, Birmingham, AL
   35226, 1993.

8

◆

Steps You'll Need to Take to Regain Your Health

◆

You can overcome your health problems and get your life back on track!

And believing that you can is the essential first step. You'll need, of course, help from others, including professionals and non-professionals. You'll also need love and support from family members, friends, networking individuals and groups. Yet, say to yourself, *"If it's going to be, it's up to me."*

The common yeast, *Candida albicans,* plays an important role in contributing to the health problems of many people—especially women. No doubt about it. Yet, I want to emphasize that "candida" isn't like a dragon that you can slay with a single thrust of a sword or with a "magic bullet."

If your health problems are yeast connected, a special diet and antifungal medication will start you on the road to recovery. Yet, such therapy is only a part of what you need to do.

Most people with yeast-related health problems resemble the proverbial overburdened camel. To regain your health, you'll need to unload many bundles of straw. This may take months—even a year or more. But then your camel can get on her feet and start walking—then running.

In this section I'll outline—in brief—the steps you'll need to take. Then in Part Seven, I'll give you more detailed instructions.

A. Clean Up Your Diet

If you want to overcome your yeast-related health problems, you must change your diet. As a first step—go to your kitchen and get rid of the sugar,* corn syrup, white bread and other white flour products, soft drinks and most ready-to-eat cereals.

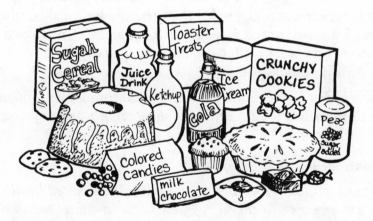

Foods and beverages containing these nutritionally deficient simple carbohydrates promote poor health. To overcome a candida-related health problem, you'll need to avoid them.

---

*To replace sugar you can use liquid saccharin (Sweeta or Fasweet) or fructooligo-saccharides (FOS), which you find at some pharmacies and health food stores. You'll find more information in Chapter 27.

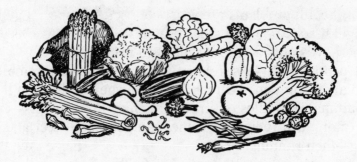

Replace them with more vegetables, including some you don't usually eat. Also, go to your health food store and buy some of the "grain alternatives"—amaranth, quinoa and buckwheat.

You'll also need to get rid of foods containing hydrogenated and partially hydrogenated oils (especially coconut and other tropical oils) and replace them with modest amounts of unrefined oils, including flax seed, canola and olive.

Avoid yeasty foods and beverages, especially dried fruits, mushrooms, condiments, alcohol, juices (except for freshly squeezed juices), leavened breads, bagels, pastries, pretzels, pizza and rolls. In two or three weeks, after you improve, you can try a yeasty food and see if it bothers you.

Diets aren't forever and after a few weeks, or months, you *may* be able to relax a bit. *Yet, until you show significant improvement, stick to your diet.*

B. Control Chemical Exposures

Almost without exception, people with yeast-related health problems are sensitive to chemicals they come in contact with during everyday life. These include tobacco smoke, perfumes, colognes, glues, carpet odors, paints, formaldehyde, insecticides, diesel fumes and other traffic odors.

Although you cannot avoid all of these things, you can "clean up your home." By getting rid of odorous bathroom and kitchen chemicals, insecticides and other volatile inhalants, you can immediately lighten your load and your symptoms will start improving. Also, do what you can to clean up your work place.

You may also react to chemicals in and on your food—even fresh foods, as well as those found in cans, plastic wrappings and other food containers. So where possible, purchase and eat organic foods and choose prepared foods in glass containers.

C. Lifestyle Changes

You'll need fresh air, sunlight (or skylight), exercise and a proper amount of sleep. Don't be a "couch potato" who spends hours looking at TV. Take a walk, do calisthenics and play outdoor games.

D. Psychological Support

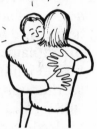

You'll need emotional and psychological nutrients, whether you are sick or well. Here are a few of them: encouragement, love, praise, touch, hugs and laughter. They'll strengthen your immune system and play an important role in helping you overcome your health problems.

E. Nutritional Supplements

Articles documenting the importance of vitamins, minerals and other supplements have been published in major medical and lay publications. Such supplements are especially appropriate for people with yeast-related health problems. They include:

- Yeast-free, sugar-free, color-free multivitamin, mineral and antioxidant preparations.
- Essential fatty acids (EFAs), including flax seed oil.* Flax seeds are the richest known source of Omega 3 fatty acids. They also contain other oils, including Omega 6 EFAs. You can mix it with lemon juice and use it for salad dressing, or take it "straight." The usual dose is one to two tablespoons a day. You can also buy flax seeds and grind them to a powder.

    Oils which are especially rich in Omega 6 EFAs include eve-

---

*Available in all health food stores or can be ordered from Allergy Resources, 800-USEFLAX (or 800-873-3529).

ning primrose oil (Efamol), borage and black currant seed oils. These oils are especially recommended for women with PMS and certain types of eczema.

F. Nonprescription Anti-Candida Substances

After you've taken steps A—E, you'll be ready to take substances which help control candida overgrowth in your intestinal tract and restore normal bacteria. These include:

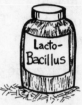

- Probiotics. Preparations of *Lactobacillus aci-dophilus* and other friendly probiotic bacteria help crowd out candida in your digestive tract. Brand names including Vitalplex, Prime-Plex, Vital-Dophilus, Kyo-Dophilus, Kala, BifidoBiotics with *Lacto-bacillus sporogenes*, Geneflora, Maxidophilus, Acidophilus DDS1, Flora Balance, GI Flora, Primadophilus, Saccaromyces boulardi and Superdophilus. Usual dose: one-quarter to one-half tsp. of powder or 1 to 2 capsules, 1 to 4 times daily.
- Citrus seed extracts (Paracan 144, Paramicrocidin and Citrici-dal). Available in capsules and liquids. Usual dose, 1 or 2 cap-sules or 2 to 6 drops of liquid, 1 to 3 times a day. The liquid preparations must be diluted in at least 4 oz. of water and stirred well. If taken undiluted, this product will irritate your mucous membranes.

    According to Drs. Leo Galland and Charles Resseger, these extracts are as effective as nystatin and caprylic acid in treat-ing patients with yeast overgrowth in the intestinal tract. They're also useful in treating patients with giardiasis and other intestinal parasites.
- Garlic cloves and/or Kyolic tablets, capsules or drops.
- Caprylic acid. Brand names include Mycopryl 400 or 680, Ca-pricin, Caprystatin and Kaprycidin A. Usual dose: 1 to 2 cap-sules with each meal.
- Mathake (Teriminalia catappa). A herbal product which is widely distributed in the tropics and introduced in the U.S. in the mid-1980s by Michael Weiner, Ph.D. According to Richard Noble, M.D.:

"Mathake is a very affordable easy to use medicine. It doesn't taste terrible, it is portable, it doesn't require refrigeration. All that it takes is boiling water and a tea bag of the Mathake herb. I often use it first in treating children and adults with mild to moderate candida-related health problems."

G. Work With A Kind and Caring Physician

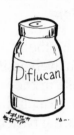

Although the measures outlined above (steps A—F) may help you improve, ideally your treatment program should be directed by a knowledgeable physician. Moreover, you can only obtain prescriptions for the antiyeast medications (Diflucan, Sporanox, nystatin or Nizoral) from your physician.

Yet, you may often experience problems in finding such a physician. Here's why: At this time, January 1995, many—and perhaps most—North American physicians regard the relationship of superficial yeast infections to chronic illness as "speculative and unproven."

What then, can you do?

- Carefully read and re-read this book.
- Copy the section in the front of this book, "A Special Message to the Physician," and send it to your doctor. You might say:

"Thank you for your kindness and your interest in helping me cope with and overcome my health problems. I've recently become interested in the relationship of superficial yeast infections to many of the symptoms which have been bothering me. Although I realize that you may feel that 'the yeast connection' is speculative and unproven, I would appreciate your help."

If you do not have a physician, or your physician isn't interested, you'll find my comments and suggestions for finding help in Chapter 6.

H. Prescription Medication

Although changing your diet and taking nonprescription medications may help you overcome your yeast-related health problems, prescription antiyeast medications can play an essential role in enabling you to overcome your health problems.

In *The Yeast Connection* you'll find information about nystatin and the azole drug, Nizoral (ketoconazole). Each of these medicines is safe and effective, and they continue to help many people. Now, two other safe and effective medications are available on prescription. Both are azole drugs and "kin" to Nizoral. *Yet, extensive tests and clinical experiences show that they are safer.* Their names are *Diflucan* (fluconazole) and *Sporanox* (itraconazole).

Diflucan   This systemic medication was developed by the Pfizer Pharmaceutical Company in the 1970s and used extensively in Europe in the 1980s. In early 1990 it was licensed for use in the U.S. for treating patients with severe immunosuppression, including cancer and AIDS. Yet, word of its effectiveness in treating patients with recurrent vaginitis, fatigue, depression and other symptoms spread to physicians around the United States.

In discussing this medication, candida pioneer Sidney M. Baker, M.D., said:

"I started using Diflucan before it was on the market in the U.S. and by now I have prescribed it for hundreds—probably over a thousand—patients. I have not seen a single significant toxic effect—even in children. It is a remarkably effective drug which is helping many, many people."

Another candida pioneer, Ken Gerdes, M.D., said:

"I'm using Diflucan more and more. I feel like it's a very positive, capable kind of drug that does a good job against yeast and sometimes it is the only drug that will help. I've had a number of patients where I've increased the dose up to 400 mgs. a day. And they gain additional benefit."

Charles S. Resseger, D.O., commented:

"I've now treated over a thousand people with Diflucan ranging up to 600 mgs. per day up to 18 months. *I've never yet seen any adverse reaction, other than an occasional mild one after over 4 months of therapy."*

Philip K. Nelson, M.D., said:

"I've been using Diflucan more than nystatin and have found that an initial dose of 200 mgs., followed by 100 mgs. weekly for several months has apparently succeeded in clearing the gut of candida when combined with carbohydrate restriction."

Sporanox   This antifungal drug, developed by Janssen, has been used in Europe for over a decade. It was licensed for use in the U.S. in early 1993 and many reports in the medical literature show that it is a safe and effective medication in treating people with a wide variety of fungal infections, including candida-related health problems.

In discussing this medication, candida pioneer George Kroker, M.D., commented:

"Sporanox seems to have an excellent tissue penetration and a longer half life than other azole drugs. It's especially good in people with fungal infections."

Albert Robbins, D.O., commented:

"I think Sporanox is a wonderful, safe medication that has been quite beneficial in treating people with fungal or yeast-related infections and a chemical sensitivity that goes along with these problems."

Elmer Cranton, M.D., commented:

"Of the azole drugs I like Sporanox the best. I've experienced no significant side effects. My patients tolerate it well. Moreover, I find it's more effective when I combine it with nystatin."

Nizoral   This effective antifungal azole drug was developed by Janssen and licensed for use in the U.S. in 1981. Although side effects may occur more frequently than with the other azole drugs, such reactions are rare, and some physicians prefer it. In their comprehensive review of the azole drugs, Como and Dismukes said:

> "Ketoconazole is less expensive than fluconazole and itraconazole—an especially important consideration for patients receiving long-term therapy."[1]

Nystatin This medication has been used for over 40 years and is the safest medication listed in the Physician's Desk Reference (PDR). It continues to be the standby of many physicians. Because it's insoluble and not absorbed into the circulation, it does not reach candida in the respiratory tract or the deeper layers of the mucous membranes of the vagina or intestinal tract.

I. Track Down Hidden Food Sensitivities

If you continue to experience significant problems after getting rid of sugar and junk food, taking antifungal medications and following other treatment measures, sensitivity to foods you're eating every day may be playing a major role in causing your symptoms. Common troublemakers include yeast, milk, wheat, corn, eggs and citrus.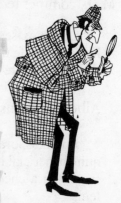

Although laboratory tests *may* help your physician identify foods you're sensitive to, the elimination/challenge diet is considered "the Gold Standard" for determining a food sensitivity. On such a diet you carefully avoid food suspects for five to seven days. When your symptoms improve, foods are eaten again, one food a day, and reactions are noted. You then avoid foods that triggered any of your symptoms for four to six weeks before eating them again.

Concluding Comments

If your health problems are yeast connected and you follow the treatment program outlined in steps A—I, you'll usually show significant improvement.

In working to regain your health, remember that you are unique. Accordingly your diet, nutritional supplements and the antifungal substances you require may differ from those needed by other people.

In addition to the measures listed in this brief summary, you'll need to *take charge of your life and your health.* Candida immunotherapy may also help you. In addition, you may need to be tested and treated for inhalant and food sensitivities. Tests may also need to be carried out to see if you are infested with giardia and other parasites.

Finally, if you're following the treatment program outlined above and aren't improving, other possible causes of your symptoms should be investigated. As pointed out by Ray C. Wunderlich, M.D., of St. Petersburg, Florida, in commenting on yeast-related health problems:

"Desirable at all times is a balanced approach that holds the healthy respect of *Candida albicans*—at the same time one does not wish to overlook the many other health problems that invite the candida syndrome. Those who suspect that they have symptoms—due to candida overgrowth—must not plunge headlong into a quest for a 'magic bullet.'

"Best and most longlasting health will be fostered by careful inquiry into yeast, but also, into psychological, nutritional, allergic, degenerative and toxic factors."

REFERENCE

1. Como, J.A. and Dismukes, W.E., "Oral Azole Drugs as Systemic Antifungal Therapy," *N. Eng. J. of Med.*, 1994; 330:263–272.

TWO

Yeast-Related Problems Which Affect Only Women

9

Recurrent Vaginal Yeast Infections

About four years ago, an area of a woman's anatomy which had rarely been talked about in public became front page news: the vagina. A major factor in prompting this publicity was a decision by the "powers that be" to allow women to purchase Gyne-Lotrimin, Monistat 7 and other antiyeast vaginal suppositories over the counter.

Unless you're blind, deaf and dumb, and never turn on your TV set or look at a magazine, there's no way you can keep from reading or hearing advertisements touting these and other remedies for "yeast infections."

Here's an example of the pervasiveness of these advertisements. I was talking to the mother of an 8-year-old boy who said, "Mama, if you have a yeast infection you won't have to go to the doctor now." And several people have sent me a copy of a cartoon of the Pillsbury doughboy talking to a physician, saying, "I think I have a yeast infection."

In spite of these advertisements, many—and perhaps most—women know relatively little about the vagina and adjacent parts of their body. I base this statement on the comments of gynecologists I've consulted and reports I've read in the press and in medical journals.

In March 1993 I attended a conference of the American Holistic Medical Association. A seminar, led by a female gynecologist, focused on health problems which affect women. Special emphasis was placed on the urogenital system. During her presentation, the seminar leader said, in effect:

> "Too often when referring to our genitalia, we're apt to say something about our 'bottoms' or 'down there' or our 'private parts.' You look at your face every day and when you see changes of one sort or another, you take steps to correct them. You need to do the same with your genitalia. So you should be able to look at and identify your clitoris and the various parts of your vulva, as well as your vagina."*

During the past several years, more and more emphasis has been placed on women's health problems. Included has been the neglect of these disorders by the still male-dominated medical establishment. And even though changes are occurring, a number of female physicians, congresswomen and other leaders are saying, "They aren't occurring fast enough."

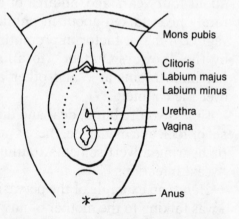

Mons pubis

Clitoris
Labium majus
Labium minus

Urethra
Vagina

Anus

Although I was trained as a pediatrician, some 25 years ago I began to see more and more adult patients, especially women with food and chemical sensitivities. Then 15 years ago, I learned about the observations of Dr. C. Orian Truss who first described the relationship of superficial yeast infections to chronic health problems which affected people of all ages and both sexes. Yet, he emphasized those which affected women.

---

*Illustration copied from McKay, M., "Vulvodynia Diagnostic Patterns, Dermatology Clinics, 1992; 10:423-33.

Why You May Be Bothered By Repeated Vaginal Yeast Infections

Based on the information I've obtained from different sources, here's why you and other women may be troubled by recurrent vaginal yeast infections:

- *The common yeast, Candida albicans, thrives in a dark, warm, moist environment:* The vagina serves as an ideal place for this yeast to live and multiply—especially when other factors encourage its growth.
- *Broad-spectrum antibiotics:* During the past 40 years, broad-spectrum antibiotics have been used freely in both people and animals. And professionals and nonprofessionals usually looked on them as "wonder drugs." These medications do save lives by eradicating the germs that cause lobar pneumonia, meningitis and other infections.

But now, professionals and nonprofessionals are becoming aware that antibiotics may sometimes cause more problems than they solve. In his 1994 book, *The Plague Makers,*[1] Jeffrey A. Fisher, M.D., feels that we may be facing "impending disaster" if we do not limit the indiscriminate use of antibiotics.

He pointed out that antibiotics could cause immunosuppression resulting in opportunistic infections with various fungi and yeast, including *Candida albicans.* In his continuing discussion, he said that elimination of the good bacteria by the antibiotic also plays a role in these infections.

In discussing vaginitis in their recent book, *Beyond Antibiotics— Healthier Options for Families,* the authors commented:

"Broad-spectrum antibiotics indiscriminately kill normal vaginal bacteria that usually keep yeast under control. Vaginal bacteria also help keep the vagina acidic, which prevents the growth of yeast. With no competition, the yeast grows unchecked."[2]

- *Suppression of the immune system by Candida albicans:* Japanese researchers in the 1970s published studies showing that candida may act as an immunosuppressant.[3] During the '80s and '90s, Steven S. Witkin, Ph.D., a Cornell University researcher, published a number of studies showing that candida infections may adversely affect the immune system.[4,5,6,7,8,9]

In a June 7, 1991, letter to me he said that the evidence is now very good that candida can be involved in the induction of immunosuppression. During the past three years, he sent me copies of a number of papers describing his research studies on women with recurrent vaginitis. Here are excerpts from his 1993 article, *Immunology of the Vagina:*

"Recent studies from our laboratories show that vaginal immune responses may cause some cases of recurrent vaginitis. IgE antibodies to *C. albicans,* seminal fluid components and contraceptive spermicides have been identified in vaginal fluids of women with recurrent vaginitis . . .

"The concentration and persistence in the vagina of orally ingested substances suggest that allergies to medications, or possibly even foods, similarly may induce an allergic vaginitis in susceptible women. By a similar mechanism, potentially allergenic substances ingested by male sexual partners, and present in their semen, may also induce an immune mediated vaginitis."[10]

- *Yeasts in the digestive tract play a role in causing vaginal yeast infections:* In the 1970s researchers at Michigan State University studied 98 young women who were troubled with recurrent vaginitis. They found that all of these women had yeast in the stool. Here's an abstract of this study published in the Journal of the American Medical Association.

"Ninety-eight young women who complained of recurrent vaginitis were selected in sequence. The results showed that if *C. albicans* was cultured from the vagina it was always found in the stool.

"*Conversely, if it was not isolated from the stool, it was never found in the vagina. These data are presented as an explanation for the recurrent nature of candida vaginitis and thus a cure for vaginitis would not be possible without prior eradication of C. albicans from the gut* [emphasis added]."

159

Recurrent Vaginal Candidiasis

Importance of an Intestinal Reservoir

Mary Ryan Miles, MD; Linda Olsen, MS; Alvin Rogers, PhD

● To test the hypothesis that all cases of vaginal candidiasis [...] ated with a "reservoir" of this organism in the bowel. [...] feces and vaginal material were cultured for [...] neously. Ninety-eight young women who were selected in sequence. The results a[...] tured from the vagina, it was always found not isolated from the stool, it was never fou[...] presented as an explanation for the recurre[...] and thus a cure of vaginitis would not be pos[...] of *C albicans* from the gut. The gut-reservoir c[...] forms of candidiasis.

(*JAMA* 238:1836-1837, 1977)

Extending the gut reservoir concept, may explain other forms of candidiasis and the immunological phenomena found in some people.

CANDID⁴ ALBICANS is found so freque[...] the gut (stools) of health[...] its presence in th[...] accepted as [...] in[...] t[...] v[...]

When C. albicans was cultured from the vagina it was always found in the stool.

a[...]
Vagin[...] become one o[...] forms of vaginitis be[...] quently a recurrent proble[...] sons that some persons present w[...] repeated episodes of vaginitis and other forms of mucocutaneous candidiasis are not known although precipitating events are known. Cellular and humoral immunological data are rapidly accumulating,[...] but as yet, [...] little knowledge in

This pap[...] evidence that the intestin[...] acts as a reservoir for *C albicans*, where it may live in harmony with the rest of the host's fecal flora. Minor alterations in the milieu [...] the host (ie, pregnancy and inges-[...] broad-spectrum antibiotics) [...] from commensal to [...] cutaneous sur-[...] ites of in-[...] n, ie, [...] per or [...] results [...] at vagi-[...] ur natu-[...] tant pres-[...] the large bowe[...] is not likely as long as [...] remains the only treatment ta[...]

PATIENTS AND METHODS

Patients.—Healthy, nonpregnant, female patients, 18 to 20 years of age, who pre-

[...]m was used for [...] C albicans. This me-[...] signated to inhibit the growth [...] ost micro-organisms but to allow the growth of *Candida* species. Yeast growth is evident as early as 24 hours after inoculation, but optimal growth may be expected between five and seven days when incubated at 24 C. Approximately 1 gm of fecal material and swabs containing vaginal specimens were inoculated directly into the media. Chlamydospore formation on cornmeal plus polysorbate-80 agar was used for positive identification of *C albicans*.

RESULTS

Ninety-eight patients were involved in the study. Fifty-one (52%) were found to harbor *C albicans* in both vagina and fecal material; 46 (47%) were *Candida* free in both sites (Table 1). Thus, there was 100% correlation between the presence or absence of *C albicans* in the feces and vagina of this population (Table 2).

A review of the patient's clinical records supported the recurrent nature of candidiasis. In approximately one third of the patients, there had been no prior laboratory confirmation

In their concluding comments, the authors of this article stated:

"Of economic importance is the knowledge that candida vaginitis cannot be cured by vigorously treating the vagina. Millions of consumer dollars are spent yearly in vain in hope of accomplishing this."[11]

A number of my other consultants have pointed out still another reason why yeast in the digestive tract leads to vaginal yeast infections: The vulva and vagina are so close to the anus that contamination from yeast to the stool can easily occur.

- *Diet: If you're troubled by recurrent vaginal yeast infections you must change your diet.*

Scientific support for this statement is presented in a recent article by Barbara D. Reed, M.D., and associates. Here's an abstract of their study:

> "The association between dietary intake . . . was evaluated in 166 women who had a history of candida vulvovaginitis in the past five years and in 207 women without such a history, as well as in 74 women with five or more episodes in the past five years and 125 women with no history of candida vulvovaginitis . . .
> "Results indicate associations between total caloric intake, carbohydrates and fiber and a history of candida vulvovaginitis. The results were not altered by controlling for age, body mass, index, smoking, use of oral contraceptives and sexual activity variables.
> "These results suggest several dietary constituents may influence susceptibility to the candida vulvovaginitis infections. A follow-up perspective study using cultured confirmation of candida infection is needed."[12]

Another study by Connecticut gynecologists Benson J. Horowitz, Stanley W. Edelstein and Leonard Lippman, supported the role diet contributes to recurrent vulvovaginitis. Here's an abstract of their study:

> "Because of the apparent increase in vulvovaginitis caused by candida species, the chronic disability caused by this infection and its stubborn resistance to current therapy, a study of 100 women was undertaken to attempt to gain insight into the role of dietary sugar ingestion in the pathogenesis of this disease. Urinary sugar patterns of glucose, arabinose and ribose were elevated. These excretion patterns correlated well with the excessive oral ingestion of

dairy products, artificial sweeteners and sucrose. Eliminating excessive use of these foods brought about a dramatic reduction in the incidence and severity of candida vulvovaginitis."[13]

Still another study[14] by Gilmore and associates showed that growing *Candida albicans* in a higher glucose medium augmented the appearance of a receptor which enhanced resistance to phagocytes . . . a white blood cell which "gobbles up" yeasts and other enemies.

Several years ago one of my adult patients, Karen, who had conquered most of her yeast-related health problems commented:

. "Dr. Crook, I was doing fine and had had no vaginal symptoms for many months. Then, just before Christmas I baked some chocolate sugar cookies for my four children. I ate four of them. Within four hours my vaginal symptoms returned and it took me three weeks to get back to normal."

Dr. Doris Rapp commented:

"Some women need only to eat a bar of candy and they develop an immediate vaginal discharge."[15]

Recently published studies by investigators at St. Jude Research Hospital, Memphis, Tennessee, provide further support for the relationship of sugar to candida overgrowth. Here's a summary of their study.

Thirty-six mice colonized with gastrointestinal candidiasis as infants were randomized into three groups. One group was allowed

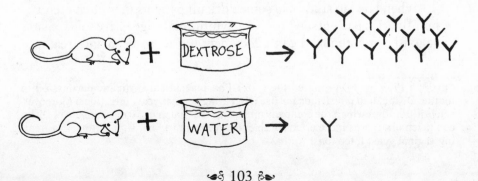

plain water; a second was given water containing dextrose; while a third was given water with xylitol.

Cyclophosphamide had been used to suppress the immune system. Stool colony counts were serially determined.

The mice were then sacrificed and cultures of the stomach wall were carried out. *The results showed that the gastrointestinal growth and invasion of candida was approximately 200 times greater in the mice receiving dextrose than in the control or xylitol group.* In their conclusion these investigators stated:

> "Results suggest that dietary dextrose may increase *Candida albicans* GI growth and invasion."[16]

Overcoming Your Vaginal Yeast Infections

Changing your diet, eating sugar-free yogurt, and/or taking oral preparations of friendly bacteria and wearing panties with a cotton crotch will lessen the chances of your developing a vaginal yeast infection. But if, in spite of such measures, you experience vaginal itching or discharge, vaginal suppositories which you can obtain without a prescription may enable you to obtain prompt relief.

Yet, if your symptoms persist, you should consult your physician to rule out other causes of your vaginal symptoms. And even if yeast is the cause, she can prescribe oral antifungal medications, including nystatin or Diflucan.*

In discussing the management of vaginal yeast infections with gynecologist John Curlin, he said:

> "When I do lab studies in some difficult patients they often aren't helpful. In patients who have symptoms suggestive of yeast vaginitis, even though I can't document it, I'll go ahead and treat it

---

*In June 1993 the FDA granted the Pfizer Pharmaceutical Company permission to market Diflucan to physicians for use in treating vaginal yeast infections. Moreover, scientific studies which the company cited, showed that one 150 mg. capsule of Diflucan taken orally was more effective than one week of vaginal suppositories in treating vaginal yeast infections.

. . . I've never seen a recurrent candidiasis that didn't improve on a low sugar diet, vaginal suppositories and oral nystatin.

"In some patients cutting down the sugar is enough to notice improvement. But if diet changes and a topical ointment don't clear the problem, I suggest that they stop the pill. I'm impressed, however, with the motivation of the women who stay on the pill despite symptoms!"[17]

In gathering material for this book, I interviewed a number of physicians, including gynecologists. I also read reports from the medical literature and a variety of other publications. One which I found especially informative was a book by Naomi Baumslag, M.D., President of the Women's International Public Health Network and Dia L. Michels, a researcher and writer who specializes in health topics relating to women.

In this book entitled, *A Woman's Guide to Yeast Infections,*[18] the authors pointed out that vaginal yeast infections are "out of the closet"; in the U.S. alone, over 22 million women each year are affected. They also said that fully one-third of all visits to gynecologists are prompted by a vaginal discharge and that a yeast infection is one of the most frequent diagnoses.

In their continuing discussion, they said that a review of the medical research on yeast infections during the past 20 years shows that *recurrence is common.* So, many women are troubled by recurrent pain, itching and discomfort and make repeated trips to the gynecologist in search of help. And in spite of creams, suppositories and ointments, infections continue to recur.

Baumslag and Michels also discuss the economic costs of these infections which can easily pass the $1000 mark in no time at all. And the cost, along with their inability to find permanent help, adds to women's frustrations.

If you continue to be bothered by recurrent vaginitis, here are my suggestions:

- First, go to your gynecologist or personal physician to make sure that you do not have an infection caused by a germ other than *Candida albicans.*

- Next, change your diet—eat more vegetables and other nutritious foods and cut way back on the sugar. Eat high quality yogurt or preparations of *Lactobacillus acidophilus* and/or garlic. Also get FOS* (fructooligosaccharides) from your health food store or pharmacy to use as a sweetener. Although it's expensive, it's worth trying because it encourages the growth of friendly bacteria.
- Then, go to your health food store or bookstore and get a copy of the Baumslag/Michels book on yeast infections. This easy-to-read and understand, 274-page book is loaded with information of all sorts. *I've never read a more comprehensive, practical book. It taught me a lot of things I needed to know!*

REFERENCES

1. Fisher, J.A., *The Plague Makers,* Simon and Schuster, New York, 1994; pp 72–73.
2. Schmidt, M.A., Smith, L.H., Sehnert, K.W., *Beyond Antibiotics—Healthier Options for Families,* North Atlantic Books, Berkeley, CA. 1993.
3. Iwata, K. and Uchida, K., "Cellular Immunity in Experimental Fungal Infections in Mice," *1978 Mykosen, Suppl.* 1, 72–81.
4. Witkin, S.S., "Defective Immune Responses in Patients with Recurrent Candidiasis," *Infections in Medicine,* May/June, 1985, pp 129–132.
5. Witkin, S.S., Yu, I.R., Ledger, W.J., "Inhibition of *Candida albicans—*Induced Lymphocyte Proliferation by Lymphocytes and Sera from Women with Recurrent Vaginitis," *AMJ Obstet. Gynecol.,* 1983; 147:809–11.
6. Witkin, S.S., Hirsch, J. and Ledger, W.J., "A Macrophage Defect in Women with Recurrent Candida Vaginitis and Its Reversal In Vitro by Prostaglandin Inhibitors," *AMJ Obstet. Gynecol.,* 1986; 155:790–95.
7. Witkin, S.S., "Immunology of Recurrent Vaginitis," *AMJ, Reprod. Immunol. Microbiol.,* 1987; 15:34–37.
8. Witkin, S.S., Jeremia, J. and Ledger, W.J., "A Localized Vaginal Allergic Response in Women with Recurrent Vaginitis," *J. Allergy Clin. Immunol.,* 1988; 81:412–416.

---

*See Chapter 27.

9. Witkin, S.S., "Immunologic Factors Influencing Susceptibility To Recurrent Candidal Vaginitis," *Clinical Obstet. & Gynecol.*, 1991; Vol. 34, pp 662–668.
10. Witkin, S.S., "Immunology of the Vagina," *Clinical Obstet. & Gynecol.*, 1993; 36:122–128.
11. Miles, M.R., Olsen, L. and Rogers, A., "Recurrent Vaginal Candidiasis: Importance of an Intestinal Reservoir," *JAMA*, 238:1836–37, October 28, 1977.
12. Reed, B.D. and associates, "The Association Between Dietary Intake and History of Candida Vulvovaginitis," *J. of Family Practice*, 1989; 29:509–515.
13. Horowitz, B.J., Edelstein, S. and Lippman, L., "Sugar Chromatography Studies in Recurrent Candida Vulvovaginitis," *J. Reproduct. Med.*, 1984; 29:441–443.
14. Gilmore, B.J. et al, "An ic3b Receptor on *Candida albicans*: Structure, function and correlates for pathogenicity," *Journal of Infectious Diseases*, 1988; 157:38–46.
15. Rapp, D.J., Personal Communication, April 1991.
16. Vargas, S.L., Patrick, C.C., Ayers, G.D. and Hughes, W.T., "Modulating Effect of Dietary Carbohydrate Supplementation on *Candida albicans*, Colonization and Invasion in a Neutropenic Mouse Model," *Infection and Immunity*, February 1993; 61:619–626.
17. Curlin, J., Personal Communication, February 1994.
18. Baumslag, N. and Michels, D.L., *A Woman's Guide to Yeast Infections*, Pocket Books, New York, 1992.

10

Vulvodynia

Common symptoms experienced by women with yeast infections include a white cheesy discharge and itching. Yet, some women complain of symptoms of a different type. During the past decade I've received letters and phone calls from women who complained of *burning* and pain. One such woman said:

> "My bottom burns. Yes, burns. It's on fire. I've been bothered by this problem for over 5 years. Suppositories, creams, cotton panties and even standing on my head with my bottom stuck up in the air haven't really helped."

The medical term for this disorder is "vulvodynia," a term which I had never heard of until early 1993. At that time, a Nashville psychiatrist called and sent me the medical records of one of his patients (I'll call her Laura). This professional woman had been troubled by persistent, intense burning of her external genitalia for several years. In looking for help, she had consulted many physicians.

In her search for answers, Laura went to her university medical library and copied many articles and reports. One of the articles was entitled, "Vulvodynia, A Multifactorial Clinical Problem," by Dr. Marilynne McKay. In this comprehensive review article published in 1989, Dr. McKay said:

> "As a first year dermatology resident at the University of Miami in 1977, I assisted in the care of a patient referred to Dr. Harvey Blank

for the problem of vulvar burning. She was especially adamant in denying pruritus, insisting, 'I don't itch, *I burn.*' She complained that although no one could tell her exactly what she had, she had been told that it was 'all in her head,' and she would 'just have to live with it.'

"Dr. Blank acknowledged the patient's distress in not having a diagnosis by suggesting that we call her problem *vulvodynia,* a term analogous to glossodynia, or burning tongue. As I subsequently became more interested in this problem, I discovered that the word *vulvodynia* was also suggested (along with pudendagra) by Tovell and Young in 1978. Other investigators have subsequently concurred with the appropriateness of vulvodynia (based on the Greek word, odynia ['pain']) as a term that is both scholarly and descriptive.

"At a conference on 'Diseases of the Vulva and Vagina' in 1980, I listened with interest to the suggested treatments for intractable pruritus vulvae, which included such modalities as subcutaneous alcohol infiltration of the entire vulva.

"When I inquired whether this had proved successful in the treatment of recalcitrant *burning,* the response was negative, 'No, we don't have any answers for that.'

"With Dr. Blank's encouragement that the best place to begin is where little or nothing is known, I declared my interest in seeing patients with *vulvodynia* when I joined the faculty of the Department of Dermatology at Emory University, Atlanta. I became chairman of the task force on 'Burning Vulva Syndrome' for the International Society for the study of Vulvar Disease (ISSVD) in 1983, at the seventh congress in Orlando, Florida, where we presented new terminology and the definition of vulvodynia.

Vulvodynia is described as chronic vulvar discomfort—characterized by burning, stinging, irritation or rawness.

"As defined by ISSVD in 1984, vulvodynia is chronic vulvar discomfort, especially that characterized by the patient's complaint of burning, stinging, irritation or rawness. Vulvodynia is different from the itch of pruritus vulvae, and the patient with vulvar burning seldom has frankly abnormal physical findings, such as might be seen with continued cutaneous rubbing, scratching, or excoriation.

"Although some patients with vulvodynia probably resign themselves to the chronicity of their problem, others become familiar to the medical community as they go from physician to physician in hopes of finding a diagnosis and 'cure.'

"Because physical signs may be subtle, many have been told that their problem is primarily psychological, especially when dyspareunia is a major component. Unrealistic expectations and unrewarding medical experiences contribute to the resentment, frustration, and anger so often expressed by these patients [emphasis added]."[1]

Yeast-related Vulvodynia

Soon after learning about the term vulvodynia, I received calls on the International Health Foundation hotline from women with this syndrome in Michigan, Georgia and North Carolina. Then as I thought about it, I realized that many of the women with yeast-related problems (who wrote and called me during the 1980s) who said, "I'm troubled by a constant yeast infection," were, in fact, troubled by vulvodynia.

In a comprehensive article published in 1992, Dr. McKay said:

"Bacterial, fungal and viral infections should all be considered in this area, occurring as either primary or secondary problems."

And she described her experiences with more than 1000 patients in "an academic referral practice." And she said:

"Candida is by far the most important infectious agent to consider in the evaluation of patients with vulvodynia [emphasis added]."[2]

> ***Consistent long term anti-candida therapy seems to be a successful treatment strategy for vulvodynia.***

Although Dr. McKay pointed out that candida organisms cannot be consistently cultured from the vagina of patients with this syndrome, consistent long term anti-candida therapy seems to be a successful treatment strategy.

I'm happy to report that Laura's story has a happy ending. On the antifungal medication Nizoral and a sugar-free, yeast-free diet, her vulvodynia, fatigue and many other health problems disappeared. Yet, after taking this drug intermittently for a number of months, she experienced sexual dysfunction. Then her physician discontinued the Nizoral and prescribed Diflucan. In a recent letter to me, Laura said:

> "Since I wrote you last, I quit taking Nizoral and took nothing for the candida for a few weeks. My orgasmic dysfunction disappeared within a few days after stopping the Nizoral. I began to have yeast symptoms again with fatigue and depression. So I started back on the Nizoral. Again the orgasmic difficulties appeared. When I discontinued the Nizoral, my ability to have a pleasurable orgasm increased.
>
> "When my candida symptoms returned, I took Diflucan. With the Diflucan I had much less difficulty with orgasm and the yeast symptoms (vulvodynia, fatigue and depression) were eliminated. I now use Diflucan every three days or so and have no yeast or orgasm problems."*

To learn more about Dr. McKay's experiences, I called her in November 1993. Here are excerpts from our conversation.

> "Patients with vulvodynia are an easily definable group. Vulvodynia, strictly speaking, means *burning*. This differentiates it from pruritus vulvae, which is just chronic itching. Some have nerve root dysesthesias. These are patients who burn 'all the time' and respond to amitriptyline therapy.
>
> "Other women have days without symptoms—'good days' and 'bad days.' Perhaps a better term to apply to women with these problems is cyclic vulvovaginitis. Women with these problems are especially apt to flare at time of their menstrual periods."

---

*You can find more about Laura's story in Chapter 34.

Dr. McKay said that initially she treated all these patients with low-dose antifungal therapy for four to six months. Some were given Nizoral, some Gyne-Lotrimin or Terazol. She said:

> "I'm now finding that Diflucan, 100 mg. once or twice a week, is very effective."

Other Causes of Vulvodynia

This disorder, like many other chronic health disorders, including PMS, endometriosis, chronic fatigue syndrome and interstitial cystitis, is rarely, if ever, due to a single cause. And I learned more about it through further networking in late 1993 and during 1994. A Michigan woman (I'll call her Louise) wrote saying in effect:

> "I've suffered from multiple health problems for many years, including PMS, fatigue, depression and vulvodynia. I've tried just about all the treatments I've read and heard about including laser surgery and antiyeast medication. Nothing has really worked.
>
> "Then a friend with similar problems told me about Joanne Yount and the Vulvar Pain Foundation in North Carolina. Why don't you get in touch with Joanne? She'll send you information about the work of Colorado researchers who have found that too much oxalate in the body plays an important part in causing vulvodynia and related problems."

So I wrote and called Joanne who sent me copies of the Vulvar Pain Newsletter and other information, including a copy of an article by the Colorado researchers, Clive C. Solomons, Ph.D., M. Herzl Melmed, M.D., and Susan M. Heitler, Ph.D. Here's an excerpt from their paper published in the *Journal of Reproductive Medicine*.

> "A woman had suffered from vulvar vestibulitis (vulvodynia) for four years. Pain from the disorder had disrupted her ability to function at work and home as well as sexually. An initial full range of treatments, including multiple operations, had produced no relief. Examination of the urine for evidence of excess oxalate, which has been shown to cause epithelial reactions similar to those found in

vulvodynia, showed periodic hyperoxaluria and pH elevations related to the symptoms.

"Calcium citrate was given to modify the oxalate crystaluria. The symptoms were significantly reduced in three months, and the patient was free of pain after one year. She was able to resume normal work, family, sexual and recreational activities. Withdrawal of the calcium citrate resulted in a return of the symptoms; reinstitution alleviated them. These findings suggest that further study of individualized metabolic factors that may underlie vulvodynia is warranted."[3]

To obtain further information, in the fall of 1994 I wrote to Joanne Yount, who sent me additional copies of the Vulvar Pain Newsletter, including the Spring 1994 issue which featured a conversation with Dr. Solomons. Here are *very* brief excerpts:

"Oxalate is an irritating material which has long been known to cause pain. It is produced by several tissues in the human body during normal metabolism . . . It causes pain on making contact with nerve fibers . . . Increased sensitivity of nerves, abnormal skin, and peaks in oxalate concentration all contribute to pain."

> **Oxalate is an irritating material which has long been known to cause pain.**

Dr. Solomons established The Vulvodynia Project in 1992 to further study the relationship of oxalate to vulvar pain. His colleagues, Drs. Melmed and Heitler, are not presently involved in this project although they collaborated with Dr. Solomons in the late 1980s. Here are excerpts from a five-page discussion I received from Dr. Solomons.

"A significant number of project participants have responded positively to the citrate and dietary treatments for vulvar pain. Research is ongoing to find other treatments that could be effective in those individuals who do not respond, and also in situations where high oxalate is not present and pain is the result of causes not yet identified."

Testing requires analyses of multiple urine specimens, the results of which are analyzed and recommendations are then made. In his discussions, Dr. Solomons said:

"Although the medication component of the treatment is an over-the-counter supplement, I do strongly urge that a health care professional in your area is involved in your overall medical supervision."

For more information write to Scientific Connections, Clive C. Solomons, Ph.D., P.O. Box 61386, Denver, CO 80206–8386 or to Joanne Yount, Executive Director, The Vulvar Pain Foundation, P.O. Drawer 177, Graham, NC 27253.

Comments About Vulvodynia and Its Management by Leo Galland, M.D.

During the past decade, I have sought the help and consultation of Dr. Galland on a variety of topics, including fatty acids, magnesium and the overall management of patients with candida-related health problems. He served as the keynote speaker at the IHF Candida Conference in Dallas (1987) and in Memphis (1988). I've also heard a number of his other presentations, including a 1992 discussion of genital problems in women.

To get an update on his thoughts about vulvar pain, I called him in November 1994. Here are excerpts from our conversation:

"I've seen a number of women with vulvar pain and their problems seem to fall in three categories. Approximately one-third of them have candida problems and allergies, and the pain is provoked by specific foods or chemical exposures.

"Another third have oxalate problems, or other metabolic disturbances that are related to the oxalates. Moreover, these two groups overlap.

"Then there's another third of patients I see in my practice where their problems have a neuromuscular cause. Those are the people who respond best to physical therapy, pelvic floor rehabilitation and possibly muscle relaxants or low doses of antidepressants."

I asked him to comment further on his experiences with oxalate and he said:

"I don't have any doubt that Solomons and Melmed have discovered an important and real phenomenon. I've found that for some women with chronic vulvar pain, as well as some with bladder pain, the treatment based on their principles has been very helpful. It rarely produces a cure, but it can significantly alleviate symptoms.

"In my opinion, the oxalate problem may be a secondary one which is associated with small bowel inflammation and with a leaky gut."

My Comments

During the past two years, since I first heard the term *vulvodynia*, I've "picked the brains" of a number of knowledgeable and experienced professionals. I also went to the medical library and read many articles which dealt with female urogenital problems. These included vulvodynia, focal vulvitis and interstitial cystitis.

An article by William M. McCormick especially interested me. It was entitled, "Two Urogenital Sinus Syndromes, Interstitial Cystitis and Focal Vulvitis." Here's an excerpt of this article.

"Forty-six young women had unusual and presumably noninfectious disorders of unknown etiology involving tissues derived from the embryonic urogenital sinus (Urogenital Sinus Syndromes). Ten women had interstitial cystitis, and 25 had focal vulvitis. Eleven women had both interstitial cystitis and focal vulvitis. . . .

"Both unusual conditions occurred in the same woman more often than could be expected by chance. This observation suggests that some, perhaps autoimmune, mechanism may be involved in the etiology of these syndromes."[4]

I also read another report by Dr. McKay in which she described her experiences in treating 20 patients with vulvodynia using low-dose amitriptyline. Although three of these patients were in their

40s, the remainder of the patients were older. Moreover, only four out of the twenty showed positive yeast vaginal cultures. In her concluding paragraph, Dr. McKay referred to the observations of Dr. McCormick and she said:

"The multifactorial nature of vulvar disease requires a multidisciplinary approach to investigation and treatment. It is intriguing to consider that vulvodynia may actually be a subset of other pelvic floor symptoms complexes and that we may actually be investigating only one aspect of 'urogenital sinus syndrome.'

"The more we know about vulvodynia, the better we will be able to help our patients. Fortunately, we're learning more each year about this frustrating problem, and new treatments for specific problems are widening our therapeutic armamentarium."[5]

Concluding Comments and Speculations

Some women with vulvodynia and/or interstitial cystitis improve when they take antifungal medications. They improve even more when they follow a sugar-free special diet and avoid foods which cause sensitivity reactions (see Chapter 13). Yet, vulvar and urethral smears and cultures for candida may be negative.

Here are possible explanations: Candida overgrowth in the gut may so disturb the intestinal membrane that food antigens, endotoxins and enterotoxins present in the gut are absorbed, and they, in turn, adversely affect the urogenital system. Or, as noted by Iwata, candida itself may form potent toxins which cause immune system disturbances. Perhaps in the not too distant future these possibilities can be investigated.

REFERENCES

1. McKay, M., "Vulvodynia—A Multifactorial Clinical Problem," *Arch. of Dermatol.*, 1989; 125:256–262.
2. McKay, M., "VULVODYNIA Diagnostic Patterns," *Dermatol. Clin.*, 1992; 10:423–33.

3. Solomons, C., Melmed, M., Heitler, S., "Calcium Citrate for Vulvar Vestibulitis—A Case Report," *J. Reprod. Med.*, December 1991; 36:879–882.
4. McCormick, W.M., "Two Urogenital Sinus Syndromes, Interstitial Cystitis and Focal Vulvitis," *J. Reprod. Med.*, 1990; 35:873–876.
5. McKay, M., "Dysesthetic [Essential] Vulvodynia Treatment with Amitriptyline," *J. Reprod. Med.*, 1993; 38:9–13.

11

Premenstrual Syndrome (PMS)

Several times each week, the average American, both male and female, hears or reads about PMS. Frequent newspaper and magazine articles and programs and advertisements on TV have now made PMS a household word. I even ran across a cartoon showing one moppet whispering to his playmate (with an irate mother in the background),

"Don't worry, Mama's PMS is making her grouchy."

PMS is "for real." No doubt about it. Because I'm the father of three daughters in their early and mid-40s, and because most of the patients I saw during the past decade are women, I'm especially interested in the subject.

The Observations of Guy E. Abraham, M.D.

Some 15 years ago this California gynecologist began publishing his observations on women with PMS.* And he noted that many women with this disorder showed significant nutritional deficien-

---

*Dr. Abraham has written a number of other articles and several booklets which document the role nutrition plays in women's health problems, including PMS and post menopausal osteoporosis. Information can be obtained by writing Guy E. Abraham, M.D., F.A.C.N., 2720 Monterey Street, Suite 406, Torrance, CA 90503.

cies. And he found that by supplementing his patients with magnesium, vitamin B₆ and other nutrients, they improved significantly.

Here are excerpts from his paper entitled, "Nutritional Factors in the Etiology of Premenstrual Tension Syndromes":

"Premenstrual symptom complex many women experience in a moderate to severe form can be divided into four subgroups. Because there is more than one syndrome, and nervous tension is one of the most common symptoms, the term premenstrual tension syndromes (PMTS) is used.

> ### Premenstrual symptom complex many women experience can be divided into four subgroups.

"The most common subgroup, PMT-A, consists of premenstrual anxiety, irritability and nervous tension, sometimes expressed in behavior patterns detrimental to self, family, society . . . Administration of vitamin B₆ at doses of 200–800 mg./day . . . results in improved symptoms under double-blind conditions. Women in this subgroup consume an excessive amount of dairy products and refined sugar and progesterone may be of value . . ."

The second most common subgroup, PMT-H, is associated with symptoms of water and salt retention, abdominal bloating, mastalgia and weight gain. Dr. Abraham pointed out that vitamin B₆ and vitamin E help patients with this type of PMS.

He noted a third type which he labeled PMT-C, which is characterized by:

". . . premenstrual craving for sweets, increased appetite and indulgence in eating refined sugar, followed by palpitation, fatigue, fainting spells, headache and sometimes the shakes."

In treating these patients, he found that magnesium replacement helped relieve symptoms.

A fourth group of PMS patients were noted to be the least common type, but:

"... most dangerous because suicide is most frequent in this subgroup. The symptoms are depression, withdrawal, insomnia, forgetfulness and confusion . . . This subgroup needs careful medical attention when the symptoms are severe. Therapy should be individualized according to the results of the evaluation."[1]

The Yeast Connection to PMS

In his superb book, *The Missing Diagnosis,* Dr. C. Orian Truss clearly describes the unique health problems of the woman between puberty and menopause. He pointed out that such women often are troubled by symptoms which affect many parts of the body, including vaginal symptoms, digestive symptoms, personality changes, impairment in concentration and a destructive loss of self-confidence. And he said that in such women:

"Premenstrual tension becomes progressively more severe and longer in duration."[2]

In my own practice, during the decade of the '80s, I saw dozens of young women with yeast-related health problems. Most of these patients experienced fatigue, headache, irritability, bloating and depression—*especially the week before their periods*. And I found that a sugar-free special diet and antifungal therapy was successful in many of these patients.

> ### *A sugar-free special diet and antifungal therapy was successful in many of these patients.*

To obtain more information and help I sought the consultation of others, including John Curlin, M.D., a gynecologist in my own community.

In the early '80s, Curlin and I visited Jay S. Schinfeld, who at that time was a research professor in the Department of Obstetrics and Gynecology at the University of Tennessee.* We told him of our experiences in treating women with PMS (and related health disorders) using nystatin and a special diet. And we persuaded him to study the problem.

The Observations of Jay S. Schinfeld, M.D.

In 1985 and 1986, Schinfeld and his colleagues enrolled several hundred women in the premenstrual syndrome unit of the medical school. Each woman underwent an extensive history and physical examination and filled out a long questionnaire. All were then interviewed for one hour by a nurse psychologist.

Women in the study were selected from the entire group because of a history of vaginal candidiasis and a failure to respond to the usual PMS therapeutic regimen. All patients received at least a one year follow up and a minimum of three visits.

In tabulating results, several study groups were set up, including some who received vitamin B_6, some who received the elimination diet and nystatin, others who received diet alone and still others who received nystatin.

Schinfeld published his observations in an article in *The Female Patient*[3] in 1987 and presented them at the 1988 Candida Update Conference in Memphis. Here's an abstract of his presentation:

"With the documentation of an apparent increase in the incidence of recurrent *Candida albicans* infections, a possible association between premenstrual syndrome might be expected. However, whether a causative link exists has been speculative until this point.

"We performed a study at the University of Tennessee in which 32 women with severe premenstrual syndrome and a history of vaginal candidiasis for whom prior standardized therapy had failed were treated with oral anticandida agents and yeast elimination diets.

"*Treated patients showed significant physical and psychological*

---

*Dr. Schinfeld is now an associate professor, Department of Obstetrics and Gynecology, Temple University School of Medicine.

improvement over untreated controls, although the mechanism for this improvement and the role of yeast in this disorder remained controversial."[4]

Comments by Other Professionals

During the past decade, I've talked to a number of professionals and read reports which provided me with additional information about PMS, including the favorable response of many women to a special diet and antifungal medication. Here are some of them.

Carol Jessop, M.D., El Cerrito, California In the spring of 1989, I met this California internist who told me of her success in treating hundreds of her patients with chronic fatigue syndrome using Nizoral and a sugar-free, alcohol-free diet.

During subsequent visits with Jessop in North Carolina (1990) and in California (1992), she told me more about her observations. Then, in the summer of 1993, I called her and asked her to tell me how important she felt the role of yeast was in contributing to PMS. Here are excerpts from our conversation:

"It's certainly significant. *I would say maybe 30–35% of the patients I've evaluated over 13 years do have yeasts as the major reason for their PMS and respond very nicely to a special diet and nystatin, Diflucan, Nizoral or Sporanox.*

> ### 30–35% of the patients I've evaluated over 13 years do have yeasts as the major reason for their PMS.

"My first introduction to yeast as a factor in causing PMS was back in 1982. I was just finishing up as chief resident at a UCSF affiliated hospital. I had been asked to host Grand Rounds to the medical students and staff and to give my thoughts on women's menstrual disorders from the point of view of an internist.

"PMS was one of the issues I talked about. I went through all the data and all the literature. Yet, all I could come up with in 1982 was that vitamin B₆ (in levels of 250–500 mg. a day) and magnesium supplementation (400–800 mg. a day), plus dietary changes, helped many women.

"Then a few days later, I got a call from the late Dr. Phyllis Saifer, a Berkeley, California, physician who specialized in allergies and environmental medicine. She subsequently sent me literature on candida and yeast problems. *Quite frankly I thought her ideas were ludicrous!*

"But because I hadn't found any great answers, and more and more women were coming to my university clinic to be evaluated, I decided to at least look at and listen to what Dr. Saifer had to say.

"So I went over and had lunch with Dr. Saifer and I came away shaking my head and saying, 'She's really, really very brilliant, or she's off her rocker!'

"Not long after that I read Orian Truss' paper and started using Saifer's protocol in treating a few of my PMS patients. *Lo and behold, out of my first ten patients, six of them responded beautifully.* They felt a lot better compared to anything else I had done.

> ## *I've found that antiyeast therapy has been incredibly helpful in most of my PMS patients.*

"I kept in contact with Dr. Saifer over the years and since that time I've found that antiyeast therapy has been incredibly helpful in most of my PMS patients. I will also say though, that since 1989 I also use the Serotonin uptake inhibitors, including low dose Prozac in combination with one of the antiyeast medications."

George Miller, M.D., Lewisburg, Pennsylvania During the last several years I've been impressed by the observations of this Fellow of the American Academy of Gynecology and Obstetrics, who has shared some of his knowledge and experiences with me.

In July 1993 I asked him how often antiyeast treatment had helped his patients with PMS—occasionally, frequently, or most of the time? Dr. Miller replied:

> "*Most of the time.* Here's what I tell them: 'I'll do my best to help you. I don't want you to live in a glass box by doing everything to the nth degree. And I know that you cannot afford everything. Yet, *if you'll clean up your diet, avoid chemicals in your environment, and take antiyeast medication, I'm reasonably certain that your PMS will show significant improvement.'*"

John Curlin, M.D., Jackson, Tennessee In early 1994, to get an update on his observations, I again interviewed Dr. Curlin. Here are excerpts from our conversation:

Crook: What do you do for women who come in with PMS?
Curlin: First I talk to them about the multifactorial concepts regarding PMS and that there is not at this time one clear cut etiology. I say to most of them, "If you work on your diet and work on your exercise, you'll improve."

Crook: What do you tell them about the diet?
Curlin: To me diet is basically just like the yeast diet. It's low in the simple carbohydrates. I also think that pyridoxine (vitamin B_6) is beneficial.

Crook: How about the yeast connection to PMS?
Curlin: *In my patients who work on the yeast regimen, which to me is still nystatin, diet and exercise, their PMS improves. There's no question about it.* Yet, my greatest limiting factor has been that I can't get people to stay on the diet. If I could, I feel that more of my PMS patients would improve.

Pamela Morford, M.D., Tucson, Arizona In a special medical report in the April 1986 issue of *Redbook Magazine*, entitled, "The Newest Mystery Illness," Dr. Morford, a gynecologist who at that time was practicing in Minneapolis, commented:

"The premenstrual problems of at least 90% of my patients can be traced to chronic candidiasis. I've found that when I give these patients anticandida therapy, they get better."

> **The premenstrual problems of at least 90% of my patients can be traced to chronic candidiasis.**

In subsequent letters to me, Dr. Morford said:

"I've probably treated 400 to 500 women with PMS. The majority came in complaining of bloating, irritability and depression before their periods. Many were very concerned about being out of control and unable to handle their anger. Some had lost their confidence. Another major complaint: spaciness and inability to concentrate.

"Within a month after starting antiyeast treatment, many of these symptoms diminish considerably and occasionally disappear. Many women, however, found that they could not vary much from their diet without experiencing a return of their symptoms."

During more recent conversations, in 1993 and 1994, Dr. Morford told me that she was able to help many more of these patients using "mini" doses of progesterone, as first described by Dr. Joseph B. Miller of Mobile, as well as by Dr. Richard Mabray. She also said:

"I also use the tiny doses of candida vaccine as described by Dr. Truss. What's more, I use the vaccine more than anything else because of its low cost . . . And it works!"

Jean Rowe, R.N., Denver, Colorado In the mid-1980s, during a visit to Denver, I met Rowe* who at that time was head of the PMS Clinic at St. Luke's Hospital in Denver. I visited with her by phone

*Rowe is now working with Ken Gerdes, M.D., and also doing consultation with women about breast cancer.

and in person on a number of occasions since that time. Here are excerpts from our recent phone conversation.

Crook: Tell me about your first work when you and Dr. Mabel Brelje started your PMS clinic in 1982.

Rowe: When we first began, we relied mainly on minor dietary changes, vitamins and progesterone. Although we helped some women using such an approach, many did not benefit.

In 1983, I read an article on hormone allergy by Richard Mabray, M.D. He had found that tiny doses of progesterone helped women with many different health problems. He led us to Ken Gerdes, M.D., and Nick Nonas, M.D., two Denver environmental physicians who told us about *Candida albicans*. Subsequently, nystatin and diet became our main way of treating PMS. Moreover, it was a vital part of managing some 90% of our patients.

Crook: Tell me a little more about your experiences in treating women with progesterone.

Rowe: Although we initially used high dose progesterone, we now use a natural micronized oral progesterone. The usual dose ranges from 50–100 mgs., twice daily. We also use progesterone neutralization, or "mini dose" progesterone. Such therapies are of particular value for women who feel bad seven to ten days before their period, and who feel well the rest of the month.

In PMS, as in all illnesses, many factors must be considered. In my contact with patients, I continue to address hormonal problems, candida, food and chemical sensitivities. I also do more work with nutrition and the psychic and spiritual aspects of healing.

My own experience with environmental illness and cancer has led me deep into an awareness of truth about the meaning of illness, healing and our very existence. In working with people with health problems of any sort, including PMS and breast cancer, I've learned the value of the cultivation of inner peace in healing.

In PMS, as in all illnesses, many factors must be considered.

Joseph Martorano, M.D., New York, New York While browsing through a bookstore in December 1993, I came across a book, *Unmasking PMS—The Complete PMS Medical Treatment Plan,*[5] co-authored by Dr. Martorano and Maureen Morgan, C.S.W., R.N., with William Fryer. As you might guess, I immediately went to the index to see if these professionals commented on the yeast connection to PMS.

I was delighted to read that they said that no discussion of unresponsive PMS would be complete without some mention of yeast infections and their role in intensifying PMS. They also said that it is "crucial" for women to develop their own histories and present them to a physician familiar with yeast infections.

In reading through the book, I learned that Martorano, a psychiatrist and psychopharmacologist and Morgan, a registered nurse and psychiatric social worker, had been working with women with PMS for a number of years. They had developed a particular interest in the importance of nutritious, low-sugar diets and natural progesterone* in helping their patients.

Women's Stories

During the early and mid-1980s, I saw dozens of women with yeast-related health problems. And many of these patients complained of irritability, fatigue, breast tenderness, depression and other symptoms. Moreover, these symptoms became much worse the week before menstruation.

Arlene's Story

"I've been married for 12 years, have two sons—ages 7 and 3—and a very loving and understanding husband . . . Like everyone else, I would often feel 'not up to par' for 7–10 days before my period. I would also at times feel upset or moody, but this was never really a problem. Gradually, over the past few years, my moodiness increased to a point where, within minutes, it could change either way, from depression to anxiety, then back again. I could feel it coming

---

*For a further discussion of progesterone and PMS see Chapter 40.

on, but I had no control over it. I found that mood swings were especially severe during the 5 or 6 days before my period.

> **I would clinch my fists, grit my teeth, wring my hands and tense every muscle in my body.**

"Increasingly, I began to have 'attacks' where I would get so upset I would clinch my fists, grit my teeth, wring my hands and tense every muscle in my body. I'd feel like screaming. I wouldn't be able to sit down or lie down. I would usually end up getting in the car and driving until I calmed down . . . Even when I wasn't having attacks, I found I could not cope without getting upset with any situation. Such as the washer or dryer going out, or my husband forgetting to call and tell me he'd be late coming home after work."

In her continuing discussion, Arlene said that prior to the development of her severe PMS she had had many urinary tract infections and had to take a lot of antibiotics. And she said that the episode which sent her to a psychologist was provoked by her husband not calling to say he'd play cards one evening. And she said:

"He didn't come home until late. By that time I was a raving maniac. This was 4 days before my period was due to start. I tried to talk to him but ended up screaming insults. When I got no response, I started hitting him. It scared me so badly that I got in my car at 1:00 A.M. and drove around till 3:00 A.M. I prayed out loud that God would give me an answer . . . Finally I called my gynecologist who referred me to the psychologist who sent me to you."

I first sent Arlene to a gynecologist for a careful checkup. Then when she came to me I put her on a sugar-free special diet and nystatin. Within three weeks she was much better and seven weeks after our first visit when she returned, she said:

"I'm much better. For the first time in three years my premenstrual period wasn't hell. I got through it without any blow ups. Although I still have a little vaginal discharge, and some of my old emotional symptoms pop up occasionally, I can deal with them. Thank you, Dr. Crook, I'll always be grateful for your help."

> ## For the first time in three years my premenstrual period wasn't hell.

Diana's Story

In the spring of 1994, during a conversation with Dr. George Miller, he told me about the response of Diana, an elementary school teacher who had been troubled by PMS. To get more information I visited with Diana on the phone. Here's what she told me.

"My symptoms really appeared after the birth of my first child and started with mild depression, irritability, and headache. I visited two different physicians who told me, 'These symptoms will go away in due time.' Although I felt a little better in six months, they still didn't go away.

"Then as I began to keep records, I noted that my symptoms followed a pattern. They began 10 to 14 days before my period. They would go away when my period started, only to return again with my next cycle. I was bothered by anxiety and lots of the other PMS symptoms which varied in severity. With diet and exercise, I showed some improvement.

"Then I had another child and right after that my symptoms really got worse. So I began to read about PMS and I knew it was something I had to deal with.

"My doctors prescribed different remedies, including progesterone suppositories which really did help. I felt wonderful for a few months—but then they stopped working and I developed constant bleeding. Finally, I decided I couldn't take it anymore.

"About that time I heard about Dr. Miller and his work with allergies. So I went to see him and he put me on nystatin, told me to tighten up my diet, especially the sweets. I took the nystatin for a year and continued to watch my diet. And my PMS symptoms went away.

> ### My health today is so much better than it was 10 years ago.

"All of these things I'm telling you about began 16 years ago (the time my first child was born) and my health today is so much better than it was 10 years ago. I wouldn't go back for anything."

More About Nutritional Factors and PMS

In his superb book, *Healing Through Nutrition*,[6] Dr. Melvyn Werbach provides readers with a comprehensive discussion of the many dietary factors which play a role in causing anxiety, irritability, sugar craving, headache and other symptoms experienced by women with PMS.

Moreover, he carefully documents his recommendations with references from the scientific literature.

In a discussion entitled, "Nutritional Healing Plans," he pointed out that PMS is not associated with evidence of B_6 deficiency. Yet, he also said that supplementation with B_6 has been found to be an effective treatment in a number of double-blind studies.

Dr. Werbach also cited other double-blind studies which showed that supplementation with vitamin E, primrose oil and calcium were effective in reducing or controlling PMS symptoms.

In discussing the importance of other supplements, he cited scientific studies which showed that almost half of a group of 105 women with PMS were found to have lower than normal red blood cell levels of magnesium. And he stated that magnesium supplements provided relief for nervous tension, breast pain and weight gain in over 90% of the patients studied.

In his continuing discussion of nutritional therapies, Dr. Werbach discussed the botanical extract, *Ginkgo biloba,* which has been shown to prevent leakage from small blood vessels (capillaries). Moreover, women in the study given *Ginkgo biloba* extract showed significant improvement in their PMS symptoms.

In managing his patients, Dr. Werbach recommends what he calls a "Basic Healing Diet" for all of his patients, regardless of their complaints. This diet features a variety of foods, and he emphasizes fruits, vegetables, whole grains and the limitation of fats. He also recommends vitamin B$_6$, 40 mg. a day; vitamin E, 300 IU twice daily; calcium, 1000 mg. daily; along with 400 mg. of magnesium; evening primrose oil, 1.5 g. twice daily; and *Ginkgo biloba,* 40 mg. three times a day.

My Comments

During the past 40 years, I occasionally found that a single therapeutic intervention solved a chronic and persistent health problem. A recent example: My wife, Betsy, told me that one of her friends (I'll call her Lucy) was bothered by chronic digestive symptoms, including bloating and diarrhea. Even though she wasn't my patient, I suggested an elimination diet. *In one week, her digestive symptoms vanished!* When Lucy added foods, one food per day, she found that wheat was the culprit.

But with most complaints, including PMS, multiple factors play a role in causing symptoms. And there is rarely a quick fix. But if you're bothered by PMS and made a high score on the yeast questionnaire, a sugar-free special diet, oral antifungal medications and nutritional supplements could change your life.

REFERENCES

1. Abraham, G.E., "Nutritional Factors in the Etiology of Premenstrual Tension Syndrome," *J. Reprod. Med.,* 1983; 28:446.
2. Truss, C.O., *The Missing Diagnosis,* P.O. Box 26508, Birmingham, AL, 35226, 1986; pp 19–31.
3. Schinfeld, J.S., "PMS and Candidiasis: Study Explores Possible Link," *The Female Patient,* 1987; 12:66–69.
4. Schinfeld, J.S., "Possible Links of Chronic Candidiasis and PMS," 1988 Candida Update Conference, International Health Foundation, Box 3494, Jackson, TN 38303.

5. Martorano, J., and Morgan, M., with Fryer, W., *Unmasking PMS—The Complete PMS Medical Treatment Plan*, M. Evans and Company, Inc., New York, 1993.
6. Werbach, M., *Healing Through Nutrition*, HarperCollins, New York, 1993; pp. 325–331.

12

---◆---

Endometriosis and the
Yeast Connection

---◆---

Because I was trained as a pediatrician, during my early years of practice most of my patients were infants and young children. Although I liked working with teenagers, I usually referred young women with menstrual and other gynecological problems to my partner, Blanche Emerson—or to a gynecologist for an examination and continuing care.

About 25 years ago, as my interest in food and chemical sensitivities increased, I began to see more adult patients—especially women—with complex health problems. My role in working to help these patients was that of a consultant. And their gynecologist, or other personal physician, provided overall care.

In 1979, after learning about yeast-related illness from Dr. C. Orian Truss, I was both excited and delighted when many of my patients improved on a sugar-free special diet and nystatin.

A year or two later, John Curlin, a gynecologist in my hometown, began using anticandida therapy in some of his patients with menstrual irregularities, pelvic pain and endometriosis. And he said:

> "Although this program doesn't relieve *all* of the symptoms in women with these problems, the response in many of my patients has been gratifying."

Then in 1983 I obtained a copy of Dr. Truss' book, *The Missing Diagnosis*. In discussing the overall pattern of the illnesses seen in many of his patients, Dr. Truss said:

"Endometriosis is found in a high percentage of women with this condition."[1]

In about 1985, my increased interest in endometriosis came from another direction. At that time I met Laura J. Stevens of West Lafayette, Indiana. Ms. Stevens was the founder of a self-help support group and had been troubled by multiple allergies and endometriosis.

Because of our common interest in children with hyperactivity and related problems, Laura and I worked together for over two years and co-authored *Solving the Puzzle of Your Hard-to-Raise Child,* which was published in 1987.

Through Laura I learned of the work of Mary Lou Ballweg and the Endometriosis Association and obtained a copy of their book *Overcoming Endometriosis.* In a chapter in this book, "The Endometriosis-Candidiasis Link," Stevens pointed out that Dr. Truss and other physicians have observed that women with endometriosis often respond to anticandida measures. And she quoted Dr. Truss who said:

> "I think it is unquestionable that there's a very high association of endometriosis with chronic candidiasis. Naturally we cannot at this time be sure whether the yeast is causing endometriosis, or whether some common factor predisposes to both. My own feeling is that the yeast is the cause of endometriosis because it is associated with so much evidence of interference with hormone function in both men and women."

> ## It is unquestionable that there's a very high association of endometriosis with chronic candidiasis.

In this same chapter, in discussing yeast-related illnesses, Ballweg described the observations of other physicians, including Drs. Wayne Konetzki, C.R. Mabray, a Texas gynecologist, and Sidney Baker, who said:

"I believe that a large portion of the endometriosis problem is candida related, and I can cite some spectacular results in patients managed in this way."[2]

In September 1988, Ballweg attended the Candida Update Conference in Memphis and shared some of her observations on endometriosis with me and others at an informal luncheon get-together. Since that time, Ballweg has sent me additional information through personal letters, the Endometriosis Association Newsletter, and telephone conversations. I also visited Ballweg at the Endometriosis Association offices in Milwaukee in 1991.

More About Mary Lou Ballweg and the Endometriosis Association (EA)

Sometimes, in fact, many times, dedicated, caring, persistent people can advance the frontiers of medicine more than physicians and other "experts."* Ballweg is one of those people.

In her ten-page introduction to *Overcoming Endometriosis*, Ballweg told how and why the Endometriosis Association was started. She said that in 1978 she was a healthy, productive business woman—

"... flying high—traveling all over the U.S.—doing wonderful assignments such as editing a speech for Buckminster Fuller; media travel tours—troubleshooting on assignments for the U. S. Department of Housing and Urban Development."

---

*As I look at what Ballweg has accomplished, I think of the seven young mothers in Franklin Park, Illinois who almost 40 years ago were concerned and distressed because the importance of human breast milk was usually ignored or given only lip service by most physicians and hospital personnel. So they did something to change things. They formed an organization which they named *La Leche League*. La Leche means "the milk." This organization has thousands of members, chapters in all 50 states and many foreign countries. And pediatric leaders, including Lee Forrest Hill of Iowa, endorsed and supported their work and said in effect, "The La Leche League International has done more to encourage and promote the optimal physical and mental development of infants and young children through breastfeeding than any other organization or group in America."

Then a series of health problems developed, including mononucleosis. Several months later, a laparoscopy showed that she had endometriosis. During the ensuing months, she was given a number of different therapies, including drugs of various sorts. Yet, no treatment was really satisfactory. Ballweg said:

> "I decided only a group of other women who had 'been there' were likely to understand and provide the emotional support I needed to come to terms with this baffling experience of endometriosis."[3]

So, in the fall of 1979, with the help and encouragement of a number of other people, including Carolyn Keith, Fran Kaplan and Dr. Karen Lamb, the Endometriosis Association was born. Here are excerpts from their statement, "Who We Are":

> "The Endometriosis Association is a self-help organization of women with endometriosis and others interested in exchanging information about endometriosis, offering mutual support and help to those affected by endometriosis, educating the public and medical community about the disease, and promoting research related to endometriosis . . .

The Endometriosis Association is a self-help organization of women with endometriosis.

> "The Association is an international organization with headquarters in Milwaukee, Wisconsin (USA), members in numerous countries and chapters and activities concentrated in North America, though developing on other continents also."[4]

In a recent statement entitled, "ENDOMETRIOSIS: A NEW PICTURE OF THE DISEASE IS EMERGING," EA director Ballweg commented:

> "Endometriosis is a disease affecting an estimated five million women in the U.S. and millions more worldwide. It is a nightmare of

misinformation, myths, taboos, lack of diagnosis and problematic hit-and-miss treatments overlaid on a painful, chronic, stubborn disease.

"Women with this disease have been much maligned—supposedly they were white, stressed out, perfectionistic, upper socioeconomic level women who brought the disease on themselves by postponing childbearing.

"Only when the Endometriosis Association began in 1980 and systematically gathered data were we able to disprove all of these myths . . . Endometriosis is, in fact, an equal opportunity disease affecting all races, personalities, socioeconomic groups, as well as all ages of females from as young as 10 or 11 to as old as women in their 60s and 70s."

The disease or disorder that we call "endometriosis" is just the tip of the iceberg.

In her continuing discussion, Ballweg pointed out that the disease or disorder that we call "endometriosis" is just the tip of the iceberg for a whole range of health problems that are related to hormonal/immune dysregulation. And she said:

"In studies of animals which had been exposed to dioxin and PCBs, toxic chemicals, those exposed were much more apt to develop endometriosis than animals not exposed. In *our Association study, 79% of the animals exposed to dioxin developed endometriosis.*"[5]

In describing what she terms as the "new picture of the disease which is emerging," Ballweg lists these traditional symptoms of endometriosis:

- chronic pelvic pain
- gastrointestinal and bladder problems
- pain with sex
- infertility

In addition, she said that it is now becoming apparent that women with endometriosis are also more apt to be troubled by—

- asthma and eczema
- food intolerances
- chemical sensitivities
- mitral valve prolapse
- autoimmune disorders, including lupus and Hashimito's thyroiditis
- a tendency to infections
- mononucleosis
- chronic fatigue syndrome (CFS)
- fibromyalgia

My Interview With Ballweg

I had been interested in chemical sensitivities and toxicities for many years. Yet, I didn't realize that toxic chemicals played such a major role in causing endometriosis until I read newsletters from the Endometriosis Association. I was impressed—truly impressed—by the work Ballweg and her colleagues were doing. And to learn more, I made an appointment for a phone interview.

During a 40-minute discussion, she pointed out that auto-immune diseases of many types, including not only endometriosis, but also possibly interstitial cystitis, thyroiditis and lupus erythematosus, appear to be related to each other. And she emphasized the close relationship between the immune system and the endocrine system. And in her comments she said:

"What's going on here? Why are these diseases affecting women more than men? . . . Based on research studies in the U.S. and Canada, we feel that toxins of various kinds are adversely affecting the immune system. These toxins include dioxin and PCBs."

In her continuing discussion, she told me that she had testified at health care hearings a number of times during the past several years. Other participants included representatives of various other groups, including interstitial cystitis, PMS and cancer. At one of these hearings, she said:

"Rather than all of these women's groups fighting each other for research funding, saying 'Who's got it worse?' let's look at the common denominators of all of these diseases that are plaguing women in modern society."

During my interview, I asked Ballweg about the yeast connection to endometriosis. And she said in effect:

"I'm not sure it's always vaginal yeast infections. Instead it may be yeast overgrowth in the intestinal tract."

She pointed out that many members of the Endometriosis Association have found that nystatin, Nizoral or Diflucan and a sugar-free special diet have helped them overcome many of their symptoms. And in following an antiyeast treatment program, she said:

"The diet is very important. If a woman just takes the antiyeast drugs, that doesn't do it."

Reports from the Endometriosis Association (EA)

During the past several years I've read and reviewed a number of the EA newsletters. Included have been research reports and information on a number of related disorders, including interstitial cystitis and other autoimmune diseases. Also, there have been letters from women whose endometriosis and other symptoms were improved following dietary changes and antifungal medication. Here are a couple of these letters:

Mindy's story

"I'm writing with good news that I hope will help others with endometriosis. I have stage 3 'endo' and have had severe symptoms for several years. I wasn't diagnosed until 1988.

"The pain was chronic and debilitating. I had many classic symptoms: walking and exercise were painful . . . I had bladder urgency and burning, irregular periods, diarrhea and painful gas. *I was also exhausted and dizzy and troubled by joint pains, sore throats, insomnia, excessive sleepiness and difficulty in concentrating. I was beginning to think I was losing my mind* [emphasis added].

"In desperation, I turned to alternative treatments and in October 1989 I went on an aggressive antiyeast diet and started oral and vaginal nystatin. Within 48 hours I started to feel better. At first, I thought this was a placebo, but luckily I can tell you that after a year and a half on this diet and antiyeast medication, it wasn't.

"One word of caution. After 4 days my symptoms started to worsen considerably. Yet, my doctor reassured me that a worsening of symptoms often occurs, particularly in severe cases. Here's the rationale: As the yeast is destroyed toxins are released that can cause symptoms to worsen temporarily.

"I made steady progress; by February 1990 I was feeling well. In March, I felt terrific. But in late April, mild bowel symptoms started to recur. My doctor took me off nystatin and put me on Diflucan which acts throughout the body.

"Within a week or so I started feeling better. I was also taking Vitalplex, a nonprescription product which contains the friendly bacterium *Lactobacillus acidophilus*, vitamins and Efamol [evening primrose oil]—an essential fatty acid. I also started taking allergy shots.

"Again I improved. Six months ago I had another flare up of bowel symptoms and added bismuth to my treatment program. [If you can't get bismuth citrate, try Pepto-Bismol.] The effects were dramatic and immediate. I'm still taking all the medications every day and in this I'm unusual. Most people with yeast-related problems are on maintenance doses or taking none at all by this time.

"So I continue to be careful with my diet and I avoid sugar, dairy, yeast products, wheat, coffee, preservatives. However, I can break the diet occasionally.

"If I'm under stress or get sick, my symptoms recur, but generally I'm functioning pretty well. Whether what I have is an allergy or part of chronic fatigue syndrome, I don't know. All I know is that I have improved."

Martha's story

"I'm writing to send you some good news . . . for a change. Through the Endometriosis Association, I met a woman with 'endo' who knew about the anticandida diet. We talked at length about the diet and since I was a long-time vaginal yeast sufferer, I decided to go on the diet.

> ## My premenstrual symptoms, pain, bloating and nausea have all but disappeared.

"It's been approximately 6 months since I began the diet. It has not only helped my candida problem—but my symptoms of endometriosis have improved greatly! My periods are much less painful and I no longer pass large blood clots. My premenstrual symptoms, pain, bloating and nausea have all but disappeared. I'm now able to work during my periods . . . with the help of a few tablets of Advil, rather than lying at home with a hot water bottle."

The Observations of Wayne H. Konetzki, M.D., Waukesha, Wisconsin

In the mid-1970s, this specialist in allergy and environmental medicine first developed an interest in health problems which affect women, including menstrual cramps, PMS and endometriosis. Konetzki described his observations at the 10th Anniversary Meeting of the Endometriosis Association in 1991.

In his presentation, "An Allergist Looks at Endometriosis," he told of his experiences in treating his patients with progesterone immunotherapy using the methods first described by Dr. Joseph B. Miller.[6]* In brief, this therapy involved the use of tiny doses of progesterone given either by injection or sublingually.

---

*See also Chapters 37 and 40.

Then in the early 1980s after learning of the observations of Dr.
C. Orian Truss, Dr. Konetzki found that he could help even more of
his patients using a treatment program which included oral antifungal medication, special diet, immunotherapy and nutritional
supplements.

In his concluding remarks, Konetzki said:

"Using these various techniques I've been able to help many
women with PMS and symptoms related to endometriosis. Some
people have even found their infertility problems have disappeared.
The hard part lies ahead of us—convincing family physicians and
gynecologists that these are valid effective treatments.

Comments by Sidney M. Baker, M.D., Weston, Connecticut

In November, 1994, as I was completing the manuscript of this
book, I sent several of the chapters to Dr. Baker for review. Here
are his comments on endometriosis:

"My first endometriosis patient to respond to antifungal therapy
(nystatin and yeast-free diet) 15 years ago surprised me to say the
least. She was a teenager who was 'too young' to have endometriosis, but had just completed a year of hormone suppression treatment when her gynecologist referred her to me. Her history strongly
suggested a connection to repeated antibiotic use and yeast infections.

**Her history strongly suggested a
connection to repeated antibiotic use
and yeast infections.**

"A dramatic response to treatment gave me more confidence to
consider the connection in other cases. In my opinion, there is almost always a connection. I think it's a good example of the yeast-
magnesium relationship. Endometriosis seems to be associated

with a kind of muscular disturbance of the uterus and fallopian tubes with a back up of the menstrual flow. Like constipation of the bowel, it is an expression of muscular disturbances found in magnesium deficiency, and magnesium deficiency is associated with yeast problems."

My Comments

Obviously candida isn't the cause of endometriosis,* PMS and (the) many other health problems which affect women. Yet, based on reports I've received from both professionals and nonprofessionals, a sugar-free special diet and antifungal medication often help women with these distressing disorders.

REFERENCES

1. Truss, C.O., *The Missing Diagnosis*, P.O. Box 26508, Birmingham AL 35226, 1986; p 39.
2. Stevens, L.J., "The Endometriosis-Candidiasis Link" in Ballweg, M.L. and the Endometriosis Association, *Overcoming Endometriosis*, Congdon and Weed, New York and Chicago, 1987; pp 198–204.
3. Ballweg, M.L. and the Endometriosis Association, *Overcoming Endometriosis*, Congdon and Weed, New York and Chicago, 1987; p 1.
4. Ballweg, M.L. and the Endometriosis Association, *Overcoming Endometriosis*, Congdon and Weed, New York and Chicago, 1987; p 11.
5. Statements for Scientific Advisory Meeting III: Women's Health and the Environment. Sponsored by the Society for the Advancement of Women's Health Research. Published in the *Endometriosis Association Newsletter*, Vol. 14 No. 4, 1993.
6. Miller, J.B., "Relief of Premenstrual Symptoms, Dysmenorrhea and Contraceptive Tablet Intolerance," *J. Med. Assoc., St. of Alabama*, 1974; 44:57.

---

*For additional information about endometriosis, including education, support and research, write to the Endometriosis Association, International Headquarters, 8585 N. 76th Place, Milwaukee, WI 53223. 1–800-992-3636 or 414–355-2200. Fax 414–355-6065. This organization has chapters throughout the world and carries out medical research. It also publishes fact sheets, brochures and a newsletter. It serves as an information clearing-house and provides technical assistance.

THREE

Health Problems Which Affect Women Much More Often Than Men

13

♦

Cystitis and Interstitial Cystitis

♦

Cystitis

During my many years of pediatric practice I saw and treated many patients—especially females—for urinary tract infections. Often such infections would respond to a short course of an antibacterial drug. Yet, when children continued to be troubled by recurrent infections, I would refer them to a urologist for examination and further therapy.

After becoming interested in adults with complex health problems, I began to receive letters and phone calls from women who were troubled by repeated urinary tract infections. And about ten years ago at a conference in the UK, I met Angela Kilmartin,* an English woman who in 1980 published a book in the States entitled, *Cystitis—The Complete Self-Help Guide.* (And it's still available here.) Here are excerpts:

> "Antibiotics are the commonest medical way of dealing with bladder troubles . . . *The action of antibiotics is to remove bacteria—all bacteria, not just the bad, but also the good . . .* On a prolonged course

---

*In the spring of 1994 I received a letter from Angela who said, "My work continues. My sixth book on cystitis will be published in the summer of 1994 in the UK. I have three titles which I expect to be published in the U.S. in the year to come, plus a video which isn't yet ready for TV in the states." If you'd like to obtain a copy, you can write to Angela Kilmartin, P.O. Box 217, Walton-on-Thames, Surrey, KT12 3YF, UK, enclosing a check for $25 payable to Kilmartin Videos, LTD.

of antibiotics lasting several weeks (which the medical profession is still fond of prescribing in cases of recurrent cystitis) . . . the patient feels washed out and lethargic and finds it immensely difficult to get out of bed.

"An even more insidious side effect of antibiotics is yeast . . . which comes first in the fight for possession of those vacated cells. After the course of antibiotics it goes in for warm moist places, such as the tongue, mouth, vagina, intestines and rectum . . . Vaginitis takes the form of a creamy liquid discharge which emerges from the vagina out along the perineum (the best word yet for that area which contains all of your body's private openings).

"Out there in that warm, washed area, vaginitis spreads around and soon finds its way back into your urethra . . . giving what seems like another attack of cystitis. So you go back to the doctor and he, often, without a perineal examination, prescribes yet another antibiotic."[1]

In her continuing discussion, Kilmartin points out that antibiotics may be needed in women with severe urinary tract infections. Yet, she suggests that urinary burning, frequency and other symptoms may not require an antibiotic if the cause proves to be non-bacterial.

In early September 1994, I received additional information from Angela who said in effect:

"I've spent most of the last 15 years castigating doctors and leading women into infallible self-help procedures for cystitis. Not so in America, which has a bad self-help image."

The Observations of Larrian Gillespie, M.D.

About six years ago, I picked up a copy of Dr. Larrian Gillespie's book, *You Don't Have to Live With Cystitis*. Here are excerpts.

"I've found that cystitis is preventable. It is not some kind of primeval female curse that we all must endure . . . Using common sense, its causes can be found and treated. *You don't have to live with cystitis.*

"Most infections could have been avoided had my patients known a few simple facts about female anatomy and how bladder infections arise. Indeed cystitis is now an ailment most women can avoid . . .

"Tragically American women continue to make more than 8.9 million visits a year to the doctor's office because of cystitis.

"Women get cystitis again and again, we are told, because women are built funny . . .

"But if you are like most cystitis sufferers, your anatomy is perfectly normal. Your infections can be traced to functional cause . . . That is, it is something you can easily prevent if armed with common sense knowledge . . ."

In her comprehensive discussion of cystitis in women, Gillespie emphasized the importance of urine cultures prior to the use of antibiotics. She also stated that antibiotics need not be given for long periods of time, saying:

"You don't want to take antibiotics if you do not have a bacterial infection . . . I steadfastly refuse to prescribe antibiotics for long periods of time except in rare exceptions . . . Why expose your entire body, as well as sensitive bladder tissue to 10 days of antibiotic therapy? . . . To me that didn't make sense."[2]

She also sharply criticized the practice of prescribing antibiotics over the phone because such practices may ultimately lead a woman to develop interstitial cystitis.

Interstitial Cystitis (IC)

Even though I had dipped into Dr. Gillespie's book, I knew almost nothing about interstitial cystitis, and I didn't realize IC could be helped—in some women at least—with a special diet and antiyeast medication.

Then, about three years ago, Michael Kwiker, D.O., Sacramento, California, wrote to me stating that he had successfully treated four patients with IC by using Diflucan.

A brief summary of Kwiker's observations was reported in the

IHF newsletter, *Healthline*. From there the information was picked up by Marjorie Crandall, Ph.D., who passed it to Terry Oldham, an Indiana woman with severe interstitial cystitis.

In November 1992, at a candida seminar sponsored by an Indiana group, *Hoosiers for Health,* I met Terry who told me about her favorable response to a comprehensive treatment program which featured Diflucan and a sugar-free, special diet. Because Terry's interstitial cystitis had improved significantly—even dramatically—on Diflucan and diet, I asked her to write me. Here are excerpts from her six-page letter.

Terry Oldham's Story

"I had lived with interstitial cystitis for 12 years and it is much more serious and involved than a bacterial infection of the bladder. I developed tiny hemorrhages in the lining of my bladder which allowed urine to leak through the wall of my bladder; this, in turn, caused constant severe burning and pain.

"I was diagnosed with IC in 1981—my symptoms at that time were urinary frequency, burning, pelvic pain, bladder spasms, fatigue and mild to moderate digestive problems.

"Prior to 1981 I had suffered on and off for several years with these symptoms. Although a urinalysis was usually clear and a urine culture was rarely done, I was always placed on antibiotics . . . One time I was given antibiotics for four straight months."

During the next four years, Terry's symptoms continued and gradually became worse. And by 1989, because of severe bladder pain, frequency, pelvic pain, bladder spasms, fatigue, muscle and joint pains and chemical sensitivities, she had to give up her position as staff nurse at the Methodist Hospital in Indianapolis.

"My pain and fatigue were so severe I could barely stand up for more than an hour at a time. I had to urinate every 20 minutes on a bad day, and at least once an hour on a so-called 'good' day . . .

"From January 1989 to June 1991 I tried every treatment for IC available at that time. These treatments consisted of various drugs (DMSO, heparin, clorpactin and steroids) being instilled into the bladder via a catheter . . . I also tried using a Tens unit for pain relief . . . I began each treatment with a positive attitude thinking, 'If I just stick with it long enough the treatment will help my symptoms.' Time and time again I was disappointed when each treatment failed.

> ## I could barely stand up for more than an hour at a time. I had to urinate every twenty minutes.

"By the beginning of 1991, I was in pain almost constantly with severe fatigue. I woke up each day feeling like I had 'the flu' . . . I could no longer enjoy a simple activity with my family such as taking a ride in the car or a long walk in the park.

"By the spring of 1991, my husband and I decided my only remaining option was to consider having my bladder removed [emphasis added]."

Yet, after weighing the pros and cons, Terry decided against that option. Then, in June 1991, after she learned about Diflucan, she sought the help of her personal physician, Stephen Heeger, D.O. He prescribed Diflucan, which she took in gradually increasing doses until she was able to tolerate 100 mg. a day. By November 1991, her bladder pain and frequency were 50% improved. Yet she said:

"I still suffered with moderate fatigue, diarrhea and joint pain and colon discomfort continued to be a problem. In November 1991, I decided the diet change was an important factor I had not yet addressed. In December I met with Martha Erickson, a registered dietician who had worked with other IC patients with multiple food sensitivities and related problems."

> ## *To maintain my improvement I must take Diflucan and adhere to my diet.*

Following dietary changes, Terry began to show further improvement. And in a June 1993 letter, she said:

> "I found that for me to maintain my improvement, I must take Diflucan and I must adhere to my diet. When I cheat on my diet I begin to develop symptoms ranging from digestive and colon problems to vaginal yeast infections and bladder pain.
>
> "I'm happy to report that most of the time I'm 75% better than before treatment with Diflucan. Some days I'm better than 75% and I hope that some day I will be well . . . I can now enjoy everyday activities with my family that many people take for granted. I can attend my children's sports activities and I can go out to dinner and a movie with my husband. I can do my own shopping, another task which was impossible when I was at my worst.
>
> "I interviewed for a nursing position last week. The job was offered to me and I accepted . . . I feel I'm finally regaining my life that was taken away from me by this disease. I can now look forward to being a wife, mother and part-time nurse. Words cannot tell you how much this means to me and my family."

Terry continued to improve and in April 1994 she called to tell me how well she was doing. Here are excerpts from our conversation:

> "I'm working in a doctor's office and doing very well with my interstitial cystitis and my yeast problems, just as long as I follow the diet. Yet, I find I don't have to follow the diet as strictly as I did the first year. But if I vary too much I will begin to have an increase in my problems.
>
> "I generally stay away from simple sugars and after reading in your newsletter that food was a problem with some patients, I began to experiment. Wheat does cause problems just as quick, if not quicker, than sugar. It not only makes my IC flare, but it also gives me problems with my joints and muscles. I also have to watch the

acidic foods. If I consume a lot of them, I will have some burning and irritation in my bladder.

"You asked about the Diflucan. I still take 50 mg. two or three times a week on an average. Occasionally I try to skip a few days in a row. But I still find that for me personally I cannot completely stop it or I'll begin to have problems.

"You asked me about urinary frequency. I can sleep 7 or 8 hours at night and not get up to void. Before starting on Diflucan and diet, 2 hours would have been fantastic for me. In the day time I may need to urinate only every 3 to 4 hours."

Terry continued to improve and in October 1994 she wrote me and gave me a report. Here are excerpts from her letter:

"I can travel in a car with no problems of pain and frequency. This is a freedom I did not think I would ever regain, but I have. Recently my husband and I, along with another couple, traveled from Indianapolis to Kentucky to an amusement park. We left early morning, spent the day at the park and arrived home at 9:00 P.M. I did not have any problems traveling; I took several rides at the amusement park and I went to work the next day, put in a busy day and did not experience any problems with my health.

"To most people this small trip would seem extremely simple. To someone with severe IC, this trip would be impossible.

"My only problem of significance is that I develop an increase in IC symptoms 3 to 5 days before and the first 24 to 48 hours after I begin menstruating. Some months the pain is quite severe, along with muscle and joint pains and fatigue. The rest of the time I'm able to keep my IC symptoms to a minimum with Diflucan, diet and rest."

Terry sent me a packet of articles, reprints and other information about interstitial cystitis, including an article by Mary Ellen Hettinger, published in the August 11, 1992, issue of *Your Health*. Here are excerpts:

"Five hundred thousand women are suffering from interstitial cystitis, an incurable chronic inflammation of the bladder that many doctors still fail to diagnose, let alone treat . . .

"Imagine being in constant pain, having to urinate every half hour, not being able to enjoy sex, dreading long car rides or plane trips and undergoing endless doctor visits only to be told, *'there's nothing wrong with you!'*

"That's what often happens to people who have interstitial cystitis (IC), which is very difficult to diagnose, especially because many doctors are not aware of it."

During one of my conversations with Terry, she told me about Kay Longworth, a friend with interstitial cystitis who improved on a treatment program which included dietary changes and Diflucan. Here are excerpts from a letter I received from Kay in March 1993.

Kay Longworth's Story

"I suffered for almost 10 years, 8 doctors, 2 laparoscopic examinations, dilatation of the urethra, etc.

"In 1989 I read Dr. Larrian Gillespie's book, *You Don't Have to Live With Cystitis*. With the help and encouragement of my husband, I saw Dr. Gillespie in February 1989. After a week of tests and surgery she confirmed that I did have a disease and it had a name, interstitial cystitis. On the downside—no cure.

"After returning home I began Dr. Gillespie's IC diet immediately. I also had six treatments with DMSO, plus bicarbonate and steroids. *Gradually*, over the next year, I improved so much I was able to go water skiing, snow sledding and enjoy all sorts of everyday activities. I still had to follow my diet. I kept a food diary for two years to test foods that increased my pain.

"Then in spite of various therapies, my troubles came back. By the second summer I was bright red in the vulva, had constant discharge and pelvic pain. Numerous trips to the gynecologist proved useless. And they'd say, 'No yeast infection.'

"So I went to the health food store and ran into Jody Taylor-Smith—a woman who had tried to help me before without too much success. She suggested an antiyeast program, including vitamins and garlic and a diet free of sugar and yeast. This time I experienced some improvement.

"Then I went to Dr. Betty Raney in Zionsville, my new gynecologist, who was very sympathetic to IC and yeast and started me on

Diflucan, 100 mg. every other day. I have improved, but sometimes I still have vaginal itching and discharge (much milder, but still there), headache and fatigue, especially 3 or 4 days before my period.

"I know that Terry and I are not alone . . . there are thousands of women suffering some of the same problems or there wouldn't be nightly commercials for Gyne-Lotrimin and Monistat 7."

To learn how Kay was getting along, I called her on February 20, 1994. She said:

"I'm doing great—terrific. I would not even know most days that I ever had IC. It's absolutely incredible. I can sleep 6 or 7 hours and never get up. The only times I still have problems are during ovulation and a few days before my period. At such times I have a feeling of heaviness or pressure or pain and sometimes I get a urethral throbbing.

"Other symptoms which once bothered me, including eczema on my hand, cleared. And my sinus/allergy symptoms are almost nonexistent.

"As far as the frequency and the pain and the pressure and just feeling like your bladder's on fire, all of the symptoms that I had in '89 and before are all so much better. It's just unbelievable. I occasionally have some vaginal problems, yet when I do I know it's because I cheated with sugar and things like that.

"I'm still taking the 100 mg. of Diflucan every other day, plus nutritional supplements, including dairy-free strains of the good bacteria Lactobacillus acidophilus. I still follow Dr. Gillespie's diet, but I've been able to add a lot of things back, including oranges, grapefruit and salad dressing, every now and then. I still drink only distilled water—no coffee, tea or other beverages. I think that helps too."

Further Observations by Dr. Larrian Gillespie

After receiving Kay Longworth's report, I bought another copy of Dr. Gillespie's book (someone had borrowed my other copy). As I re-read it, I found that she included a 57-page discussion entitled, "Interstitial cystitis—the real story."

Dr. Gillespie pointed out that IC is not a *new* disease and that it was first described by a French physician in 1836. Yet, she said that even today the disorder is often misunderstood and that as recently as 1979 a major urology textbook stated that it may be caused by an emotional disorder. In responding, Dr. Gillespie said:

> "This was the first disease I'd ever heard about in which the mind could cause an organ to burn, ulcerate and shrink. It was the first psychiatric disease that could mysteriously cause tissue to scar."

She also cited the stories of some of her patients, including Pamela Sue Martin, who, after her successful response to therapy, appeared with Dr. Gillespie on a television talk show, "Hour Magazine." Following the program, Dr. Gillespie's office received more than 20,000 letters from women around the country who said they had the same problem.

In describing the symptoms of IC Dr. Gillespie said:

> "If you pay close attention, you probably will notice some hallmarks of this disease. The pain in your bladder feels worse after you urinate. It hurts both before and after you go to the bathroom. In fact, the only time you get relief is during those few moments when you are voiding.
>
> "You probably also have noticed that some foods make your symptoms worse. Perhaps you've eliminated coffee, tea and orange juice from your diet, but you continue to have unexplainable bouts of pain.
>
> "Moreover, your doctor is as baffled as you are. She or he knows you're in pain, but can't find anything to explain it. When the doctor looks into your bladder in the office with a cystoscope . . . everything appears normal. Your urine cultures turn up negative. You do not have a bacterial infection."

In her continuing discussion, Dr. Gillespie said:

> "Don't let them tell you it's all in your head . . . If you, as a reader, recognize this as the story of your life, then I would like to assure you, you don't have a psychiatric disorder. You're not crazy. Your childhood mishaps have nothing to do with the constant pain you're coping with every day of your life."

In late 1993, after seeing Dr. Gillespie on "Good Morning America," I wrote to her and she sent me additional information, including a copy of the 1993 article in the *British Journal of Urology** which dealt with some of the metabolic factors that contribute to symptoms in patients with hypersensitive bladders. In summarizing her findings, she said:

"The response to dietary management of patients with chronic bladder hypersensitivity offers a cost-effective therapeutic approach for clinicians who are frustrated with current pharmaceutical and surgical approaches . . . However, it should be emphasized that dietary restriction alone will not result in complete relief of the symptoms of this disorder."[3]

In this article and in her book, Dr. Gillespie lists foods which she has found cause bladder irritation in patients with interstitial cystitis and related disorders. Included are fruits and other acid foods and foods high in several amino acids.

If you'd like to know all about cystitis and interstitial cystitis, I urge you to get a copy of Dr. Gillespie's book.

Comments by Charles W. Lapp, M.D.

In a September 29, 1993 letter, Dr. Lapp said:

"We recently hospitalized a patient with severe chronic fatigue syndrome, encephalopathic headaches and multiple chemical sensitivities. She had terrible problems with frequent daytime and nighttime urination, as well as pelvic discomfort and urinary burning. She had consulted several urologists and cystoscopy with biopsy confirmed a diagnosis of interstitial cystitis.

"She did not respond to dietary manipulation, nor was she able to tolerate . . . therapy with prednisone, DMSO, or cytoxic agents. She was so miserable that we tried using long term Diflucan. On 50 mgs. daily, the IC symptoms were reduced well below 50% of what they had been . . . I hope someday we will understand the mechanism of how this therapy works."[4]

---

*For more information on pelvic pain and interstitial cystitis, write to The American Foundation for Pain Research, 120 S. Spalding Dr., Suite 210, Beverly Hills, CA 90212.

My Comments

In talking to one of my consultants, I said:

"Based on information I've received from various sources, including Dr. Gillespie's book, interstitial cystitis is more apt to develop in people who have taken repeated or prolonged courses of broad-spectrum antibiotic drugs."

As noted elsewhere in this book, long-term antibiotic use creates an imbalance of the normal bacteria in the intestinal tract which, in turn, leads to yeast overgrowth. As a result, a cascade of other symptoms may develop, ranging from multiple sclerosis to chronic fatigue syndrome to asthma.

Although I fully realize that yeast isn't THE cause of interstitial cystitis, I hope that funds will be provided to support studies on the yeast connection to IC.

One group of women could be treated in the customary manner, including dietary changes. In addition they would be given a systemic antifungal drug such as Diflucan or Sporanox. Alternate patients could be treated in the same manner and be given a placebo instead of azole drug.

Based on the reports of Terry Oldham and Kay Longworth, I feel that this study could lead to helping many women with this often devastating disorder.

REFERENCES

1. Kilmartin, A., *Cystitis—The Complete Self-help Guide*, Warner Books, New York, 1980.
2. Gillespie, L., *You Don't Have to Live with Cystitis*. Avon Books, 1986.
3. Gillespie, L., "Metabolic Appraisal of the Effects of Dietary Modification on Hypersensitive Bladder Symptoms," *British Journal of Urology*, 1993, 72, 293–297.
4. Lapp, C.W., Personal communication, September 29, 1993.

14

Sexual Dysfunction

During the past decade I've received tens of thousands of letters and phone calls from people seeking information and help. Some 85 to 90% have come from women—and most were women between 25 and 45.

Complaints have been multiple and varied and usually included fatigue, headache, depression, digestive problems and PMS. Most (but not all) also gave a history of genito-urinary problems, including vaginitis, vulvitis and/or burning or discomfort on urination. Also pain or discomfort during sexual intercourse (the medical term is *dyspareunia*). Yet, many, many women reported other types of sexual problems, including loss of interest and drive and inability to have an orgasm.

The Story of Patty's Sexual Nightmare

In a discussion of sexual dysfunction in the third edition of *The Yeast Connection*, I included the story of 35-year-old Patty (not her name). She had written me a long letter describing her "sexual nightmare." Her symptoms included:

> ". . . bizarre homosexual feelings, or intense heterosexual feelings that would persist for hours—even days . . . This consistent state of sexual arousal became an obsession with me. I could not concentrate on anything else.
>
> "Keep in mind that during this time most of my severe inner conflicts were religious ones. I was raised in a Catholic church with very

strict moral standards. Moreover, I was a virgin until after I married at the age of 22. So I found the anguish of these uncontrollable urges and thoughts to be emotionally destructive.

"During times of anger, my body and my emotions would respond inappropriately with intense feelings of sexual arousal. Bear in mind that this sensation was insatiable. Even 'satisfactory,' regular intercourse did nothing to control or reduce this constant sexual frustration . . .

I went to dozens of doctors, including psychiatrists, all to no avail.

"I went to dozens of doctors, including psychiatrists, all to no avail. Finally I found a doctor to help me with the yeast problem and my terrible nightmares began to improve."[1]

In her 1986 letter, Patty reported she was 95% better, no longer suffered from "horrifying sexual abnormalities" and required no more psychotherapy or mood changing drugs. And in her concluding paragraph, she said:

"My fantastic husband and super kids have supported me through the years and my life is now gratifying and I'm working with a doctor who is helping others avoid much needless suffering."

I've stayed in touch with Patty, who now works as an executive of a nonprofit health organization. In a recent letter to me, she said in effect:

"I'm happy to report that I'm healthy and happy and my sexual nightmare is now only an unpleasant memory."

During the past eight years, I have received hundreds of letters and calls from women whose major complaints included sexual dysfunction. Among these letters and calls were some who said that reading Patty's story made them feel better because they weren't alone. Then others wrote describing their own problems. Here are excerpts from two of these letters:

Elisa: "I was glad to read Patty's story because she shared the same agonies which I still have. It was the closest thing to finding God at this time in my life. I'll go 20 to 25 minutes of thinking that I'm going to be okay, then bingo, I get these unbearable sexual feelings every one to two minutes. My body feels heated up and my vision gets blurry and my skin itches. I get dizzy. The sensations in my genitals seem to build up and go to other parts of my body.

"The sensations are focused in my clitoris and I react clitorally to things that are obviously not sexual . . . At times I feel like I'm in a freak show and every sound and movement is coming at me and focusing on my genitals.

"Sometimes there's a desire to gouge out my genitals, but I don't know that it would help. I worry sometimes that one day I will lose control of keeping it all in check and of somehow being found out. My reactions to certain things seem so hard I can't believe it. And that scares me.

"Yesterday I went to buy my 5-year-old daughter a dress. I knew I'd have about 5 to 10 minutes looking at the clothes before the tension that builds up in my genitals would be beyond comfort. When this happens I must breathe slowly to avoid an outright panic attack . . . Please understand I'm just writing down my thoughts, I feel vulnerable having them on paper. I've left out the weirdest things—believe it or not.

> ## Sometimes these awful sensations come on without cause.

"Sometimes these awful sensations come on without cause. Even when I'm doing housework or talking to my daughter, I can feel myself becoming angry, scared. My vision is blurred. I leave the room and stop what I'm doing. Sometimes this gives slight relief. I guess I just want reassurance that I'll get better. Then perhaps I'll be able to see life more clearly. Now my vision and expectations are tainted by my arousal symptoms."

Arlene: "Patty's experiences prompt me to write. I am researching the cause of nymphomania, in association with yeast infections and allergies. I have my own ideas about the situation. I feel it occurs genetically in susceptible families. I also feel it's yeast-related.

"Our whole family has been affected by my monstrous yeast overgrowth and my daughter has had yeast problems since the age of 9. I asked my gynecologist about medical literature and he said there is none. But if I can find out what causes it, he wants to know the answer too. If you have any ideas to offer, I will share them with him.

"I feel we must have a medical understanding of what causes this sexual madness because it can affect whole families."

Comments by Professionals

In discussing "the clinical picture" in women with candida-related health problems in his book, *The Missing Diagnosis*, Dr. C. Orian Truss said:

> "In addition to . . . symptoms that result from yeast growth in the vagina and gastrointestinal tract, numerous manifestations result from the effect on other organs, as yeast products enter the bloodstream . . . Many patients experience wide fluctuations in weight as a result of fluid retention, especially premenstrual. *Diminution or total loss of sexual feeling and responsiveness is frequent.*"[2]

In an article in *The Female Patient*, gynecologist Jay S. Schinfeld described a study of 340 women who enrolled in the PMS unit at the University of Tennessee College of Medicine in Memphis. All were followed for at least one year and had a minimum of three visits. Questionnaires were sent to each patient to obtain additional data. In discussing symptoms in these patients, Schinfeld commented:

> "All were long term PMS sufferers (with) severe symptoms dominated by and frequently accompanied by anxiety and anger. Headaches, described as menstrual migraines were common, as were food cravings, bloating and *significant decreases in libido* [emphasis added]."

The patients in Schinfeld's study were divided into several groups, including a control group. And he stated:

"A combination of anticandida medication and yeast elimination diet produced improvement in 10 or 15 patients."[3]

In a subsequent presentation at the 1988 Candida Update Conference sponsored by the International Health Foundation, Memphis, Tennessee, September 16th to 18th, Schinfeld provided further information on his studies. And he stated:

"Treated patients showed significant physical and psychological improvement over untreated controls, although the mechanism for this improvement and the role of yeast in this disorder remains controversial."[4]

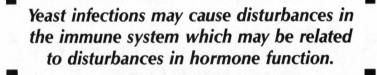

Yeast infections may cause disturbances in the immune system which may be related to disturbances in hormone function.

Steven S. Witkin, Ph.D., in an article, "Defective Immune Responses in Patients with Recurrent Candidiasis,"[5] pointed out that antibiotic therapy can create conditions conducive to *C. albicans* proliferation by several different mechanisms. He also pointed out that these yeast infections may cause disturbances in the immune system which may be related to disturbances in hormone function.

Although he did not mention sexual dysfunction, he stated that reports that endocrine abnormalities have been reversed following successful antifungal therapy for candida infections "lend credence to the idea that these abnormalities can arise as secondary consequences of fungal infections."

A number of physicians I have consulted, including gynecologists Richard Mabray, George Miller and Pamela Morford, have also told me of the frequent occurrence of sexual dysfunction in their patients with yeast-related health problems.

Women's Stories
A Typical Letter

In 1991 Loretta (not her name), a public health nurse, wrote me to obtain information about yeast-related problems. She was concerned about some of the patients she worked with every week. Subsequently she told me about her own story and her improvement on diet and antifungal therapy. Here are excerpts from her letter:

"Over the past four or five years I began developing severe PMS. A week before my menses I became irritable, with little things upsetting me that normally would not. I was also depressed and had no sexual desire for my husband.

"After my menses ended, the irritability, breast pain and water retention resolved. The depression, difficulty thinking clearly, decreased libido and vaginal candidiasis remained . . .

"When Mama's not happy, ain't nobody happy."

"My decreased libido was beginning to affect my marriage. I was just not interested in sex. I had no desire for it, which really caused problems for my husband. He felt I didn't find him pleasing to me, which caused him to be depressed. The old saying goes, 'When Mama's not happy, ain't nobody happy.' This was so true at our house [emphasis added].

"Fortunately for me, I was introduced to *The Yeast Connection.* I've been following the treatment program for almost a year now. With the diet modification, addition of vitamin supplements and nystatin almost all of my symptoms cleared, except the vaginal candidiasis. Then I was able to obtain Diflucan, which completed the cure. I took a 200 mg. tablet for two days, and have not had a recurrence. Finally, the cycle was broken.

"Now at my house, everybody's happy, because Mama's happy. Our lives have most definitely been changed for the better."

A Report On One of My Patients

In March 1993, I saw 33-year-old Marjorie in consultation. Her main complaints included "Always tired and drained and loss of sex drive (4 years duration); yeast infections/vaginitis (2 years duration)." Here are excerpts from a letter Marjorie sent me prior to our first consultation:

"All of my life I've been troubled by many nose and throat infections and have taken many antibiotic drugs. In 1988 my son was born, after a difficult labor. After that it seemed my health went downhill. Although I went back to work I had to quit after three months. I just couldn't do it. I didn't have the energy. *I also had a marked loss of sex drive* [emphasis added].

"Then came the yeast infections, vaginal dryness, urinary frequency, PMS, cramps, depression, sleep problems, abdominal pain and *very* poor memory. I saw a number of doctors who gave me different medications, including antidepressants. One doctor said, 'I can't find anything physically wrong' and my tests were all negative.

"I know that I look terrible, feel terrible and act terrible and have absolutely no sex drive. If I didn't have such a loving husband I don't know what I would do. Please, I need help for me and my son."

Because of the severity of Marjorie's symptoms, I recommended Diflucan, a sugar-free diet and nutritional supplements. During the succeeding months, Marjorie improved and on April 14th, she reported:

"The vaginitis and bladder pain are gone. Yet, I still have some rectal itching. I still have good days and bad days, especially when I overdo. Sex is better. I'm not as irritable or moody. I wake up rested most of the time and exercise daily. My memory is a lot better. I still have a way to go and I miss my coffee and sandwiches."

Three weeks later, on May 2nd, Marjorie said:

"I'm improving every day, yet I have had some problems. I took the yeast challenge and the reaction was a rash all over my body which itched excessively. So I'll really stay off yeast now. I've also found that formaldehyde, perfumes, exhaust and diesel fumes also bother me."

Then on August 23, 1993, Marjorie said:

"I'm feeling much better now. I'm just a new person altogether! My patience, memory, energy level, depression, sex drive and sleeping have improved 100% since the first time I saw you . . . But I really have to stay on my diet. I also have to exercise, which I do three or four times a week. It really helps. I can actually do a day's work without feeling give out. My PMS is much better, but it's still there . . .

My patience, memory, energy level, depression, sex drive and sleeping have improved 100%.

"In spite of these problems, my life and my marriage are much better. Thank God for the help I've received. I know I still have a ways to go before I'm well, but it's closer than before."

On September 29, 1993, Marjorie came in for a brief visit and she said:

"I'm feeling great, absolutely great! As I told you last month, I really am a new person. Something I haven't told you before. I really felt so bad that life really wasn't worth living and suicide was an option I thought about from time to time.

"Another factor that added to my load was the problem I had coping with my hyperactive, irritable, inattentive 4-year-old son. Nothing I had done for him helped . . . until you put him on the diet, Diflucan and nutritional supplements. And the changes in his behavior and ability to learn have truly been remarkable. Thank you, thank you, thank you."

My Comments

Based on the observations of both professionals and nonprofessionals, sexual dysfunction (including decreased libido and orgasmic dysfunction), occurs frequently with yeast-related problems. And in many women, a sugar-free special diet and prescription and/or nonprescription antifungal medication help. Yet, as I have expressed elsewhere in this book, such treatment will not be a quick fix and should be combined with other therapies which may include nutritional supplements, control of environmental pollutants and thyroid and other endocrine therapies.

REFERENCES

1. Crook, W.G., *The Yeast Connection*, Third Edition, Professional Books, Jackson, TN and Vintage Books, New York, 1986; pp 339–340.
2. Truss, C.O., *The Missing Diagnosis*, Birmingham, AL, 1986; pp 37–42.
3. Schinfeld, J., "PMS and Candidiasis: Study explores possible link," *The Female Patient*, July 1987; 12:66–69.
4. Schinfeld, J., Candida Update Conference, International Health Foundation, Memphis, TN, September 16–18, 1988.
5. Witkin, S., "Defective Immune Responses in Patients with Recurrent Candidiasis," *Infections in Medicine*, May/June 1985; pp. 129–132.

15

Infertility

One American couple out of every six is troubled by infertility and the causes are multiple and complex. Some are known—as for example, problems with sperm or Fallopian tubes blocked by endometriosis. Yet, others are unknown and a woman may fail to conceive even when sperm are active and normal, and a comprehensive infertility investigation comes up empty-handed.

Over 10 years ago James Brodsky, M.D., a Chevy Chase, Maryland internist interested in yeast-connected health problems told me about the successful outcome of two patients who had been troubled with an "infertility problem."

One patient had been trying to conceive for seven months and the other for ten months. On diet and nystatin, one woman became pregnant in 30 days and the other in 60 days. About the same time, I learned of another woman (I'll call her Evelyn) with yeast-related infertility.

Evelyn's Story

"I was unusually healthy as an infant and young child. My mother tells me I was rarely sick and I wasn't troubled by allergies. During my teen years I was bothered by menstrual cramps—nothing unusual. I married early and my son was born when I was 19. No significant problems on through my twenties except for moderate menstrual problems and occasional yeast infections.

"Four years ago I married again and beginning three years ago my husband and I decided we would like to have a child. Although we used no contraceptives, nothing happened.

"I seemed to think that some of my health problems began to develop about 2½ years ago. At that time I began low mileage running and over a period of months I lost about 15 lbs. I also developed other symptoms, including fatigue and lower back pain. I visited my family doctor who said, 'You seem to have a kidney infection,' and he prescribed Bactrim for 10 days. Now as I think about it, I was premenstrual at the time and the disappearance of my symptoms may have been related to my cycle rather than to the supposed urinary infection.

"Nevertheless, I agreed to have IVP (intravenous pyelogram), which showed no abnormalities. However, I developed a reaction to this test with symptoms of extreme nausea, hives and swollen eyes.

"During the next six months, while attempting conception, I developed increasingly severe dysmenorrhea, continuing lower back pain and general fatigue. So I sought further help from a gynecologist who specialized in studying patients with infertility. About the same time I began to have more acute pain on my right side with a lot of pelvic and abdominal bloating.

"A laparoscopy revealed 'mild/moderate endometriosis with a few adhesions' and chromotubation—which was attempted three times—showed that my right tube was closed.

I decided to seek a second opinion in regard to surgery.

"I was placed on Danazol and surgery was recommended. So I decided to seek a second opinion in regard to surgery and the quality of my husband's semen.

"The following month I began to have chronic uterine cramping, severe bloating, lower back pain, mood swings, nausea, occasional very painful right lower quadrant pain, insomnia, taut, dry skin (my skin was usually oily) and dizzy spells. I had so much pain that it scared me.

"So I went back for further studies and a hysterosalpingogram revealed that both of my tubes were open. Yet my symptoms continued. I was sick and emotionally and physically exhausted so my husband and I took a wonderful, but exhausting, two weeks vacation.

"Then in June 1983, I went to a university center and went through the infertility clinic. The head gynecologist thought I was 'hyperestrogenic,' which he said was not uncommon following a rigorous trip. Various studies were negative, including a test following intercourse.

"When my symptoms continued, my doctor decided I was 'severely depressed' and that she doubted that there was any organic basis for my symptoms. So she suggested I see a psychiatrist. I took her advice, yet, at the end of his evaluation, he said, 'You aren't severely depressed and I don't think you need psychotherapy.'"

"I was then seen by another infertility specialist at the same university center. He insisted that I be 'scoped' again. This time they found 'moderate endometriosis, but no adhesions.' He recommended six months of Danazol. I developed a urinary tract infection following the laparoscopy and I was treated with Bactrim and then ampicillin.

"I felt *horrible* for several weeks following this course of antibiotics. I attributed my continuing pain to endometriosis. Yet my doctor couldn't understand why Danazol hadn't eased the pain after I had taken it for over a month. (I think by this time he, too, decided I was an overanxious, depressed hypochondriac.)

"Finally my pain abated and I began treating myself with vitamins and 'friendly bacteria.' I continued to have symptoms, including terrible headaches, bloating, junky discharge and vaginal itching. I was given Vibramycin although my cultures for chlamydia and herpes were both negative.

"Then in August 1983 I went back to the second university center for further studies and again received the diagnosis of mild endometriosis. They also said it was possible that I was hypersensitive to ovulation.

I read The Yeast Connection and took the quiz.

"About that time I read *The Yeast Connection* and took the quiz. My score was 181, which indicated the 'candida almost certainly was playing a role in causing my health problems.' Among the items in my history which added significantly to my score were repeated courses of antibiotics, birth control pills, worsened symptoms on damp days and sugar craving. Also fatigue, the feeling of being drained, depression, abdominal pain, and PMS.

"Based on this history, a physician consultant interested in yeast-related health problems said, 'Your immune system and endocrine problems may be related to *Candida albicans*. And I think a therapeutic trial of nystatin, diet and nutritional supplements may help you.

"In discussing my problem with me, he said, 'Although candida is not *the* cause of your reproductive problems, it may be playing a significant role. And many women with hormonal dysfunction and reproductive organ symptoms will improve significantly on a simple, but comprehensive antiyeast program extending over a period of six months to two years.'

"So I began on the nystatin, at first one-quarter tsp., 4 times a day and after a week I increased it to one-half tsp., 4 times a day.

"During the first two weeks I showed a little lessening of my symptoms. Not a lot, but I was encouraged. After I'd been on the program 4 weeks, I was literally 'a new woman.' My depression, fatigue, bloating, mood swings, urinary symptoms and vaginal burning had all but vanished. I talked to my doctor, who said, 'Keep on with your nystatin. You can even cheat on your diet occasionally and see if it makes any difference.' And he said that because of my history of vaginitis, that a vaginal antiyeast suppository would be advisable.

Evelyn, you're pregnant!

"Then the exciting news. Because I missed my period, I went back to my gynecologist who, following the examination, said, '*Evelyn, you're pregnant!*' Then I began to wonder if it was safe to continue the nystatin.

"One of my gynecologists said, 'Stop it, you could develop complications.' Yet, my own gynecologist said to continue. I also called Dr. Orian Truss who said that in his experience nystatin during pregnancy was safe. Yet, he said, 'The decision to continue it will be up to you and your obstetrician/gynecologist.' So I kept taking it.

"When I tried to reduce the dose of nystatin to one-quarter tsp., 4 times a day, some of my symptoms returned. I also found that the amount of sugar I ate made a difference.

"My pregnancy proceeded uneventfully and nine months and 3 weeks after starting on nystatin, my husband and I became the proud parents of a beautiful, healthy 8 lb. 9 oz. son. And in the birth announcement I sent to the open minded doctor who advised my gynecologist to put me on nystatin, I said, 'Thanks seems like too little to say for your part in helping us have this baby—we felt he should be named for you!'

"He is a beautiful healthy boy and I am feeling good physically. I still have trouble believing my good fortune."

To learn more about the yeast connection to infertility, I talked to several of my physician consultants. Here are their comments:

James Brodsky, M.D., Chevy Chase, Maryland   "During the past decade several of the women I've seen in my practice have conceived after starting on the diet and nystatin. Yet, I want to point out that I'm not trying to say that yeast causes infertility. Instead, I feel that any illness may be a factor. Sick people, whether due to stress, or just not being well for any reason, may be unable to conceive."

Elmer Cranton, M.D., Yelm, Washington   "I can recall at least two female patients who had undergone multiple infertility work-ups over as long as 15 years. Both became pregnant within a few months of anti-candida therapy."

Charles Resseger, D.O., Norwalk, Ohio   "I've treated dozens of patients with an infertility problem who, following a comprehensive treatment program which included anti-candida therapy, became pregnant. What I do with these patients is to tell them, 'Don't get yourself pregnant until I get you squared around.' If they do become pregnant, I put them on caprylic acid and friendly bacteria and FOS and try to maintain them.

"It has become quite obvious to me that candida overgrowth has an anti-estrogenic effect on the body. This is probably the mechanism for the infertility."

George Miller, M.D., Lewisburg, Pennsylvania "In my obstetrics and gynecology practice I currently have 40 or 50 patients on nystatin. I also have a bunch of others that aren't on nystatin anymore because they've gotten better. They're following the diet and watching what they do. During the past several years I've also had two infertility patients who conceived while following the program."

Richard Mabray, M.D., Victoria, Texas *"Candida albicans* is a very important part of many women's problems. It isn't just a vaginal thing. Candida contributes to many other major health problems, including endocrine dysfunction, PMS, infertility, dysmenorrhea and all sorts of abnormal bleeding.

"It also contributes to psychiatric symptoms, including depression and mood changes and still other symptoms, including skin problems of various sorts, bursitis and tendinitis.

"Having said all that, I do not regard candida as the real cause of most of these problems. Instead, I see it as a major trigger and part of the vicious cycle that appears to start with immune dysfunction. So it's not so much the candida itself, but rather the initial immune dysfunction that starts the people on the road for getting candida."

In summarizing his experiences, Dr. Mabray said:

"I cannot base my life and practice on 'the yeast connection.' However, this is an extremely common problem with interaction and multiple facets for a large portion of my patients. Therefore, even though it is not the total answer, to practice good medicine without this understanding, would be impossible . . . I simply would fail to meet the needs of a large proportion of my practice."

My Comments

Yeast overgrowth is certainly not "the cause" of infertility. Yet, for a couple struggling in vain to solve the problem, anti-candida therapy is a safe option worth considering. Such therapy should be comprehensive and should feature oral nystatin and a sugar-free special diet. I would especially recommend such a treatment program if either or both partners gave the typical history.

FOUR

*Still Other Health Problems
Which Affect Women More
Often Than Men*

PART

FOUR

Still Other Health Problems
Which Affect Women More
Often Than Men

16

Chronic Fatigue Syndrome (CFS) and Fibromyalgia Syndrome (FMS)

In an October 1990 publication, *Chronic Fatigue Syndrome—A pamphlet for physicians,* appeared the following comments:

> "Most investigators studying CFS believe that the syndrome has many possible causes . . . Preliminary research also shows a variety of immunologic disturbances in some patients . . . Many patients have a history of allergies years before the onset of CFS and occasionally allergic symptoms worsen after these patients become ill.
> "Preliminary evidence suggests that several latent viruses may be actively replicating more often in CFS patients than in healthy (control) subjects . . . Most investigators believe reactivation of these viruses is probably secondary to some immunologic disorder."[1]

I developed an interest in food-related chronic fatigue, headache, muscle aches, irritability and other symptoms over 30 years ago. At that time an alert mother convinced me (against my will) that her 12-year-old son Tom's fatigue, weakness, inability to get out of bed in the morning and other symptoms vanished when he stopped drinking milk.*

A short time later, I read several articles[2,3,4] in the medical literature which described food-related fatigue and other symp-

---

*See also Chapter 35.

toms. After reading these articles, I put a number of my patients on 5 to 10 day elimination diets, followed by challenge.

Although I didn't help all of these tired, irritable, unhappy patients, I was excited when I received reports from mothers who said, "Susie's like a different child. But when I give her chocolate milk, corn chips, wheat or eggs, her symptoms return."

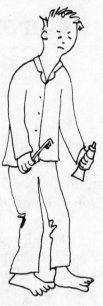

I collected and summarized my findings on 50 of these patients and reported them in the medical literature.[5] I published further observations on food-related fatigue in the 1970s[6,7] and other physicians made similar observations.[8,9,10]

During the 1970s, I began to see more adult patients—especially women—who complained of fatigue and other symptoms which made them feel "sick all over." Some of these patients were helped by changing their diets and cleaning up the pollutants in their home. Yet, many remained ill.

One such patient, 35-year-old Linda,* I saw a number of times in 1976. Although she improved on the treatment program I outlined, she continued to experience many symptoms. Linda moved away and I lost contact with her until the fall of 1979. At that time she told me that a special diet and antiyeast medication had helped her overcome her chronic fatigue and other symptoms. And she gave me a copy of an article by Dr. Truss published in a little known Canadian medical journal.[11]

And now—as Paul Harvey would say—"Here's the rest of the story": I called Dr. Truss who provided me with additional information. Soon thereafter, I began to treat and help other patients—especially women between 25 and 45—who complained of fatigue, muscle aches, poor memory, mental

---

*You'll find a further discussion of Linda's story in Chapter 17.

confusion and other symptoms. My treatment program in working with these patients featured a sugar-free special diet and the antifungal medication, nystatin.

During the 1980s, information about Truss' observations spread to physicians all over the world. And a small but growing number of physicians found that a special diet and nystatin, Nizoral or Diflucan, helped many of their patients, including some with chronic fatigue syndrome.

Chronic Fatigue Syndrome—An Enigma

During the mid-1980s, reports began appearing in medical journals and in the press about CFS and professionals and nonprofessionals were seeking answers to these questions:

"How does it start? Is there more than one cause? Is it contagious? What makes it persist? and, What is the best treatment?"

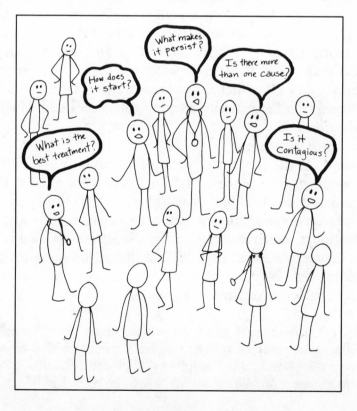

Many physicians, including researchers, emphasized the role of one or more viruses in causing this disorder. And for a time it was thought that the Epstein-Barr virus was the culprit. Yet, laboratory and other studies showed that this virus was not the causative agent. Although in many people CFS developed suddenly following a viral infection, in other individuals it seemed to come on more gradually.

As I read the reports in the medical and lay literature about CFS, it seemed to me that the symptoms in many people with this illness were similar to those experienced by my patients with yeast-related problems.

Observations of Drs. Carol Jessop, Jorge Flechas, Michael Goldberg and Philip Nelson

During the late 1980s, following the suggestion of Agnes Jonas of Enfield, Connecticut, I began going to CFS conferences. And between 1988 and 1993 I attended conferences in Rhode Island, California, North Carolina, Florida, New York and Georgia. Although the great majority of the speakers focused their attention on viral infections, two CFS clinicians and researchers, Drs. Carol Jessop and Michael Goldberg, discussed other causative factors including *Candida albicans*.

Dr. Jessop At the conference in San Francisco in April 1989 and in a subsequent conference in Charlotte in November 1990, Dr. Jessop discussed her findings in working with 1324 patients with chronic fatigue syndrome she had seen between 1984 and 1990. Her treatment program featured the use of a restricted diet (no alcohol, sugar, fruit or fruit juice) and the antifungal medications Nizoral and Diflucan.

At the Charlotte conference, she said:

"I don't believe we're going to find one single virus that causes this illness. However, I do think that genetic predisposition and environmental factors such as antibiotics, birth control pills, toxins in the environment and infections all have to be considered.

"Eighty-four percent of my CFS patients have recovered to a level where they can remain working 30 to 40 hours a week and 30% have fully recovered. Yet, 44% of the patients experience some recurrence of their symptoms with premenstrual stress, surgery or other infections."

Dr. Flechas   The relationship of CFS to *Candida albicans* was also noted by this North Carolina physician in an article in the summer/fall 1989 issue of the *CFIDS Chronicle*. In his comments, in an article entitled, "Yeast and the CFIDS Patient," Dr. Flechas said:

"In our CFIDS population we found an overgrowth of *Candida albicans* on the mucous tissues of the body to be a common occurrence . . . Based on the work in our office we hypothesize that the T-cell defects of CFIDS allow *Candida albicans* to grow . . .

"Candida is not the cause of CFIDS, but it can make a bad situation worse. It is important that an aggressive antiyeast program be in place for the CFIDS patient until his/her immune system returns to its normal state."[12]

Dr. Goldberg   In 1992 during a conversation with Nancy Smith, a "networking" friend and co-author of a book on chronic fatigue syndrome, Nancy said in effect:

"I'm quite aware that most of the CFS/CFIDS leaders are more interested in viruses than they are in any of the other causes of this often devastating illness. Yet, one of these leaders, Dr. Michael Goldberg of Tarzana, California, will be talking about the experience of treating some of his CFS patients with nystatin and elimination diet. Moreover, he is one of the leading speakers on a program at the Suncoast CFIDS Conference being held in Sarasota, Florida."

I went to the conference in Florida and to another conference in Bel Air, California, which was co-hosted by Dr. Goldberg and Dr. Jay Goldstein. And in August 1992 Dr. Goldberg and I gave presentations to members of a CFS/CFIDS support group in San Diego. Because of his knowledge, experience and interest in yeast-related health problems, I interviewed him in February 1994. Here are excerpts from our conversation.

Crook: Michael, tell me something about your experiences in treating your CFS patients with antifungal medication.

Goldberg: My focus has been primarily with Nizoral and occasionally with Diflucan. I've liked Nizoral because it does affect the immune system and I preferred it to some degree. However, I've recently seen patients who do not respond to Nizoral who respond better to Diflucan.

Crook: What kind of patient are you giving Diflucan to?

Goldberg: They're primarily CFS/CFIDS patients who are showing evidence of yeast problems. Often they are patients who show thrush, upset stomach, abdominal pain, leg and arm aches and who are not responding as I expect them to. Those are the patients I find myself turning to Diflucan. One reason it may be effective is that it is less sensitive to stomach acids.

Crook: Do you have a ballpark figure about how many patients with CFS/CFIDS you've treated with one of the antifungal drugs?

Goldberg: Probably hundreds at this point.

Crook: How do you make a diagnosis of CFIDS?

Goldberg: I look in two directions. First at the history, including a history of endocrine dysfunction. Next, I look at the lab work, including evidence of immune dysregulation, either up or down. Increasingly, I've been looking for confirmation using the SPECT scan.

Dr. Nelson   At the Sarasota conference, I met Dr. Philip Nelson, a Florida gynecologist who, along with his wife Marion, serves as professional advisor for the Florida CFS group. I saw him again at the Bel Air conference and we began to correspond. I was especially delighted to learn of his interest.

In a letter to me in the spring of 1993 he told me that initially he had been skeptical about the yeast connection, but that he had found that a sugar-free diet and Diflucan helped a number of his patients with CFS, as well as women with other health problems.*

---

*See also A Special Message to the Physician.

Exciting Stories

Like all physicians, I acquired a lot of information during medical school, internship and residency. I learned even more from reports in the medical literature and conferences and seminars. Yet, much of my knowledge about yeast-related problems has come from my own patients and people who have written and called me.

Although skeptics may put down clinical experience and anecdotal reports, I continue to rely on them. Here are several examples.

Anita's Story

This major in the U.S. Marine Corps wrote me a long letter in July 1992. She told me that she had been troubled with yeast-related chronic fatigue syndrome for several years. Although she had improved on a comprehensive treatment program which included nystatin, nutritional supplements and other therapies, she was still experiencing problems.

In responding, I sent her a packet of information including comments about Diflucan. She took this information to her physician and obtained a prescription for this new antifungal medication. She also tightened up on her diet.

A few weeks later, during a trip to California, I met Anita and she told me she had improved significantly. As I gathered material for this book, I asked her to give me a summary of her story. Here it is.

"I was the 'typical' CFS profile: Female; 30s; educated; a workaholic. I hold two law degrees and was a Major in the U.S. Marine Corps. I never took sick leave, and I often took antibiotics for a chronic urinary tract infection.

> **I slept 14 hours a day, my head felt as though it would burst and I ached all over.**

"In January 1985 I became desperately ill. I slept 14 hours a day, my head felt as though it would burst, I ached all over, especially my joints. Just getting dressed exhausted me.

"My allergies were so bad I took up to 15 antihistamines a day. Doctors could find nothing wrong. First there was concern from the Naval establishment, then nonchalance, then disdain. I considered suicide. I didn't know how I would ever be able to perform my job, but I had to work to support myself.

"I began reading everything I could find on diseases with my symptomatology and in March 1987 I ran across an article written by Arthur Kaslow, M.D., in *Let's Live Magazine* discussing Epstein Barr/CFS. I made an appointment with Dr. Kaslow, who offered not only superb medical care, but concern and compassion as well.

"He started me on nystatin, daily injections of B_{12}, plus other nutrients. I changed my diet to one of whole foods, supplemented with vitamins and minerals. I added acidophilus and a colon cleanser. Changes did not occur overnight, but I slowly turned the corner back toward the living.

"Dr. Kaslow passed away some time ago, leaving those of us whose lives he changed with a great void. He was a fine man who made a positive contribution to others. He is sorely missed.

"I have continued to read and study about CFS and yeast infections and this year I had all my mercury amalgams removed. I've modified my diet over the last few years so I eat mostly organically grown whole grains and vegetables, limited fruit and a small amount of fish, fowl and meat.

"Do I eat this well consistently? No. I still crave sweets and still adore coffee. I try to do the best I can under all circumstances and not worry too much. One thing is certain. In my case, there's no hope of ever controlling CFS unless the underlying yeast condition is treated . . .

"I am in control again, but all my priorities have changed. I no longer sleep in the office because I have so much work to do. I have a good laugh every day. I always have time to share a nice meal with a friend. I don't cling too tightly to security because good health is the only true security.

"I resigned my commission I held with the Marine Corps for 13 years to open a private practice in Texas. I want to live in the country and ride the horses I've always loved.

"Like other crusaders with a cause, I want to help other people with CFS. There's a great deal for me to do."

Virginia's Story

Because of acne, this teenager was put on tetracycline early in 1991. A short time later, Virginia said:

> "I became extremely tired. I ached all over and developed severe headaches. In the 18 months since that time I've been tired, weak and depressed."

Virginia saw a number of physicians and various medications were tried, including antidepressants. Because of her persistent symptoms, she was unable to go to school and the school provided a homebound teacher. Weakness and daily severe headache were her worst symptoms.

I saw Virginia the first time in September 1992. And at the conclusion of my office history, I made the following diagnostic impression:

> "Chronic fatigue syndrome triggered by a combination of circumstances. My first bet would be yeast overgrowth triggered by broad-spectrum antibiotics. There may be secondary nutritional deficiencies, food sensitivities and reactivation of latent viruses."

I recommended a sugar-free, dairy-free special diet, preparations of *Lactobacillus acidophilus*, and nutritional supplements. After 10 days I prescribed Diflucan, 200 mg. a day for three days, then 100 mgs. a day.

Virginia improved steadily and by Thanksgiving she was able to return to school. And in a letter I sent to Virginia and her mother on December 7, 1992, I said:

> "Dear Friends. I'm delighted at Virginia's improvement and I commend you both for following the treatment program. I feel the diet, Diflucan and nutritional supplements made a difference . . . Even though some of your doctors may be skeptical!
> "Virginia, I look upon you as a normal, healthy young woman.

Continue to eat a good diet and don't cheat too often. Cut your dose of Diflucan to every other day, then if you do well, discontinue it after Christmas.

"You can walk and carry on your usual activities, yet do not take vigorous exercise—such as running or jogging long distances—for at least three months. If you're having problems of any type which relate to your previous illness, and you feel I could help, please call me."

I called Virginia in January 1994 to get a follow up report. She told me she was doing great and that she hadn't missed any school. No headache, no fatigue. When I asked her about her diet and medication she said:

"Of course, I cheat on my diet at times, but I still consume a much better diet than most teenagers. I take the vitamins you prescribed, Kyolic odor-free garlic and a preparation of *Lactobacillus acidophilus.*"

In the spring of 1994, Virginia ran into problems. She developed a urinary tract infection and was put on antibiotics. A short time later, many of her symptoms returned. I renewed her prescription for Diflucan and told her to tighten up on her diet. Yet, because she continued to be depressed, her family physician gave her Prozac to take along with the Diflucan. Again she improved.

After three weeks, Virginia was able to taper off the Prozac and then stop it, and she remained symptom free. Then, in another two weeks, nystatin was substituted for the Diflucan. Here's another therapeutic intervention which helped her: a thyroid supplement. Because Virginia's morning oral temperature readings were low (96.8–97.4 degrees), I prescribed 32 mg. of USP thyroid once a day, in addition to other treatment measures.

In September 1994, I spoke to Virginia's mother, who said:

"Virginia is doing great. She's back in school and doing well and has an after school hours job."

In November 1994, Virginia's mother called. Here's a report.

"Virginia is a healthy, happy young woman. She's a senior in high school and has recently been selected to represent her class in a course which will be held in Jackson. She continues to follow her diet—most of the time—and she takes her nutritional supplements and nystatin and acidophilus once a day. I really feel like she's out of the woods."

Observations and Reports on CFS
by C. Orian Truss

Almost ten years before chronic fatigue syndrome began to be talked about in medical journals and in the press and media, this Alabama internist and allergist published an article describing mental and nervous system manifestations caused by superficial yeast infections. The symptoms in these patients included:

fatigue	low grade fever
lethargy	insomnia
memory loss	cervical node enlargement
poor concentration	headaches
chronic sore throat	muscle or joint pains

These symptoms are identical to the symptoms described subsequently by physicians studying patients with chronic fatigue syndrome. Truss also noted the common occurrence of hormone problems (decreased libido, acne, PMS, menstrual abnormalities), intolerance to chemicals, foods and drugs and allergies (hives, headaches, asthma and rhinitis).

In an article published in the fall 1992 issue of *Journal of Advancement in Medicine,* Dr. Truss reported on his continuing experiences in studying women with superficial *Candida albicans* infection of the vagina and gastrointestinal tract, accompanied by generalized symptoms.

In this report, Truss compared the response of 25 premenopausal women with yeast vaginitis who were treated for 26 weeks with nystatin, diet and immunotherapy, with a control group of patients. He found that the treated patients showed a highly significant improvement for vaginal symptoms, as well as generalized symptoms.

He again emphasized the relationship of yeast to the chronic fatigue syndrome and made references to his 1978 article. He also referred to the observations of Dr. Carol Jessop who had reported:

"... clearing of these (CFS) symptoms with ketoconazole therapy in 84% of 1100 patients selected by the criteria set forth in the initial 'chronic fatigue' syndrome paper. Lending objectivity to these results was the fact that 685 of 1100 patients were on disability prior to treatment, with only 12 remaining on disability after several months of ketoconazole therapy. It was concluded the *C. albicans* was the cause of these symptoms in 'a great majority of cases.' "[13]

Fibromyalgia Syndrome (FMS)

In an article, "Fibromyalgia—An Emerging But Controversial Condition," Don L. Goldenberg, M.D., of the Boston University School of Medicine, described the clinical manifestations, laboratory findings, and treatment results of 118 patients with fibromyalgia. Here are excerpts from his article.

"Fibromyalgia is one of the most common diagnoses in ambulatory practice. Recent estimates of the instance of fibromyalgia in the United States have ranged from 3 to 6 million ... Common symptoms noted in our series and other recent reports have included neck and shoulder pain, morning stiffness, sleep disturbances and fatigue. *Seventy to 90% of patients have been women and the mean age for diagnosis has varied from 34 to 55 years* [emphasis added].

"The Gold Standard for diagnosis ... has been the presence of a minimum number of tender points ... from four of 40 to 12 of 14 possible tender points."

In discussing natural history and treatment, Goldenberg said:

"Fibromyalgia is a chronic condition. The average duration of symptoms at the time of diagnosis has been five years ... Most patients reported little change in their symptoms (while taking various medications) and 90% of patients were symptomatic after three years of follow-up. Most patients continue to have symptoms whatever medication is used."[14]

At several conferences on chronic fatigue syndrome, professionals who discussed this disorder expressed varying points of view and different treatments were recommended. *The general consensus seemed to be that FM and chronic fatigue syndrome were closely related—if not the same disorder.*

In discussing terminology, Kristin Thorson, publisher, *Fibromyalgia Network*, said:

> "Dr. Don Goldenberg made the following comments during an interview in 1989: 'What you call it [FMS or CFIDS], depends on the eyes of the beholder.' I'm convinced that Dr. Goldenberg is correct. FMS could be another name for CFIDS . . . or vice versa . . . depending on which diagnosis you happen to have."

During the past several years, I've been fascinated by much of the information I've read in *Fibromyalgia Network* about the immunological and metabolic changes found in people with FMS. And recent issues of the newsletter highlighted a number of abnormalities, including reduction in cerebral/brain blood flow (by SPECT scan analysis), low magnesium levels and growth hormone deficiency.

The April 1994 issue of *Fibromyalgia Network* included a further discussion of metabolic abnormalities, including disturbances in tryptophan, serotonin, norepinephrine, DHEA and much more.

I was also especially interested in the references to the research studies of Xavier Caro, M.D., who found "significantly decreased natural killer (NK) cell activity in FMS patients." In discussing the various metabolic changes, *FM* editor Thorson commented:

> "But what about patients who can clearly trace their FMS symptoms back to a flu-like onset, or some other infectious trigger? . . . How can these infectious type onsets relate to a problem with serotonin? The friendly bacteria that commonly reside in your stomach

are routinely digested and their cell wall constituents . . . are absorbed into the blood to activate serotonin receptors in the brain . . .

"Any infectious agent that disrupts your friendly bacteria could also interfere with the necessary activation of serotonin receptors in the brain, leading to disturbed sleep and perhaps the onset of symptoms in genetically predisposed individuals. *This may be relevant in the case of Lyme disease when antibiotics are prescribed to destroy the Lyme bacterium and in the process, the antibodies kill off the friendly bacteria in the gut as well* [emphasis added]."[15]

My Comments

Based on the letters I've received and the people I've talked to during the past decade, CFS/CFIDS and FMS are related disorders. People with these disorders seem to develop them because their immune systems are disturbed. When their immune systems are weakened, viruses are activated, candida yeasts multiply, food and chemical allergies become activated and nutritional deficiencies develop.

Each person is unique. Some individuals will be bothered more by fatigue, headache and depression; others will experience more muscle aching; still others will be bothered especially by cognitive dysfunction and/or other symptoms.

In discussing these disorders, I'm reminded of the comments of Drs. E. Cheraskin and Sidney Baker in *The Yeast Connection*.[16] Cheraskin, who at that time was chairman of the Department of Oral Medicine at the University of Alabama, in an article entitled, "The Name of the Game is the Name," said in effect:

"We physicians are taught to diagnose, classify and label 'diseases.' And most of us feel if we can put a diagnostic label on each patient who comes to us, we've done our duty. Then we prescribe drugs, surgery or psychotherapy. Yet, there's a better way."[17]

In his numerous publications, including his book *Predictive Medicine*,[18] co-authored by W. M. Ringsdorf, Jr., Cheraskin pointed out that many disabling health disorders could be treated—even prevented—by helping patients make appropriate changes in their lifestyle and more especially in their diets.

Labeling diseases isn't the way we should go.

In his book, *The Missing Diagnosis,* Truss commented on the pitfall inherent in dividing human illnesses into "diseases." Sidney Baker expressed a similar point of view in one of his lectures, in which he said in effect:

> "Labeling diseases isn't the way we should go. Rather than using up so much of our time and energy trying to put labels on diseases, we should look instead at the multiple factors which play a role in making people sick."

I'm not claiming that the common yeast *Candida albicans* is THE cause of CFS/CFIDS, FMS, MS or other disorders which affect so many people—especially women. As Dr. Carol Jessop pointed out in her foreword to my book, *Chronic Fatigue Syndrome and the Yeast Connection:*

> "I've been working with CFS patients for almost ten years. I believe this illness may simply represent the 10 to 15% of our species who have not yet adapted to the rapid and startling changes in the environment, and the subsequent changes in our internal intestinal environment.
>
> "Since 1950 we've seen the development and overuse of antibiotics; the use of hormones and birth control pills; the development of immunosuppressive drugs; the introduction of various toxins and chemicals into our environment; and significant changes which have occurred within our diets, leaving us foods tainted with pesticides and depleted in nutritional value and loaded with sugars and dyes.
>
> "Can we really continue to believe these incredible changes have not affected the well being of some, and eventually perhaps all of us?"[19]

If your health problems resemble those experienced by people with CFS/CFIDS and FMS, there's no "magic bullet" to shoot down a villain making you sick. What's more, as you've already found out, there is no single cause for these health problems. As Jessop pointed out, there are many causes.

But regardless of these causes, like Anita and Jinnifer, you can get your health and life back on track. As a first step, change your diet and clean up the pollutants in your home and workplace. Then, you can follow the treatment measures you'll find described in Part Seven of this book.

REFERENCES

1. *Chronic Fatigue Syndrome—A pamphlet for physicians*, National Institute of Allergy and Infectious Diseases, Bldg. 31, Room 7A32, 9000 Rockville Pike, Bethesda, MD 20892. (301-496-5717)
2. Rowe, A., "Allergic Toxemia and Migraine Due to Food Allergy," *California and Western Medicine*, 1930; 33:785.
3. Randolph, T., "Allergy as a Cause of Fatigue, Irritability and Behavior Problems in Children," *J. of Ped.*, 1947; 31:560.
4. Speer, F., "The Allergic-Tension-Fatigue Syndrome," *Ped. Clin. of N. Amer.*, 1954; 1:1029.
5. Crook, W.G., "Systemic Manifestations Due to Allergy," *Pediatrics*, 1961; 27:790.
6. Crook, W.G., "The Allergic-Tension-Fatigue Syndrome," *Pediatric Annals*, October 1974.
7. Crook, W.G., "Food Allergy—The Great Masquerader," *Ped. Clin. of N. Amer.*, 1975; 22:227.
8. Deamer, W.C., "Some Impressions Gained Over a 27 Year Period," *Pediatrics*, 1971; 48:930.
9. Oski, F., *Don't Drink Your Milk*, Castle Hill Australia, Beta Books, 1983.
10. Tunnessen, W., "An Eight-Year-Old Boy With Lethargy and Fatigue," *Clini-Pearls*, 1979; 2:6. Published by Creative Medical Publications, Dista Products, Division of Eli Lilli & Company, Indianapolis, IN 46205.
11. Truss, C.O., "Tissue Injury Induced by *C. Albicans:* Mental and Neurologic Manifestations," *J. of Ortho. Psych.*, 1978; 7:17–37.
12. Flechas, J., "Yeast and the CFIDS Patient," *CFIDS Chronicle*, Summer/Fall 1989; pp 40–42.

13. Truss, C.O., Truss, C.V., Cutler, R.B., "Generalized Symptoms in Women with Chronic Yeast Vaginitis: Treatment with nystatin, diet and immunotherapy versus nystatin alone," *J. of Advan. in Med.*, 1992; 5:139–175.
14. Goldenberg, D.L., "Fibromyalgia Syndrome—An emerging but controversial condition," *JAMA*, 1987; 257:2782–2787.
15. Thorson, K., *Fibromyalgia Network*, 5700 Stockdale Hwy., Suite 100, Bakersfield, CA 93309–2554.
16. Crook, W.G., "Labeling Disease Isn't the Way We Should Go," in *The Yeast Connection*, Third Edition, Professional Books, Jackson, TN, and Vintage Books, New York, 1986; pp 161–162.
17. Cheraskin, E., "The Name of the Game is the Name," in Williams, R.J. and Kalita, B.K., *A Physician's Handbook of Orthomolecular Medicine*, Pergamon Press, New York, 1977; pp 40–44.
18. Cheraskin, E. and Ringsdorf, W.M., Jr., *Predictive Medicine*, Keats Publishing, Inc., New Canaan, CT, 1973.
19. Jessop, C., Foreword in Crook, W.G., *Chronic Fatigue Syndrome and the Yeast Connection*, Professional Books, Jackson, TN, 1992; pp xi–xii.

17

◆

Multiple Chemical Sensitivity Syndrome (MCSS)

◆

If your health problems are yeast connected, you'll have a better chance of overcoming them if you "clean up" your diet and track down your hidden food allergies. You'll also need to "clean up" your home. When I say "clean up," I'm not talking about keeping a neat, tidy, spick-and-span apartment or house. I'm referring, instead, to steps you should take to avoid "outgassing" (volatile) chemicals of all sorts. Most of these troublemakers you can smell—yet some may be odorless.

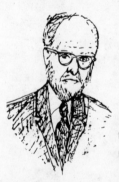
During my years in medical school and residency training and during my early years in practice, I knew little about food allergies and absolutely nothing about chemical sensitivities. And my ignorance was shared by most other physicians. During the 1940s, Theron Randolph, a Chicago internist/allergist, found that he could help many of his allergic patients by getting rid of house dust and animal danders and administering allergy vaccines. He also found that many of these patients improved even more when they avoided several of their favorite foods, including corn, wheat and dairy products. Yet, there were other patients who continued to experience problems.

To come up with answers, Randolph began to spend more time

studying his difficult patients and listening to them. One patient commented:

> "I seem to get along fine when I stay at home, but just as soon as I visit my daughter, who lives in an apartment in the city, I develop a headache and muscle aches. There's just something about the 'smell' of her apartment which bothers me."

He then began to question other patients about their possible reactions to chemical fumes of all sorts, including plastics, perfumes, paints, soaps, shaving lotions, fabric odors, gas cooking stoves and tobacco smoke.

As Randolph questioned his allergic patients, especially those with chronic problems, he noted that the symptoms in over half of them would be triggered or aggravated by chemical exposures.

The symptoms in over half of Dr. Randolph's allergy patients were aggravated by chemical exposures.

I first learned about Randolph's observations many years ago. While browsing through a medical library, I came across his paper describing fatigue, headache and other symptoms caused by sensitivities to common foods.[1] So I wrote to him and asked him for further information, which he generously sent to me.

Several years later, during a visit to Chicago, he invited me to accompany him while he visited his patients in the hospital. So, as was my usual custom, I bathed, shaved and doused my face with cologne. I met Dr. Randolph in the lobby of the hospital and then we proceeded to make "rounds."

The first patient was a woman who had been hospitalized because of asthma. She was convalescing and was sitting comfortably in a chair. Dr. Randolph introduced me, and I moved over and shook her hand. Within a minute or less, she began to cough; then, she began to wheeze because my cologne had triggered her symptoms. Dr. Randolph rushed me out of her room and sent me back to my hotel to take a bath and put on fresh scent-free clothing.

During the ensuing years, I learned more and more about Dr. Randolph and his observations and I read a number of his publications, including his 1962 book, *Human Ecology and Susceptibility to the Chemical Environment.*

In the preface to this book he said:

> "Most illnesses were originally thought to have arisen within the body. Only recently has this age-old concept been challenged."[2]

In his continuing discussion, Randolph pointed out that the importance of the environment as a cause of illness first began to be recognized in the ninteenth century. Yet, few physicians were aware of the role chemicals could play in making people sick.

Gradually, during the past 30 years, a handful of other physicians began to recognize and treat patients with chemical sensitivities. Yet, most members of the medical "establishment" weren't interested.

In spite of this attitude, awareness of chemical sensitivities gradually increased. An article published in the *New York Times* in 1980 was entitled, "Chemicals Cited as People Have More Allergies."

This article told about a woman who was "exiled" because of her sensitivities to plastics, pesticides, petrochemicals and other environmental pollutants. She had once lived in a metropolitan California community where she enjoyed a successful professional career and personal lifestyle. Then, because of chemically-induced debilitating weakness, respiratory distress, failed memory and mental confusion, she had to retreat from the twentieth century.

She thought she was dying but, since doctors didn't come up with a diagnosis, she couldn't get relief or even sympathy.

She thought she was dying but, since doctors didn't come up with a diagnosis, she couldn't get relief or even sympathy. Finally an allergist traced her symptoms to a violent reaction to a new carpet and adhesive in the bedroom. Following this exposure, she became sensitive to dozens of foods and chemicals. Although she expressed bitterness over the reasons for her devastating health problems, she said, "At least I now know what my problem is."

In its discussion of chemical allergies, the press report pointed out that most allergists, including members of the prestigious American Academy of Allergy and Immunology (AAAI), expressed skepticism over the role of chemicals in causing illnesses of various sorts.

Yet, in spite of this attitude, a number of AAAI Fellows have become knowledgeable and interested in MCSS. Included among these physicians are several academicians: John W. Gerrard, Professor of Pediatrics (Emeritus), University of Saskatchewan; William T. Kniker, Head of Allergy and Immunology at the University of Texas (San Antonio); and, Robert M. Stroud, Clinical Professor of Medicine, University of Florida (Gainesville) and a former member of the editorial board of the *Journal of Allergy and Clinical Immunology.*

My Observations in Practice

During the 1970s, I became more and more interested in food and chemical sensitivities. Word of this interest spread to many people in the West Tennessee community and I began to see more and more patients who developed symptoms when exposed to perfumes, household cleaners, soaps, gas stoves and other volatile indoor chemicals.

Most of these patients improved when they "cleaned up their diets," tracked down and eliminated hidden food allergens and got rid of home pollutants. Yet, many continued to be bothered by chemical exposures and some had to avoid social gatherings and public meetings.

One such patient (I'll call her Linda), came to my office seeking help in 1976. Chemical exposures of many types caused devastating symptoms, including headaches, flushing, numbness, tingling and a feeling of being "spaced out." Linda was, in fact, "sick all over."

Because I was unable to provide Linda with significant help, she moved away from West Tennessee and I lost contact with her. Then, in the fall of 1979, I learned from one of her former neighbors that she had moved back to West Tennessee and that she was healthy, active and energetic.

A short time later she came to my office and handed me a copy of Dr. Truss'[3] first article which described the relationship of superficial yeast infections to chronic illness. After reading the paper, I called Dr. Truss to obtain additional information and I soon found out that I was able to help many of my chemically sensitive patients by adding antifungal medications to their treatment program.

I reported my observations to my colleagues at medical rounds at the Jackson Madison County General Hospital on several occasions, and in an article in my state medical journal entitled, "The Coming Revolution in Medicine."[4] In this article I referred to the observations of Rowe,[5] Gerrard,[6] Sandberg,[7] Miller,[8] Rapp[9] and Hedges[10] on food allergies, and the observations of Rea[11] and Randolph[12] on food and chemical sensitivities. I also cited Truss' comments in his 1978 paper in which he said:

"One of the subgroups of patients with chronic candidiasis consists of those with severe intolerance to virtually all chemicals . . . One third of these patients have been found to have low T-cells . . . It has become increasingly apparent that these chemical sensitivities are disappearing and the T-cells are returning to normal (following treatment with nystatin) . . . indicating that the low T-cell counts were caused by *Candida albicans*."[13]

Shirley's Story

This 45-year-old woman first came to see me in the mid-1970s. She and her husband lived in a home on a country road a quarter of a mile from any of their neighbors. Like Linda, she was bothered by many chemicals. Here are excerpts from her history.

> "I've been bothered by hay fever for many years, especially during April, May and June. Yet, I have many other problems, including chest pains, bloating, frequent urination, muscle soreness, backache, fatigue and trouble concentrating. I guess you'd say that I'm 'sick all over.'
>
> "Anything that has an odor bothers me. I'm so sensitive to perfume that I can't even go to church or to the grocery store. So my husband—bless his heart—does the shopping because going down the supermarket aisles and smelling the fumes from soaps and detergents spaces me out.
>
> "If I put on new clothing of any sort, especially if it isn't all cotton, my skin itches, tingles and burns. In fact, I burn all the time."

Shirley's problems were difficult and complex. And sometimes the treatment measures I recommended to help her did not seem to be very effective. Here are examples of how sensitive she was:

- Her husband worked at a shoe factory and when he came home, the fumes that emanated from his clothing triggered many of her symptoms. So he began taking a shower and putting on fresh cotton clothes before coming home. This helped to some extent, but he was so saturated with chemicals that intimate contact with him still triggered her symptoms.
- Shirley's sensitivity was such that riding in a car 35 miles to my office made her acutely uncomfortable. Then, to make matters worse, sitting in the waiting room in my office, or even in my personal office, aggravated her symptoms because of chemicals in the carpet.

How did we handle things? On several occasions when Shirley came to see me, I would leave the building and visit with Shirley on a bench in a grassy plot outside the building. More often, we conducted our consultations by phone.

In working to help Shirley, my staff and I tried many things. We helped her change her diet and she took many courses of oral and vaginal nystatin on through the '80s. Because of her severe chemical sensitivity, she was unable to eat supermarket foods. And when she shifted over to home grown organic foods and chlorine-free well water, her symptoms lessened. Here are excerpts from a letter Shirley sent me in September 1990.

"I was doing better for quite a while, but I still had symptoms. My treatment program included occasional nystatin, no antibiotics, Vitaldophilus and CoQ10. I also avoided sugar, wheat, corn and other foods which triggered my symptoms. Then, I moved out of the house into a little shack in the back yard that I heated with an electric heater. All in all, I was better than I had been in years.

"Then, six weeks ago, I went to Chattanooga and visited a cousin whose house had been sprayed for termites. I developed red cheeks and the old burning of my skin. Ever since then, I've had other symptoms, including more gas and constipation and a feeling of fullness. And at night I wake up feeling like I can't get a good breath.

"Then, to make matters worse, twelve days ago I was stung three times by a wasp and had to go to the emergency room. They gave me five shots of adrenalin and a shot of cortisone."

To check on how Shirley was getting along, I called her in September 1994. Here are excerpts of what she had to say:

"I'll be 65 next month and I'm a lot healthier than I was 10 years ago. I continue to eat vegetables from my own yard and fruit from my trees. During the summer months, I stay busy canning and freezing things and we eat these foods all winter. My chemical sensitivity is a lot less and I'm even able to take trips.

"Yet, I'm very careful about where I stay. I also take my nutritional supplements, including a multiple vitamin/mineral preparation and extra vitamin C and Vitaldophilus. And from time to time I refill my nystatin prescription and take it if I feel I'm getting a yeast build up."

Other Stories

During the past 15 years, I've received countless letters, phone calls and reports from people of both sexes whose health problems developed after exposure to chemicals in their home or workplace. Yet, most of these came from women. I'm including here two typical stories.

About 13 years ago, a couple of years after I learned about yeast-related health problems from Dr. C. Orian Truss, I came across an article by Diane C. Thomas published in *Atlanta Magazine*. In this article, Diane told about Dr. Truss' work and how he had learned about the relationship of superficial yeast infections to chronic illness.

Subsequently, Diane's article was published in the Holiday Inn magazine, *Inn America*. So the yeast story spread to people all over the world.

Several years later on a visit to Atlanta, I met Diane and we have visited by phone and by mail ever since. Then, in 1986, when a *Redbook* editor told me they would love to do a story about yeast-related health problems, I immediately thought of Diane and suggested her name to the *Redbook* editor.

Some six months later, Diane's special medical report, "The Newest Mystery Illness," was published in *Redbook* and countless people read it. Moreover, almost 10,000 of them sent letters to the International Health Foundation (IHF) seeking further information.

In the summer of 1994, as I gathered material on chemical sensitivities, I again thought of Diane. I felt her story would illustrate the combined effects of chemicals and yeast in causing debilitating health problems. Here is an abbreviated report of what she told me.

Diane's Story

"Except for bad allergies to grass and ragweed as a young child, I was generally healthy. Yet, I was bothered from time to time with urinary problems and my mother, who had been a nurse, was sure they were allergy related. Every time my bladder would get upset, she would take me off citrus fruits, colas and tea, then I'd get better.

"Although dietary changes would sometimes help, on other occasions I'd be put on antibiotics. Then, in my mid-30s, things began to get worse and when I was 36 I was told I had interstitial cystitis. I was also bothered by recurring vaginal yeast infections.

"Then about that time I bought an old house and began restoring it. The restoration involved knocking out a lot of plaster and using odorous chemicals. And one of my neighbors a couple of times a month would spray malathion to kill the weeds along his fence, which was about ten feet from one of my windows.

"Although I didn't realize the connection between the chemical exposures and my health problems, I developed many new symptoms, including fatigue and PMS. My uterus felt like someone had taken it out, jumped up and down on it real hard and then put it back. It was very, very tender."

In her continuing discussion, Diane told me that she had repeated bladder problems and took more antibiotics. She also had a hysterectomy, after which her doctor prescribed Keflex. Then she developed panic attacks and she said:

"I emerged sensitive to everything. I cried every day because every time I took the Keflex I had more panic attacks that made me sick. The nurses wouldn't let me talk to the doctor and they told me to stay on the Keflex because that's what the doctor had prescribed. So I stayed on it like a good girl, and it made me horribly ill.

"In the next several years I did all sorts of things, including going to a conventional allergist and then to a doctor who diagnosed me as having multiple chemical sensitivities. Then, about 13 years ago, I learned about Dr. Truss. He put me on his program, including a special diet and nystatin and I began to improve. I also began taking acidophilus and many nutritional supplements.

"Yet, some of my symptoms still bothered me, including cystitis and postnasal drip. Although it's been an uphill battle, I'm now a reasonably healthy, productive person. I have a good job, a good marriage and when I compare my health to what it was ten years ago, I realize that I'm really well off."

Every day I learn something I didn't know before. And although I thought I knew a lot about multiple chemical sensitivity syndrome, I learned even more when I read Lynn Lawson's superb book, *Staying Well in a Toxic World.** After reading it, I called Lynn and she sent me additional information. Included was the story of Kristen (not her name) which clearly illustrates the sick building syndrome (SBS) or building related illness (BRI).

Kristen's Story

"As a child I was healthy . . . and because I grew up in the '30s, before the days of antibiotics, I never received them. I was a healthy teenager and my good health continued during my twenties and thirties.

"Of course, I had occasional little problems that might be expected from any woman who births and rears five children.

"About ten years ago, I went to work for a new company and the building I worked in was loaded with what I now realize were chemical pollutants. Included were odorous carpeting, copy machines and particle board. I gradually developed nasal congestion, sinus infections, fatigue, headache, muscle aches and other symptoms.

"A number of my co-workers experienced similar problems. When we would get together for lunch and coffee breaks, we'd often share experiences about our doctor visits, what antibiotics we were taking, etc.

"I can't begin to tell you how many courses of antibiotics I took. Probably in the course of the last three years before I quit the job, I took them at least 15 times. Sometimes it was for a week or ten days, but on other occasions it was much longer. Finally, for a variety of reasons, I left the company about a year ago and my health immediately began to improve.

"Yet, I continue to have some symptoms, including intermittent nasal congestion (in spite of sinus surgery) and troublesome arthralgia involving a number of joints and symptoms of chronic fatigue syndrome and fibromyalgia."

My Comments

In reviewing Diane's and Kristen's stories, their health problems are obviously related to chemicals. And if we compare their

---

*You'll find more information about this book in Chapter 29.

health problems to the proverbial "overloaded camel," the chemical bundles of straw were the heaviest ones. Yet, because Diane and Kristen took many courses of antibiotics, yeast overgrowth was an added-on factor.

REFERENCES

1. Randolph, T.G., "Allergy as a Causative Factor for Fatigue, Irritability and Behavior Problems in Children," *J. of Ped.*, 1947; 31:560.
2. Randolph, T.G., *Human Ecology and Susceptibility to the Chemical Environment*, Charles C. Thomas, Springfield, IL, 1962.
3. Truss, C.O., "Tissue Injury Induced by *C. Albicans:* Mental and Neurologic Manifestations," *J. of Ortho. Psych.*, 1978; 7:17–37.
4. Crook, W.G., "The Coming Revolution in Medicine," *J. of Tenn. Med. Assoc.*, 1983; 76:145–149.
5. Rowe, A.H., "Allergic Toxemia and Migraine Due to Food Allergy," *California, West Med*, 1930; 33:785.
6. Gerrard, J.W. (ed.), *Food Allergy: New Perspectives*, Charles C. Thomas, Springfield, IL, 1980.
7. Sandberg, D., McLeod, T.F. and Strauss, J., "Renal Disease Related to Hypersensitivity to Foods" in Gerrard, J.W. (ed.) *Food Allergy: New Perspectives*, Charles C. Thomas, Springfield, IL, 1980; pp 144–168.
8. Miller, J.B., "The Management of Food Allergy" in Gerrard, J.W. (ed.), *Food Allergy: New Perspectives*, Charles C. Thomas, Springfield, IL, 1980; pp 221–285.
9. Rapp, D.J., "Hyperactivity and the Tension-Fatigue Syndrome" in Gerrard, J.W. (ed.), *Food Allergy: New Perspectives*, Charles C. Thomas, Springfield, IL, 1980; pp 186–208.
10. Hedges, H., Letters, *J. Arkansas Med. Soc.*, 1982; 78:336–337.
11. Rea, W., "Cardiovascular Disease Triggered by Foods and Chemicals," in Gerrard, J.W. (ed.), *Food Allergy: New Perspectives*, Charles C. Thomas, Springfield, IL, 1980; pp 99–143.
12. Randolph, T.G., Rinkel, H.J. and Zeller, M., *Food Allergy*, Charles C. Thomas, Springfield, IL, 1951.
13. Truss, C.O., "Restoration of Immunologic Competence to *Candida albicans*," *J. of Ortho. Psych.*, 1980; 9:287–301.

18

Headaches

According to Jerome B. Posner, Professor of Neurology, Cornell University Medical College, headache ranks ninth among the causes of visits to physicians and is a major source of both time lost from work and of medical diagnostic procedures. In discussing common migraine, he said:

> "It is often characterized by recurrent headaches, often severe . . . the disorder often begins in childhood, affects women more often than men and runs in families."[1]

Headaches, Food Allergies and Sensitivities

In my pediatric and allergy practice during the past 35 years, many of my patients (including children and adults) gained relief from their headaches when they avoided one of their common foods. I published my observations for the first time in a report of 50 patients in 1961. The title of the article was "Systemic Manifestations Due to Allergy."[2] Although fatigue and mental and emotional symptoms were present in 49 of the 50 patients, some 26 complained of headaches. In ten it was a major complaint and in 16 it was a minor complaint.

In a subsequent article in the *Pediatric Clinics of North America* in 1975, I said:

> "I see a lot of youngsters who complain of headache. Not infrequently some of them have been to family physicians, ophthalmolo-

gists, otorhinolaryngologists and neurologists. And when such children have been found to have normal blood pressure, normal sinus x-rays, normal skull x-rays and electroencephalogram, normal vision and normal findings on physical and laboratory examinations, either the mother or physician is apt to conclude, 'Johnny's complaining of headache to get attention. He must be suffering from an emotional problem.' "[3]

In this article, I cited the observations of several leading allergists, including the late Jerome Glaser who published an article in 1954 entitled, "Migraine in Pediatric Practice,"[4] and John T. McGovern and T. J. Haywood who wrote a chapter on allergic headache in Frederic Speer's classic book, *Allergy of the Nervous System.*[5]

Several years later in a commentary in *The Lancet* entitled "Food Allergy," a British physician, Dr. Ronald Finn said:

"The concept that certain foods can produce abnormal reactions in susceptible individuals has a very long history."

In his discussion, Finn referred to the Lucretius statement, "One man's meat is another man's poison."

Indeed, food allergens are usually favorite foods which are eaten regularly— often in excess.

He also reviewed reports in the medical literature beginning in 1919 by researchers who noted that food allergens can be absorbed through the alimentary tract. He also referred to the pioneer observations of Albert Rowe and Theron Randolph. And he said:

"Immediate edematous and urticarial reactions to particular foods are easily recognized by the patient and the offending food is avoided. *Food allergy reactions are usually more subtle and the pa-*

tient does not realize the cause of these symptoms. Indeed, food allergens are usually favorite foods which are eaten regularly—often in excess [emphasis added]."[6]

In 1979 another British physician, Dr. Ellen Grant, published the findings of her study of 60 migraine patients.[7] The majority of her patients were women and their average age was 39. The mean length of migraine history was 18 years.

Most patients showed other symptoms, including lethargy, depression, anxiety, dizziness, abdominal pain and menstrual problems. Others gave a history of recurrent infections, especially cystitis.

In studying her patients, Grant noted that migraine was sometimes precipitated by amine containing foods, especially cheese, chocolate, citrus fruits and alcohol. When her patients discontinued these foods, there was a highly significant decrease in the number of headaches. Yet, only 13% were completely headache free.

In studying 186 migraine patients, she advised them to use elimination/challenge diets. Some 126 attempted it and 85% became headache free. The most common foods causing reactions were wheat (78%), orange (65%), eggs (45%), tea and coffee (45% each), chocolate milk (37%), beef (35%), corn, cane sugar and yeast (33% each).

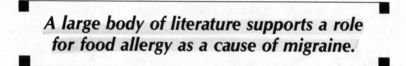

A large body of literature supports a role for food allergy as a cause of migraine.

Another British researcher, Dr. Joseph Egger,[8] placed his headache patients on a limited food diet and found that 93% of 88 patients experienced relief.

Drs. Jean Monro, Jonathan Brostoff and associates studied a group of British patients with severe migraine which they said affects about 20% of the population, with more women affected than men.[9] They found that two-thirds of the people with migraines/

severe headaches were allergic to certain foods, shown by dietary exclusion and subsequent challenge.

U.S. investigators who have noted the diet/migraine connection include O'Banion,[10] Bahna[11] and Mansfield. In a 1986 article, Mansfield said:

> "A large body of literature supports a role for food allergy as a cause of migraine."[12]

He cited reports in the medical literature as early as 1977. He also reviewed clinical reports by Vaughn,[13] published in the *Journal of the American Medical Association* in 1927 and reports of others published in subsequent years. I was especially struck by this paragraph from Mansfield's report.

> "In 1952, Unger and Unger published a manuscript in the *Journal of Allergy* entitled, "Migraine is an Allergic Disease." Thirty-two years later Monro, Carini and Brostoff would publish an article entitled, "Migraine is a Food Allergic Disease." *Such is the pace of progress.*"

Headaches and the Yeast Connection

Several years ago when I analyzed the histories of 100 consecutive women with yeast-related problems, fatigue, headache and depression were at the top of the list. And during these past 10 years, I've received countless letters from people with the major complaint, *headache.*

I've also met and talked to many people who have described yeast-related headaches. On a trip to California in 1992, I met a television personality (I'll call her Reba) who told me that her headaches were yeast-related. And I was naturally pleased when she said that my book, *The Yeast Connection,* had played a major role in helping her regain her health and her life. So I asked her to write me a letter summarizing her story.

Reba's Story

"I moved to Los Angeles in 1979 and started developing headaches even though I'd never been a headache sufferer before. I went to every doctor at UCLA—every allergist. No one could find the source of my allergic rhinitis, which they said was my problem.

> *I took all sorts of over-the-counter medications. Nothing helped.*

"Two years later I moved to New York and I continued to have debilitating headaches. I took all sorts of over-the-counter medications. Nothing helped. So I kept on seeing specialists who were convinced I was crazy and were prescribing mood elevators—but I wouldn't take them.

"Finally I happened upon a nutritionist who said that I was a classic candidate for the yeast connection and told me to go out and buy your book. He immediately told me to stop eating bread and dairy. He also put me on vitamins, minerals and acidophilus.

"I improved some, but he said, 'As long as you keep drinking coffee and insist on eating sugar, you'll never get rid of your headache.' So I followed his instructions and today, five years later, I can tolerate wheat and bread in limited quantities and take occasional sugar. I continue to stay away from dairy.

"I never did have to take prescription yeast drugs. I did it mainly with a diet and acidophilus and lifestyle changes.

"I also had a secretary working for me last year who had headaches all the time. We were standing in my kitchen and she was going to housesit for us and she started describing her symptoms to me. Her father thought she was a hypochondriac and told her to stop being hysterical and told her she needed to see a shrink.

"Because her symptoms were so much like mine, I felt she had yeast problems. I'm happy to report that she found a naturopath here in L.A. and he started treating her for yeast. She's fine now."

In the summer of 1992, as I was gathering material for a presentation in the Chicago area, I called my good friend, Dr. George

E. Shambaugh, Jr., and asked him if he could give me the names of patients he had helped using antifungal medications and a special diet. He responded with several dramatic stories, four of which I cited in Chapter 6. Here's another story which I received from Kathleen, the mother of one of Dr. Shambaugh's patients.

Kathleen Pawalczyk's Story

"My daughter, Rachel, started having headaches and stomach aches after a bout with the flu in December 1986. She also had the urge to urinate all the time and complained of being tired. She developed asthma and would get bronchitis every October. The doctors treated her with numerous antibiotics and other medications. She gradually became worse and worse.

> ### No doctor could find a medical reason for all her complaints.

"We took her to numerous specialists . . . No doctor could find a medical reason for all her complaints. In the 1989–90 school year, she missed 97 days of school. *She would lie on the couch all day and dunk her head in a bowl of ice water for relief from her headache.*

"She was so weak the doctor suggested we take her to a special headache clinic. I made an appointment with them—but luckily I saw a doctor on TV talking about the yeast connection and how it could make people 'sick all over.'

"I ran out and bought your book and stayed up until 4:00 in the morning reading. It seemed as though you were writing about Rachel. The next morning I called her neurologist and pediatrician and asked them about it, but they were skeptical.

"Then we learned about Dr. George E. Shambaugh, and the rest is history. On a comprehensive program which included a sugar-free diet and avoidance of food allergens and environmental pollutants, and oral antiyeast medications (nystatin and Diflucan), plus nutritional supplements, my daughter is a healthy young woman. She attends school full time and her headache and other symptoms are a thing of the past."

My Comments

How and why are headaches yeast connected? Probably there are several mechanisms, as described elsewhere in this book. But it seems to me that a principal one is the disturbance in the balance of normal bacteria in the intestinal tract which leads to a "leaky gut" and the absorption of food antigens and toxins.

REFERENCES

1. Posner, J.D., M.D., *Cecil's Textbook on Medicine*, W.B. Saunders Co., Philadelphia, PA, 1988; p 2129.
2. Crook, W.G., Harrison, W.W., Crawford, S.E. and Emerson, B.S., "Systemic Manifestations Due to Allergy," *Pediatrics*, 1961; 27:790–799.
3. Crook, W.G., "Food Allergy—The Great Masquerader," *Ped. Clin. of N. Amer.*, 1975; 22:227–238.
4. Glaser, J., "Migraine in Pediatric Practice," *Am. J. Dis. Child*, 1954; 88:92–94.
5. Speer, F., *Allergy of the Nervous System*, Charles C. Thomas, Springfield, IL, 1970.
6. Finn, R., "Food Allergy," *The Lancet*, February 3, 1979.
7. Grant, E.C., "Food Allergies and Migraine," *The Lancet*, 1979; 1:986-988.
8. Egger, et al, "Is Migraine Food Allergy? A double-blind control trial of oligoantigenic diet treatment," *The Lancet*, 1983; 2:865–868.
9. Monro, J., Carini, C., Brostoff, J., "Migraine Is a Food Allergic Disease," *The Lancet*, 1984; 2:719–721.
10. O'Banion, D.R., "Dietary Control of Headache Pain, Five Case Studies," *Journal of Holistic Medicine*, 1981; Vol. 3 No. 2, pp 140–150.
11. Bahna, S., "Food and Additive Sensitivity Present Diagnostic Dilemma," *Consult—A Forum for Physicians*, The Cleveland Clinic Foundation, 1988; Vol. 7 No. 3, pp 8–9.
12. Mansfield, L.E., "The Role of Food Allergy in Migraine: A review," *Immunology and Allergy Practice*, 1986; Vol. 8 No. 12, pp 406–411.
13. Vaughn, W.T., "Allergic Migraine," *JAMA*, 1927; 88:1383–86.

19

◆

Depression and Manic Depression

◆

According to a cover story in *Newsweek*, 15 million Americans suffer from clinical depression. Physicians are writing or renewing 650,000 Prozac prescriptions every month and many people who went years without relief are receiving help.

Yet, in spite of the benefits provided by Prozac and other psychotherapeutic drugs, these medications, like many others, have the potential for adverse reactions. These include flu-like symptoms, impaired liver function and a loss of motor control. In addition, a small minority of patients fail to improve on Prozac and related medications—and some become worse. And in rare cases, Prozac users have become manic, violent or suicidal.

Because of these possibilities, many therapists point out that Prozac shouldn't be the treatment of "first resort." And according to the article, *"Prozac should not be given to people without looking for the underlying physical and psychological causes of the person's depression."*[1]

Like headaches, joint pains, abdominal discomfort or any other chronic complaint, depression may develop from many different causes. Moreover, such causes are often multiple and among them *Candida albicans* ranks high on the list—especially in women between 25 and 45. Here's supporting data.

Observations of C. Orian Truss, M.D.

In his lectures and medical reports, Dr. Truss discussed the many and varied manifestations of patients he had seen with candida-related health problems. And in his book, *The Missing Diagnosis,* he discussed many complex health problems which he had found to be yeast-related. Included were hormone dysfunction, depression and manic depression. And he said:

> "The mechanism of depression is poorly understood. Certain chemicals are known to be involved in normal brain function. It is thought that depression occurs when some factor upsets their proper balance or interferes with their proper function."

In his continuing discussion, Dr. Truss pointed out that *depression in some patients responds to anticandida therapy—often dramatically.* But he cautioned:

> "Depression is a serious and potentially dangerous condition and one deserving care by a competent psychiatrist; self-diagnosis and treatment should never be attempted. *It is perfectly reasonable to look for some correctable cause of depression, but even when found, its treatment should not immediately and abruptly replace the psychiatric program.*
>
> "Drugs prescribed by the psychiatrist should be gradually withdrawn, preferably under his supervision. Their use should not be discontinued suddenly or prematurely."[2]

Medical Support for the Relationship of Candida to Depression

Several years ago, John W. Crayton, M.D., Professor of Psychiatry, Loyola Medical School, described his laboratory findings in a group of patients with fatigue, weakness, depression and many other symptoms. The 28 subjects who were studied ranged in age from 18 to 45; 20 were women and 8 were men. All gave a convincing history of exacerbation of symptoms following ingestion of food.

Antibody studies to candida in these patients showed "higher levels of candida antibodies than asymptomatic controls."[3]

In studies carried out at the University of Tennessee several years ago, Jay Schinfeld, M.D., studied a group of women with severe premenstrual syndrome (PMS) and a history of vaginal candidiasis. And he noted that *"depression was often found in women with severe PMS."*[4]

Patients who received anticandida therapy showed significant physical and psychological improvement when compared to controls.

Various treatment programs were tried in managing these patients, including oral nystatin and yeast elimination diets. *Although Schinfeld's study was a small one, patients who received anticandida therapy showed significant physical and psychological improvement when compared to controls.*

Ten years ago, I reviewed the records of 100 of my own patients with candida-related health problems. *Depression, fatigue and headache were the most frequent presenting symptoms.* Eighty-five percent of these patients were women and the majority of them were between 30 and 45.

Other symptoms in many of these patients included recurrent vaginitis or cystitis, abdominal pain, bloating, sexual dysfunction, constipation, diarrhea, poor memory and a feeling of being "sick all over."

Although antifungal medication and a sugar-free special diet did not provide a "quick fix" for these patients, 85% of them improved significantly following such therapy.

Letters I've Received from Women with Manic Depression

I had read Dr. Truss' comments on depression and manic depression and had received hundreds of letters from women with depression. Yet, only within the past several years did I receive reports from women with yeast-related manic depression. I found the story of a New Zealand woman (I'll call her Martha) especially dramatic.

Martha's Story

"Until I was 38 I never knew what depression was apart from a couple of very brief bouts. I remember once coming out with those terrible words, *What on earth has she got to be depressed about?*

"Then it happened. I developed a pattern of manic depression—swings of mood from extreme highs to extreme lows—it lasted nine years and ultimately nearly cost me my life, did smash up my career and could easily have finished my marriage. It caused me unspeakable suffering.

"It was like I imagined it would be having both legs amputated or losing an adored child—I often thought if it were to go on like this I'd rather be dead. But in the end, the prisoner without hope *was* rescued from the dungeon, so this tale has a happy ending."

Martha's illness started with a viral infection which caused liver damage. Although she apparently recovered from this illness, she developed recurrent episodes of mood swings. "Two and a half weeks up, two and a half weeks down"—that completely took over (her) life. Describing how she felt when depressed, she said:

"Imagine the whole world spray painted gray or being in a small windowless cell or in a tunnel. I had no energy or drive whatsoever. I used to feel that I had 50 pound weights on each foot and—thirty pound weights on each wrist. All my favorite things suddenly became meaningless and sterile.

All my favorite things suddenly became meaningless and sterile.

"If someone had given me two round trip air tickets to London and Paris and $15,000 spending money, I would have been completely unmoved. Nothing could trigger a flicker of interest or enthusiasm . . .

"If Yul Brenner himself had purposely moved over to my side of the bed, I would have rebuffed him! I was sexually 100% dead."

Then, after a week or two of this hell, Martha would swing into a manic world of exhaustion and even delirium.

"I was king of the castle, drunk with joy, bursting with crazy schemes, on the go literally 22 hours a day, talking nonstop, constantly interrupting, spending money like water, issuing dinner and party invitations, smashing up the car. You'd have to have seen it to believe it . . .

"I was diagnosed from the beginning as a 'textbook case of manic depression.' Over the whole depression period, I had been sent to a string of different specialists for what seemed quite unrelated conditions."

After struggling with this problem for eight years, Martha began to deteriorate rapidly and was put in a psychiatric hospital. Following discharge, she received therapy outside of the hospital, including medication and group therapy for many weeks and months.

In her continuing discussion, Martha said:

"In spite of all the tears and the new insights, the manic depression didn't go away . . . Then came the great breakthrough I'd waited so many years for. My general practitioner prescribed eight nystatin tablets a day for the candida, plus large doses of the B vitamins and calcium. The bouts of mania stopped immediately, the depressions became briefer and much less severe; within three months, they disappeared."

In addition, Martha found that a number of foods, including sugar, white flour and eggs played a part in causing her symptoms. In her concluding comments she said:

"I can hardly believe it's really over. I feel tremendous gratitude that I've been saved from this living death. But I also feel angry that I wasn't properly diagnosed earlier . . . Of course, I can only assume that the *Candida albicans* and its treatment with nystatin was the critical thing in my case. I can hear the doctors say, 'You would have recovered anyway.' But to me it is beyond a reasonable doubt that candida/nystatin was the answer. It was the only new factor after nine years of illness.

"Now that I have been completely free of manic depression for a year, I plan to visit all the psychiatrists and specialists involved in my treatment over the past nine years to tell them what happened to me. Please, God, my sufferings might help others even in a small way . . . the medical profession should get this sort of feedback."

Rebecca's Story

In the summer of 1993, I received a letter from a woman in a neighboring state who reported episodes of manic depression which responded to a comprehensive program which featured nystatin. Here are excerpts from her letter.

"To say that your book, *The Yeast Connection*, has saved and changed my life, renewed my mind and revived my spirit is an understatement. I am a 36-year-old professional woman. As a child I had kidney infections, yeast infections, depression, attention deficit disorder, confusion and a severe lack of energy. I had many upper respiratory infections and pneumonia and took countless antibiotics.

"*By the age of 26 I had been diagnosed as having manic depression.* I had had a nervous breakdown, acne, gastrointestinal problems, more yeast infections and bladder infections. I also had been troubled by abdominal pain, sinus problems, chronic fatigue, insomnia, confusion, processing problems, poor memory and distractibility.

"But that's not all. I was also troubled by joint pains, rashes, menstrual problems, craving of sweets and overeating, chronic cough, repeated upper respiratory infections and purple inflamed gums (even though I'm a dental hygienist and have near perfect plaque removal! I was a real anomaly in my college class).

"I went on lithium at age 26 because of a nervous breakdown following the birth of my son. Surprisingly, this medication took care of some of my symptoms and made others more tolerable.

"I muddled through the next nine and a half years with the lithium, being very slowed down and bothered mostly (but more mildly) by confusion, attention problems, poor memory, lack of energy and efficiency, acne, cravings. Also, I continued to have the rash and cough during the winter months.

"At the age of 35 I decided to try and go off of the lithium and within a few weeks many of my symptoms returned. In addition, my hands and feet were crawling and going numb, my eyes bothered me constantly, sinuses poured, ears felt full and I had constant yeast and bladder infections. I also had kidney and back pain and related leg pain that was almost disabling, abdominal pain and an itchy, scaly red rash.

"One day a wonderful girl I knew, named Lisa, came to my back door and handed me your book. She said, 'You need to read this.' And I did.

Within four days after starting nystatin I was getting relief.

"I went to my physician and told him what was wrong with me and after a pause with his head down, he graciously agreed to treat me. *Within four days after starting nystatin I was getting relief and after ten days the disabling symptoms were diminished.* I stayed on the nystatin for five months. Yet, when I tried to go off of it, my ghastly symptoms would immediately return. My doctor said, 'I don't think it's a good idea to stay on nystatin for an extended period of time and I don't know what else to do. This is out of my field.'

"I then went to an allergist in March 1993. He tested me and gave me dust, mold and candida injections. When I first started them they made me sick, sick, sick. Gradually, however, by taking tiny doses, I started feeling so much better that it was astonishing. Now my symptoms are all gone. This is profound!

"I have none of the aforementioned yeast symptoms as long as I take the nystatin, receive the injections, get proper amounts of sleep, exercise and stay away from sugars and foods that bother me. I have no attention problems, confusion, distractibility or poor memory. The nystatin alone eased all of my symptoms, but it did take the rest of the above measures to give the quality of health and mental well-being that I now have. I have tremendous mental and physical energy and am experiencing a type of life I didn't know existed.

"My days are organized now, and I'm on time. I run in the mornings, finish things I start and am proficient in handling stress. Within months I was naturally able to apply rational principles that counselors had tried to teach me in years past and I was astonished that I, all of a sudden, understood why 'other people' worked, thought and performed the way they did. I was not doing the same things! Life used to be a painful chore (*all* my life it has been) and things that always appeared easy to others have stressed me to the max.

"Even with the other things that I do, I still have to take six nystatin tablets a day or I get bladder and yeast infections, nervousness and most of my old symptoms."

My Comments

Depression and manic depression, like CFS, MS and other disorders described in this book, can develop from many different causes. These include genetic factors, nutritional deficiencies, endocrine disturbances, viral infections, chemical sensitivities and toxicities and psychologic stress or trauma.

I do not want you (or anyone) to think I'm saying that *Candida albicans* is *the* cause of depression. Yet, if you suffer from depression and/or any other disabling disorder and give a history of—

* repeated or prolonged courses of antibiotic drugs
* persistent digestive symptoms
* and/or recurrent vaginal yeast infections—

a comprehensive treatment program which features oral anti-fungal medications and a special diet may enable you to change your life.

REFERENCES

1. *Newsweek*, March 30, 1990.
2. Truss, C.O., *The Missing Diagnosis*, P.O. Box 26508, Birmingham, AL 35226, 1986; pp 73, 75–76.
3. Crayton, J.W., "Anticandida Antibody Levels in Polysymptomatic Patients," Candida Update Conference, International Health Foundation, Memphis, Tennessee, September 16–18, 1988.
4. Schinfeld, J., "PMS and Candidiasis: Study explores the possible link," *The Female Patient*, 1987, Vol. 12, pp 66–70.

20

Multiple Sclerosis

In his observations on candida-related health problems, Dr. C. Orian Truss described the response of a number of his patients with severe autoimmune diseases to nystatin and a low carbohydrate diet. Included were brief descriptions of several of his patients with multiple sclerosis.

One of these patients was a 30-year-old woman who showed many of the symptoms and signs of MS, including numbness, tingling, reflex changes, visual defects and a slight elevation of her spinal fluid protein. In addition, she gave a history of receiving many antibiotics, digestive problems, vaginal symptoms and other health problems. She was placed on diet and nystatin therapy and after two years on such therapy a neurological examination was "entirely normal."[1,2]

When this therapy was discontinued, a number of her symptoms began to return. She was again placed on nystatin and in a subsequent report, Dr. Truss stated:

"She is entirely well now seven years after nystatin was begun."

In this same report, Dr. Truss described the response of another young woman with MS who was given nystatin and diet.

"She started improving immediately and was asymptomatic by eight months unless ... she would go 'on a carbohydrate binge.' This would induce abdominal bloating, diarrhea, and faint suggestions of tingling in her extremities."[3,4]

In discussing multiple sclerosis and other autoimmune disorders in *The Yeast Connection,* I said:

> **Candida is not THE cause of MS . . . but there's growing evidence . . . there is a yeast connection.**

"Candida isn't THE cause of these often devastating disorders—but, there's growing evidence based on exciting clinical experiences of many physicians that there is a yeast connection."[5]

Reports of My Patients

In my discussion of MS, I told about several of my patients who improved on anticandida therapy.

Bobby Carter's Story

In 1982 this 42-year-old businessman developed numbness, weakening and tingling in his left arm and similar symptoms in his left leg. His symptoms progressed to such a degree that he needed a cane for support.

Bobby was seen by many physicians, including a neurologist who noted an ataxic broad-based jerky gait, muscle weakness, spasticity and impairment of vibratory and joint sense in both upper and lower extremities.

Because I had known Bobby for many years and had served as the family pediatrician, he told the neurologist that he would like to see me in consultation. Bobby's history suggested the probability of yeast overgrowth, so I recommended an anticandida program. After taking nystatin and a yeast-free, sugar-free diet and nutritional supplements, Bobby improved promptly. Within six weeks he reported:

"I can now play golf. All of my symptoms are gone except for a little numbness and weakness in my left hand. I'm fine until I cheat on my diet. Even one bite of a sugar-containing food will immediately trigger my symptoms."

During the past 13 years Bobby has continued an active, productive life and in 1986 he was elected the Jackson, Tennessee, "Man of the Year." He also serves as a member of the Board of Directors of the International Health Foundation and in November 1994 he was elected to the Tennessee State Senate. During a recent conversation Bobby said:

"I'm doing great as long as I stay on my diet and take my anti-fungal medication. I take nystatin every day and during the past six months, from time to time, I have taken Diflucan. I also feel that a vegetarian diet has helped a lot.

"I put cauliflower, broccoli, cabbage, celery, carrots, an apple and half a lemon in a juicer I bought for $29. This mixture makes a pint drink and I don't have to add water. Since adding this to my program, my strength has improved and I can now do push ups, which I hadn't been able to do for some years.

"Skeptics might say my MS would have gotten better without the diet, nystatin and Diflucan, but I know what I'm talking about."

Dorothy's Story

This 48-year-old office worker took antibacterial drugs continuously beginning in 1969. In a letter she sent to me she said:

"Beginning in 1975 I noticed that I was losing strength. My head hurt most of the time and I developed problems with my vision that would come and go. In 1977 I began to have joint pains. Yet, these, too, would come and go. I was able to keep on working, but I seemed to get weaker each year. In 1980 an eye doctor said I had scars in both eyes and in 1981 my left eye 'went out.' The doctor said it was optic neuritis."

In 1982 Dorothy developed many other symptoms, including joint pains, numbness, tingling and a feeling of "electricity" in her legs. She was also troubled by mental confusion, mood changes, headaches, bladder problems and eye symptoms. In addition, Dorothy commented:

"At times I felt I'd scream if I couldn't get out of my legs. I felt like a person with boots on who needed to take them off. I also felt drugged and weak."

Dorothy was seen by several physicians, including a neurologist who said:

"It's possible you may be developing multiple sclerosis, although my findings on examination do not warrant making such a diagnosis at this time."

I first saw Dorothy in June 1982 and her history of long term antibacterial drugs made me feel her health problems could be yeast connected. I prescribed a comprehensive program of management including nystatin, a yeast-free, sugar-free diet and nutritional supplements.

Seven months after beginning treatment, Dorothy commented:

"Most of my major symptoms have disappeared, including mental confusion, headaches, numbness and weakness. I'm also pleased that most of the electricity feeling in my arms and legs have gone away. I still tire easily but this is getting better."

Most of my mental confusion, headaches, numbness and weakness disappeared on antiyeast therapy.

Regarding Dorothy's progress, I thought to myself, *Wouldn't it be great if patients with early MS-like symptoms could be turned around and made well before an actual disease developed?*

Dorothy—A 1994 Update

"Twelve years ago in 1982, I came to you with many symptoms. My doctors had said, 'You probably have multiple sclerosis.' I took the nystatin which you recommended and for 4½ years I stayed rigidly on the diet. Also, during the last year, because wheat and other gluten-containing foods caused problems, I eliminated these foods from my diet as well.

"I also took the vitamins and minerals and I soon began to feel better. During the past five years, I have not followed the diet quite as strictly, although I still take the supplements. I also take the nystatin off and on. Yet, when I get too far off the diet, my old symptoms return. When this happens, I tighten up on my diet and get back on the nystatin.

"I really believe I would now be an invalid if I had not gotten your help. I'm still working as a speech therapist and I drive to ten West Tennessee counties every month. I'm now 60 years old and I feel confident that I'll be able to work until I can take full retirement in 1996 when I'm 62."

Comments of Neurologist
R. Scott Heath, M.D.

In January 1993, I received a letter from Dr. Heath who expressed an interest in the relationship of *Candida albicans* to neurological problems, including MS. In December 1993, I had a two-hour visit with Dr. Heath and he told me about his experiences. Then in January 1994, I interviewed him. Here's what he had to say.

"Sometimes I've felt sort of like a voice in the darkness . . . just as you have felt. Yet, I have seen a number of people who have unusual symptoms, including fleeting numbness, transient speech problems and vision complaints. In such patients, I often can't find anything wrong neurologically. Obviously my concern is simply this: do they have MS or don't they?

"I've been impressed over the years that people with MS who do not have spots on their brain generally do well on the antifungal treatment. Also, when people DO have spots and we make a diagnosis of MS, they do better too. They have fewer exacerbations . . . [emphasis added].

"Here's another treatment step I've taken: If these people do get put on antibiotics by their primary physicians, I tell them to let me know. In such cases, I switch them from nystatin to Diflucan for a couple of weeks. What I've seen happen on a number of occasions is that one of these patients will get treated for a bladder or a respiratory infection. Then they'll come in to see me several weeks later with an exacerbation of their MS.

"I think there's definitely a link there between upsetting the internal milieu and getting yeasts sort of revved up which follows treatment with the antibiotics.

"Here's another interesting point. Some recent studies came out on the use of prednisone in patients with optic neuritis. If prednisone or Solumedrol or similar drugs work for exacerbations, why can't you keep people on them indefinitely? The answer is possibly that these drugs promote yeast overgrowth.

"Today if a person is seriously ill with an exacerbation, I'll put them on Diflucan. Then once they're off the prednisone or ACTH, I'll switch them back over to nystatin. The problem is it's kind of hard to judge exactly what I'm doing . . . I'm sort of a lone wolf in my group of 15 neurologists. None of my colleagues give it a whole lot of credence."

Crook: I've read a lot in the CFS/CFIDS literature about the "up and down" regulating of the immune system. Would you comment?

Heath: "I think it parallels your story about the yeast, that a flare up of candida will upregulate the immune system if you will. I think that as long as people are sort of in a balance that they will get along pretty well. But if something causes the yeast to flare up, I think it revs up the immune system and in patients who are prone to MS, it may flip them into an exacerbation. I don't think it's just the yeast, but I think that somehow it's symptomatic of something that's going on with the immune system . . .

"The body was designed to tolerate certain things in the system and most people tolerate yeast without problems. But there's something peculiar about MS patients and/or some of these CFS/CFIDS patients, as well as people with other autoimmune diseases. In such patients, whatever the reason, the immune system is very sensitive. I don't yet think we have the answers. I do believe that the yeast factor is at least part of the answer . . .

"I tell people who have little faith that medical science doesn't necessarily have all the answers and there are certain things, in particular like candida, that we cannot at this time necessarily measure. Yet, it would be interesting to see if some of the immunologists would get excited about this.

"Perhaps they could demonstrate that people's T-cells are more activated in the face of non-yeast treatment as compared to those who received antiyeast therapy. I mean that one way to do this would be to try to prove it in a test tube."

Crook: Dr. Heath, I was interested in what you had to say about vitamin B_{12}. Could you elaborate?

Heath: "In studying chronic patients with MS, I've found that a certain percentage of them, maybe 10 to 20%, will have documented low B_{12} levels. I think such deficiencies may relate to possible colonization of the gut and with the yeast and their inability to absorb or transport B_{12}.

"I've had a number of those people whose MS, to some extent, is immunologically burned out. Yet, they still have ataxia, numbness and so forth. In such patients, their B_{12} levels are often low; then when you treat the yeast and get them on replacement B_{12} they seem to function at a better level."

A Scientific Study Begins

For over a decade, since the first edition of *The Yeast Connection* was published, critics, including the American Medical Association (AMA) and American Academy of Allergy and Immunology (AAAI), have said in effect:

"Where is the scientific proof of Dr. Truss' hypothesis that superficial yeast infections can make people 'sick all over'? Where are your double-blind studies?"

In responding to these challenges, I began "knocking on doors" of the National Institute of Health (NIH), the AMA (and other medical organizations) and the Squibb and Lederle pharmaceutical companies. I said in effect:

"Your product, nystatin (Mycostatin, Squibb and Nilstat, Lederle), given orally along with a low-sugar special diet can help countless people with chronic illnesses. It provides women who suffer with fatigue, recurrent vaginitis, cystitis and other symptoms with help unobtainable from other therapies."

Yet, my pleas fell on deaf ears for a number of reasons. Here's one of them: nystatin, which was first developed and marketed in the 1950s became a generic drug in the 1970s. This meant that any company could manufacture it. So there was little incentive for these pharmaceutical companies to invest the time and money required to carry out double-blind studies on yeast-related health disorders. In the mid-1980s, I also wrote letters and made phone calls to people at Janssen. This pharmaceutical company had developed and marketed another effective anti-yeast oral medication, Nizoral (ketoconazole). Yet, they, too, showed no interest.

Then, in 1990, fluconazole (Diflucan, Pfizer) became available in the U.S. This oral antifungal medication had been found to be safe and effective by researchers and practicing physicians in Europe.

This drug was released in the U.S. initially for the treatment of patients with severe immunosuppression, including AIDS, cancer and other life-threatening diseases. Yet, through networking, word of its effectiveness in treating patients with fatigue, headache, depression, PMS and other yeast-related symptoms spread to physicians throughout North America.

So in the fall of 1991, I began knocking on the door of the Pfizer Pharmaceutical Company and I urged them to fund studies on the relationship of superficial yeast infections to chronic illness.

In October 1993, eight candida clinicians (Sidney M. Baker, M.D., Ken Gerdes, M.D., Pamela Morford, M.D., Patricia Noah, Ph.D., Keith Sehnert, M.D., Robert M. Stroud, M.D., C. Orian Truss, M.D. and I) met in New Orleans for four hours to discuss ways of carrying out the studies.

Also included in the four-hour workshop were John Bennett, M.D., National Institute of Allergy and Infectious Diseases; John Edwards, M.D., Professor of Medicine, UCLA (Harbor/Torrance); Jack Sobel, M.D., Professor of Medicine, Wayne University; and,

Douglas Webb, Ph.D., Director, Anti-Infectives, Medical Department, Pfizer, Inc.

Although a useful dialogue ensued, the group experienced difficulties in coming to a consensus as to what should be done and how it should be done.

Since people with yeast-related problems develop symptoms which affect every part of the body, defining the type of patient to be studied wasn't easy. And no consensus was reached.

Another problem was the absence of laboratory tests which could identify the candida organism and clearly document that this organism is in fact a major cause, or *THE* cause, of illness in these people.*

In early 1994, as discussions continued, several knowledgeable consultants concluded that studying a single, easily identifiable disorder such as multiple sclerosis, asthma, Crohn's disease or endometriosis would be the best way to proceed.

In June 1994, the Pfizer Corporation made an initial grant of $60,000 to the International Health Foundation to support studies on the relationship of superficial yeast infections to chronic illness, and multiple sclerosis was the first illness selected. Here are excerpts from a news report by Sue McDonald, published in the Wednesday, September 14, 1994, issue of the *Cincinnati Enquirer*.

YEAST CONNECTION, REVISITED

Is there a connection between multiple sclerosis and an overgrowth of yeast in the body?

A tri-state neurologist who's teaming with a Tennessee physician who has written several books on the health effects of *Candida albicans* . . . to test whether an overgrowth of yeast can affect symptoms in people with multiple sclerosis.

"I think this is something where we should at least consider the possibility," says neurologist Dr. Scott Heath, who is recruiting five

---

*Although *Candida albicans* is the organism in question to be studied, it is found normally in many people. And, up to this point, most physicians working with these patients have found that the typical history, followed by the response of the patient to a comprehensive program which features a sugar-free special diet and oral antifungal medication is the best way to make a diagnosis.

men and five women, ages 18 to 45 with MS, to participate in a year long study.

In his 17 year practice, Heath has found that MS symptoms—numbness and weakness, for example—frequently worsen or reappear after patients have been treated with antibiotics. Antibiotics can upset the natural balance of microorganisms of the body and cause yeasts to multiply.

Dr. William G. Crook, author of *The Yeast Connection*, will help coordinate the pilot study from his International Health Foundation offices in Jackson, Tennessee. Heath and Crook will test whether an antiyeast drug, Diflucan, can influence the severity and frequency of symptoms in people with MS. Crook will educate patients about controlling yeast through diet and other lifestyle changes.

Patients also will be monitored monthly and undergo blood tests and an MRI (magnetic resonance image) at Northern Kentucky Rehabilitation Hospital in Edgewood.

REFERENCES

1. Truss, C.O., "Tissue Injury Induced by *C. Albicans:* Mental and Neurological Manifestations," *J. of Ortho. Psych.*, 1978; 7:17–37.
2. Truss, C.O., *The Missing Diagnosis*, P.O. Box 26508, Birmingham, AL 35206, 1983 and 1986; pp 137–138.
3. Truss, C.O., "The Role of *Candida albicans* in Human Illness," *J. of Ortho. Psych.*, 1981; 10:228–238.
4. Truss, C.O., *The Missing Diagnosis*, P.O. Box 26508, Birmingham, AL 35206, 1983 and 1986; p 172.
5. Crook, W.G., *The Yeast Connection*, Third Edition, Professional Books, Jackson, TN and Vintage Books, New York, 1986; pp 211–215.

21

Other Autoimmune Diseases

In his book, *The Missing Diagnosis*, Dr. C. Orian Truss commented on the relationship of *Candida albicans* to many serious illnesses which he had observed over the years. Among the illnesses that he noted were the autoimmune diseases. In commenting on them, he said:

"As with many illnesses, the diagnosis of . . . an autoimmune disease is difficult in the early stages when some symptoms are mild and some not yet present, and when useful laboratory and x-ray diagnostic criteria are lacking. The frequency with which such diagnoses as . . . lupus, multiple sclerosis, etc. have been entertained in patients with chronic candidiasis, i.e., in patients who have become well with antiyeast therapy, suggests that in such patients we may perhaps be seeing the mildest manifestations of these more serious diseases."

In his discussion of autoimmune diseases, Dr. Truss described his experiences in treating a woman who developed systemic lupus erythematosus at age 41 years. And he said:

"In this disease, one measurable abnormality that may be present is antibody against material in the nuclei of the cells of the body. This is termed 'anti-nuclear antibody' and exists in several forms that are customarily included in the abbreviation 'ANA.'

"Many symptoms occur in this disease. Severe fatigue, skin rashes, muscle and joint symptoms, nephritis, pleurisy and pericarditis are among the most common. This patient had a history of all but pericarditis. Her ANA had fluctuated between 1:80 and 1:320 . . .

"Significantly she had a history of much yeast vaginitis starting at age 19 years, aggravated by antibiotics and by pregnancy . . . Thus chronic candidiasis had preceded the onset of the lupus by many years.

> ## Her response to diet and nystatin can only be described as dramatic.

"Her response to diet and nystatin can only be described as dramatic [emphasis added]. In two days the bowel movements were normal and the bloating had cleared."

Many other symptoms and manifestations of her illness also improved, including arthritic symptoms, muscle soreness, bloating, fluid retention and pleurisy. Moreover, her ANA which had been elevated became negative. According to Truss the only setback this patient experienced came following antibiotic therapy in association with the removal of a kidney stone.

Truss also told of his experiences in treating a 44-year-old woman with Crohn's disease—another autoimmune disease.

"At age 29 years this woman developed intestinal bleeding followed by severe diarrhea . . . During the next several years three operations removed approximately eight feet of small intestine, despite which diarrhea, bleeding, and abdominal pain continued chronically.

"Twelve to fifteen bowel movements daily were usual, accompanied by extreme weakness and many infections . . .

> ## She reported immediate improvement within one week of beginning nystatin together with a low-carbohydrate diet.

"She reported immediate improvement within one week of beginning nystatin together with a low-carbohydrate diet . . . The third week she reported having one to two formed stools daily, and soon thereafter one formed stool 'daily or every other day.'

"After receiving treatment for three months, she was temporarily without nystatin. Her abdominal pain and diarrhea recurred immediately, and persisted for the ten days that she was not taking this drug. . . .

"Two days after resuming nystatin therapy the bowel function had changed to two formed stools, and the abdominal discomfort had ceased. . . . This normal intestinal function has been maintained during the six months that have elapsed from then until the present."[1]

During the years 1993 and 1994, I've had a number of phone visits with Dr. Truss and we've exchanged many letters. In discussing the type of patient who would be suitable for study, he said in effect:

"I feel that Crohn's disease would be an ideal one to investigate. All patients in the study could be put on the same special, low carbohydrate diet. Then, one group could be given nystatin in capsules, while a control group could be given a placebo. And their response could be easily followed by counting the number of stools."

To gain more information about the yeast connection to autoimmune diseases, in 1993 and 1994 I interviewed a number of candida clinicians. I asked them especially to comment on their experiences in treating patients who had symptoms suggestive of autoimmune diseases, yet in whom a specific diagnosis had not been made.

Sidney M. Baker, M.D., Weston, Connecticut This board certified, former member of the clinical faculty of Yale University Medical School was among the first physicians to learn about Dr. Truss' observations. And at three conferences on the candida/human interaction (1982, 1983 and 1985) Sid served, along with Dr. Truss, as conference co-leader.

During the past 13 years, I've repeatedly asked him for information and help in a variety of areas, including candida-related disorders and nutrition. Moreover, with his permission I featured many of his concepts in *The Yeast Connection*.

As I gathered material for this book, I interviewed him on several occasions. In one of our conversations, I asked him what his thoughts were about the relationship of *Candida albicans* to autoimmune diseases. Here's an excerpt of his comments.

"Autoimmune conditions are part of a general problem of illness related to a state of immune activation. Various triggers are capable of involving the immune system in an inappropriate overactivity. When the overactivity is directed at one's own tissues, it is called autoimmunity. When the overactivity is directed at foods, pollens, mold, dust, chemicals or animal products, we call it allergy. The only difference is whether the target of the immune system's activity is in the outside world (allergy) or the inside world (autoimmunity).

"Triggers include physical and emotional injury, nutritional stress and infection. Bear in mind that the trigger is not "the cause" of the autoimmune condition. It simply is the spark that lights the fire. The material for the fire is made by genetics and other preexisting conditions in the person. Addressing the influences of the trigger can, however, be very helpful in controlling symptoms. This is rarely more true than it is in the case of chronic fungal overgrowth. Antifungal strategies are often very helpful in alleviating autoimmune problems, as well as allergies.

"The key generalization I would make about the management of autoimmune problems is that it is generally helpful to reduce the overall load on the immune system."[2]

Constance Alfano, M.D., Ridgewood, New Jersey I met this New Jersey physician at a medical conference in 1992 and I was, of course, delighted to learn of her interest in my books. Because of her experiences in treating patients with yeast-related health problems, I asked her about candida-related autoimmune diseases.

"Using Diflucan and a special diet I've helped several patients with lupus—their symptoms definitely improve. And some have been able to stop taking Plaquenil. I also have two patients who are diagnosed as myasthenia gravis who showed significant improvement."

Ronald Hoffman, M.D., New York   During the last several years, I've visited with Ron and his wife, Helen, on several occasions. Moreover, at the 1990 CFS/CFIDS Conference in Charlotte, North Carolina, they took me to dinner. Subsequently, I ordered his books, *Seven Weeks to a Settled Stomach* and *Tired All the Time*, and his newsletter.

People sometimes keep looking for stronger and stronger medications to use, instead of taking a look at their diet and lifestyles.

To learn more about his observations and experiences, I interviewed him in the spring of 1994. In our discussion, he said that he had used antifungal therapy in helping many of his patients. Yet, he also said:

> "We, as clinicians, have to alert our patients that candida is not some sort of scourge in the modern world that has to be eliminated through the use of very, very powerful medications. Too often, patients and physicians, too, think all diseases are caused by a bug and all we have to do is find a drug to knock it out. People sometimes keep looking for stronger and stronger medications to use, instead of taking a look at their diet and lifestyles."

However, in our continuing conversation, he told me about a woman with a lupus-like disorder that he treated with anticandida therapy as part of his comprehensive treatment program. Within three to six months her facial rash went away, her arthralgia improved and her ANA returned to normal. In discussing patients with MS-like symptoms, he said:

> "You have out there a group of patients who have MS-like symptoms and even the neurologists can't agree on the diagnosis. Yet, they leave the patients with the impression that they have an auto-

immune neurological disease, not at this time diagnosable as MS. But just wait until the other shoe drops.

"This group is very amenable to therapy for allergies and therapy for candida. By reducing the antigen challenge to their systems, we can actually shape the course of their disease."

James Brodsky, M.D., Chevy Chase, Maryland Like Sid Baker, this board certified internist and member of the clinical faculty at Georgetown University Medical School became interested in yeast-related health disorders over 10 years ago. During this time, I've visited with Jim and his wife, Mindy, on many occasions. I've also "picked his brain" on the phone when I needed an authoritative answer.

You may recognize his name because he wrote the foreword to this book and to the third edition of *The Yeast Connection*, which included a succinct, but comprehensive, review of the medical literature. Here is an excerpt.

"Many patients with yeast-related health disorders are being treated ineffectively just because their problem has gone unrecognized. If one reviews the literature carefully, the supporting research is well documented."[3]

Recently, I asked Jim if he had seen any patients with lupus, or lupus-like symptoms, who had been helped by anticandida therapy. Here's an excerpt from his response.

"The patients with full blown lupus are few and far between and I don't see many of them. Some of these patients have been on steroids and immunosuppressants and at times they feel awful. In such patients, I've found they often get better once they get on the yeast program.

"I'm not ready to say that the yeast caused the lupus. Instead, I think that the treatment for the lupus and the weakened immune system from the lupus may be causing yeast overgrowth. So, if we can control the yeast and reduce these toxins and their effect on the immune system, we can certainly make these patients feel better.

"I also see a lot of people with ANA's 1:80, 1:160 and 1:320 who generally don't feel well, but who do not meet the criteria for lupus. These people with nonspecific autoimmune disorders often do very well on the program. Most frequently a major complaint is fatigue and joint pain, even though they do not have active synovitis. Such patients often respond very well."

Other physicians who commented included:

Elmer Cranton, M.D., Yelm, Washington I first met this graduate of Harvard Medical School over 20 years ago when we were both serving as members of the Advisory Board of Nathan Pritikin's Longevity Research Institute. In the years since that time, we've kept up a running dialogue on subjects of mutual interest, including nutrition and food allergies. Elmer, a medical pioneer, served as the second president of the American Holistic Medical Association and is the author of several books, including *Bypassing Bypass* and a book which was introduced by double Nobel Laureate Linus Pauling entitled *Textbook of EDTA Chelation.*

I cited Dr. Cranton's comments elsewhere in this book, as well as in *The Yeast Connection* and several of my other publications. Included was a reference to his 1984 book (co-authored by Richard A. Passwater, Ph.D.) *Trace Elements, Hair Analysis and Nutrition.* Some of the things I learned from him for the first time dealt with free radical pathology and antioxidants—subjects which are now coming into the public and medical mainstream.

In commenting on his experiences in treating autoimmune diseases with antifungal medicine and diet, he said:

"Almost anyone with a chronic debilitating disease can be helped to varying degrees by such a program. Yet, I'm always cautious to tell them I don't think such treatment is a cure. Yet, it's another thing they can do to take the stress off their immune system. It relieves symptoms."

Allan Lieberman, M.D., North Charleston, South Carolina Since the early 1980s, this board certified pediatrician has treated thousands of chronically sick patients, including both children and adults. On many occasions when I wanted to obtain sound timely information I called him. Moreover, I cited his comments in the third edition of the *The Yeast Connection*.[4] In commenting on his success in treating patients with autoimmune diseases, he said:

"Many patients respond dramatically to antifungal therapy, no matter what the diagnosis is. These include MS, Crohn's disease, rheumatoid arthritis, myasthenia gravis and other autoimmune diseases.

> ## The best way to find out if a patient has the yeast-related problem is through a therapeutic trial of antifungal medications.

"The best way to find out if a patient has the yeast-related problem is through a therapeutic trial of antifungal medications. I start out by giving the patients Diflucan or Nizoral for a couple of weeks. If they improve, I then work on the diet."

Geraldine Donaldson, M.D., Livermore, California   I met Dr. Donaldson for the first time several years ago and I was impressed by some of the things she told me. So when I began gathering material for this book, I sought her help and she sent me a tremendous amount of information.

In early 1994, I interviewed her and she told me about a woman in her mid-40s who had been diagnosed as having lupus many years ago and had taken prednisone on a regular basis. On a comprehensive treatment program, which included management of food allergies, immunotherapy and a nonprescription antifungal medication (Pau d'Arco), this patient showed significant improvement.

I also read the comprehensive instructions she gives to her patients. She listed chronic, unwarranted depression, extreme fatigue, weakness, asthma, colitis and a number of other complaints which she felt were yeast-related. And she said:

"Treatment of yeast has resulted in dramatic improvement in a variety of symptoms."

Heiko Santelmann, M.D., Mandal, Norway   In 1988, I was both surprised and delighted when this physician wrote me and asked for permission to translate *The Yeast Connection* into the language of a country with only four million people. During our conversation, he said, "Many, many people in my country are troubled by yeast-related problems. Although some speak English, I can help more people by translating your book into Norweigian."

In 1990, I received a copy of a 243-page book. My name appeared in English across the top and the title was *Candida Syndromet*.

Then in the summer of 1992, I spent four hours with Dr. Santelmann. I asked him about his experiences in treating a variety of patients, including those with autoimmune disorders. Here's a brief excerpt from our conversation.

"One of my patients with MS-like symptoms showed a remarkable improvement on nystatin and diet. He then went to a neurologist and told him, 'The diet makes me free of symptoms.' The neurologist said, 'The diet must be wrong because it is not possible for MS to get better using a diet!'"

Myasthenia Gravis (MG)

What is myasthenia gravis? How can it affect you? And what causes it? Does it affect women more often than men? And can it be yeast connected?

Although I knew that this disease caused severe muscle weakness and other symptoms, I had never seen a person with MG. Yet it seems to fit into the group of "autoimmune diseases." I also recalled that Dr. C. Orian Truss reported that he helped a patient with MG using a special diet and nystatin.

The Almost Unbelievable Story of Joyce Frederick

In August 1992, this 35-year-old woman called me on the IHF Hotline. She said:

"I've had severe MG for over 20 years and have been troubled by many other symptoms. I recently obtained a copy of your book, *The Yeast Connection,* and began to change my diet. I'm already improving! I'm off all MG medication and gaining back my strength."

Joyce also told me she had taken many, many antibiotics, and that she had been troubled by recurrent vaginal yeast infections in childhood and early adolescence.

At the age of 13 she began to show symptoms which led to the diagnosis of MG. Her symptoms at that time included: completely nasal voice—air came out of her nose instead of her mouth when she spoke; she was unable to swallow and had to wash down food with liquid. Joyce had no control of muscles in her face. She was unable to smile and her eyes remained open when sleeping—she was uncoordinated and troubled by double vision, migraine headaches, and stomachaches.

In subsequent letters, Joyce sent me further details about her illness. She said:

"I was tired all the time and slept a lot and was unable to wake up in the morning for school. I was also troubled by sinus drainage and mucus.

"During the years following the diagnosis, many therapies were tried, including removal of my thymus gland three weeks after diagnosis; prednisone, 100 mgs. on alternate days for 7 years.

"Then at the age of 21, following a positive blood test for MG, I was placed on Mestinon and a year later I began taking Mytelase. Between ages 21 and 32, my symptoms of MG improved, yet I was troubled by recurring yeast infections, constipation, depression, recurrent colds and flu, and constant eyelid weakness.

"In 1990, at the age of 32, my MG became full blown with severe body weakness. I took additional medications, including daily prednisone and gamma globulin by intravenous drip, once a week. Also the dose of Mytelase was increased from 20 mgs. to 40 mgs. daily."

In spite of these therapies, in 1992 Joyce continued to be troubled by many symptoms, including PMS, headache, irritability, panic attacks, poor memory and "indescribable" body weakness and fatigue.

"I had to be vertical most of the day. I could not carry on normal duties, including cooking and cleaning. I had to quit my job. Some days I had to stay in bed all day—folding a load of clothes required too much energy.

"My right eye drooped in various degrees and the right corner of my mouth felt numb or weak. My right eye remained open at night causing extreme pain.

"After reading your book and talking to you in August 1992, I began a sugar-free, yeast-free special diet. I also eliminated most fruits, white rice, white pasta, white flour, and all refined processed dairy products, with the exception of real butter. Any of the above foods would bring back my symptoms, especially the sweets, which caused weak days to return.

"Within a week or so my constipation and fatigue began improving and I had more good days than bad days. In addition, my memory began to improve, so did my PMS and depression. My panic/anxiety attacks disappeared completely. However, my right eye continued to droop, so did the right corner of my mouth and I was still bothered by my right eye staying open at night."

Because of Joyce's history of recurrent yeast infections, improvement following dietary changes and Dr. Truss' success in treating patients with MG using nystatin and diet, I wrote to her and said, "Call or write Dr. Truss. I feel he may be able to help you."

Early in 1993, Joyce went to Birmingham to see Dr. Truss. Following a careful history and examination, he prescribed nystatin, 1/2 tsp. four times a day, along with vaginal nystatin twice daily. He also stressed the importance of carefully following a restricted diet.

Within a short time, she reported greater improvement, including 100% more energy; no more 'weak' days. She said, however, "I had symptoms if I ate any of the foods I had been avoiding—especially fruits and sweets.

"In March 1993, I went on a ski vacation and skied from 7:30 in the morning to 4:30 in the evening! By contrast, seven months earlier, I couldn't sit up or do other normal household duties. My memory

showed remarkable improvement—100% better—especially with recall. My depression also improved 100%.

"I actually felt happy. My PMS disappeared and so did my yeast infections. I still have some mucus in my nose, but no more bronchitis or sinusitis.

"I also noticed my double vision which is present 100% of the time is improving and I am able to pull the two images together. Prior to the diet and nystatin I was unable to do this. I noticed a tremendous improvement in the weakness and numbness in the corner of my mouth and my right eye no longer stayed open at night.

"Symptoms that still bothered me included droopiness of the right eye, some irritability at times and cold hands and cold feet."

August 1993 Progress Report

Joyce wrote that she was continuing to do well, yet she was still troubled by weakness in her eyelids and right corner of her mouth. She also said that with these symptoms still present, MG specialists would question the success of the diet, even though their method of treatment had also failed in controlling this symptom. She also said:

"Prior to avoiding sugar and fruits and making other changes in my diet, I had constant problems with colds and flu. For example, I had 11 spells of colds, flu, sinusitis, bronchitis in a 12 month period. Now, since being on the diet, I have recovered without antibiotics for the first time. And I've had only *one* flu attack in the 12 month period since starting the diet. That attack happened four days after drinking a glass of punch with sugar in it."

October 1993 Progress Report

Here are excerpts from Joyce's letter.

"An exciting update. Dr. Truss increased my dose of nystatin and I now have days where my eyelids are completely balanced and my mouth feels fine—in other words, the treatment is working!!

"The only thing is—I absolutely have to get the oral and vaginal doses done as instructed. I ran out of nystatin and lost the improvement. Now I'm getting it back. I also *have to* do the vaginal dose. If I miss even one time, the improvement lessens.

"I also tested fruit and lost the improvement. I also tested frozen Rice Dream (sweetened with brown rice syrup) and lost the improvement. The loss is only temporary, but confirms what is taking place.

"*Conclusion: Taking the proper dose of nystatin regularly, orally and vaginally, restricting carbohydrates, and staying away from all sweets, as well as junk food, white flour, white rice, and all refined foods is crucial to the recovery of a myasthenic.* Sweets (even so-called 'healthy sweets' like fruit, honey, rice syrup, maple syrup, etc.) are my number one enemy. I'm sure other MG victims will experience this also.

"In *The Yeast Connection* you mentioned a positive attitude being important and faith in God. I feel that my belief in God and my faith in Jesus gave me the strength to be committed to the diet and stay on it strictly.

"As a former sugarholic, I would not have had the strength on my own. God healed me through *The Yeast Connection* diet, and I will eat a healthy diet the rest of my life."

July 1994 Progress Report

During the past winter, due to financial problems, Joyce was unable to obtain nystatin. She continued to do well for about six weeks on diet alone. Then, many of her symptoms began to return, including drooping of her mouth and eyes, fatigue and weakness.

She obtained compassionate supplies of Diflucan in May 1994, and again she improved. Subsequently, she received further nystatin. For a time she took them both.

Here are excerpts from Joyce's July 1994 letter.

"• My memory remains good.
• The vision problems I was having prior to the Diflucan have gone away.
• I'm no longer struggling with constipation.
• I feel a lot of my strength returning.
• I'm not having the problems urinating that were bothering me."

September 1994 Progress Report

In letters I received from Joyce in September, she told me that she had visited Dr. Jacob Siegal, a kind and caring physician in Houston, Texas. She said:

> "He discussed food allergies/sensitivities with me and recommended a rotated diet. He really helped me."

In her continuing discussion, she said that the Diflucan helped for a while but then it seemed to lose its effectiveness. So she went back to the nystatin, 1/4 tsp., twice daily. And she said:

> "Along with my diet and nutritional supplements, I'm doing reasonably well."

November 1994 Progress Peport

Here are excerpts from a letter I received from Joyce.

> "I'm no longer as dependent on the nystatin to control symptoms and I'm certain that my continuing improvement is diet related. I eat only organic products, including vegetables, organic whole grains (wheat, limited amount; kamut; spelt; millet; and, quinoa), organic fruits, mostly apples; organic sprouts of all beans and grains, organic beans (pinto, red, lima, northern, black and black-eyed peas); organic tofu; organic nuts (limited amount); olive oil, only extra virgin, unrefined. My diet would now be considered 'vegan' and similar to the macrobiotic diet without using sea vegetables . . .

> *My energy level is on the rise and everything else is falling into place.*

> "My energy level is on the rise and everything else is falling into place. I'm now doing 21 push-ups each day—2½ years ago I could

barely lift a clothing item to fold and had no more energy than to lay flat all day!

"I am now doing great and am going from strengths to strengths—glory to glory—victory to victory. I can say that the Lord and I have truly beaten myasthenia gravis and all the other related problems that have attacked me through the years."

My Comments

Joyce Frederick's story is an exciting one and the longest one in this book. Yet, I left out many of the things she told me. At the same time, I included many, many details as I felt, in so doing, I would provide many of my readers with courage and hope.

Are all autoimmune diseases yeast related? I don't really think so. Yet, the observations of Dr. Truss and those of other physicians suggest that many of them are, and that a comprehensive treatment program which includes an appropriate diet and antifungal medication can help many people.

Joyce's story illustrates many points which are relevant to the person with a chronic health disorder, including those which are yeast-related. Here are a few of them which I would like to reiterate and to emphasize.

- Although many chronic health disorders are yeast related, antifungal medications alone do not provide a "quick fix" or a long term answer.
- *An appropriate diet is essential for any person who wishes to regain, her/his life and health.* Based on scientific studies that I have read in major medical journals and reports from the press and media, such a diet should feature plant foods. They should also be diversified and as free as possible of insecticides, chemicals and toxins.
- Faith in God, courage, persistence and determination are key ingredients in any treatment program.

REFERENCES

1. Truss, C.O., *The Missing Diagnosis*, P.O. Box 26508, Birmingham, AL 35226, 1983 and 1986; pp 83–95.
2. Baker, S.M., personal communication, November 1994.
3. Brodsky, J.H., Foreword, *The Yeast Connection*, Third Edition, Professional Books, Jackson, TN and Vintage Books, New York, 1986.
4. Lieberman, A., As quoted in *The Yeast Connection*, Third Edition, Professional Books, Jackson, TN and Vintage Books, New York, 1985; pp. 195–361.

FIVE

Yeast-Related Disorders Which Affect Both Sexes Equally

22

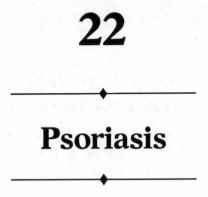

Psoriasis

In June 1982 at a medical conference in Dallas, Sidney M. Baker, M.D., who at that time was a member of the clinical faculty of Yale University School of Medicine, described the favorable response of several of his patients with psoriasis to oral nystatin.[1]

Word of Baker's observations spread to E.W. Rosenberg, M.D., Professor and Chairman, Division of Dermatology, University of Tennessee Center for Health Sciences in Memphis. And in a letter to the editor published in the *New England Journal of Medicine*, Rosenberg said:

> "We have been aware . . . of improvement of both psoriasis and inflammatory bowel disease in patients treated with oral nystatin, an agent that was expected to work only on yeast in the gut lumen. We've now confirmed that observation in several of our patients with psoriasis. We suspect, therefore, that gut yeast may have a role in some instances of psoriasis."[2]

Subsequently, Crutcher, Rosenberg, Belew, Skinner and Eaglstein of the Division of Dermatology at the University of Tennessee College of Medicine, and Baker, published a report on the treatment of psoriasis in the Archives of Dermatology.[3] They described the response of four patients with longstanding psoriasis to therapy with oral nystatin.

Their case reports were especially fascinating and impressive as the psoriasis had been present in each patient for 10, 25, 30 and 40 years. The duration of nystatin treatment ranged from 2 to 4 months.

Further Reports from the University of Tennessee

In a presentation at the September 1988 Candida Update Conference in Memphis entitled "The Role of Yeast Seborrheic Dermatitis and Psoriasis," Robert Skinner, M.D., Associate Professor of Dermatology, stated:

"Studies at the University of Tennessee indicate that the pathogenesis of seborrheic dermatitis and scalp psoriasis are related to yeast. Double-blind studies indicate improvement of seborrheic dermatitis and scalp psoriasis with antiyeast agents.

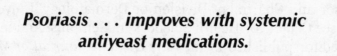

Psoriasis . . . improves with systemic antiyeast medications.

"Other forms of psoriasis, including psoriasis of the palms and soles, erythrodermic psoriasis, plaque psoriasis and intertriginous and seborrheic psoriasis, improve with systemic antiyeast medications."

I was especially fascinated by the slides Dr. Skinner showed of infants and young children with generalized skin rashes who responded dramatically to oral nystatin.

During the past several years, Drs. Rosenberg and Skinner and their colleague, Patricia Noah, Ph.D., have continued their studies on psoriasis, including its relationship to *Candida albicans*. In a 1994 report, they said:

"Patients seen in our psoriasis clinic are studied for the possible presence of microbial factors that might be activating the disease . . . Here we report 14 patients in whom palm and/or plantar psoriasis was associated with the recovery of *Candida albicans* on culture from their throat and/or dental plate.

"Patients were treated with oral nystatin, fluconazole or keto-conazole. Nine patients were evaluated following treatment. Of these, seven were cleared or substantially improved."[4]

To obtain additional information about the experiences of the University of Tennessee researchers, I called Dr. Rosenberg who told me that if a patient has a dental plate, it will always be loaded with candida and that you cannot help it without an ultrasonic cleaning machine. I also interviewed Dr. Noah in February 1994. Here are excerpts.

Crook: Dr. Noah, tell me more about the experiences of your group in studying patients with yeast-related psoriasis.

Noah: Psoriasis develops from many different causes, including strep infections. Yet, some 10 to 20% are helped by antifungal medications, including Sporanox and Diflucan. Patients with palmar and plantar psoriasis are especially apt to be yeast-related. Moreover, they seem to have heavy intestinal yeast and as pointed out by Dr. Rosenberg, dental plate involvement.

Crook: Have you seen significant systemic symptoms in your patients with psoriasis?

Noah: We haven't really tabulated these symptoms. Yet we've noticed that patients with yeast-related psoriasis all complain of severe itching—even though they don't have an active yeast infection of the skin.

Crook: How do you identify the organism?

Noah: We do throat, dental plate and gluteal fold cultures. We also culture the urine and the intertriginous folds of the body.

Crook: Do you get good correlation between the people in whom you find positive yeast cultures and those who respond to antifungal drugs?

Noah: Yes. And we presented our observations of the response of patients with plantar psoriasis to Diflucan at an international conference in Trieste.

Further Observations on the Relationship of Yeast Infections to Psoriasis and Other Skin Disorders

In the fall of 1993, I received a letter from David R. Weakley, M.D., of Dallas, Texas, a Diplomate of the American Board of Dermatology. Here are excerpts.

"In my opinion, many cases of infectious eczematoid dermatitis are, to use Bill Rosenberg's terminology, 'yeast driven' and respond dramatically to antiyeast therapy. I've now seen and treated at least 30 patients who responded promptly and well to Diflucan. I've used anywhere from 200 mg. daily to 100 mg. every three days.

"In addition to the skin problems, a number of these patients also are troubled by migraine headaches, GI symptomatology, chronic arthritis and chronic fatigue.

"In addition to anticandida therapy, I've found it important for patients to adhere to a diet which restricts alcohol, vinegar and other yeast containing foods. They must also avoid sugar which fertilizes the little beasts."

Concluding Comments

Is the common yeast, *Candida albicans,* **the** cause of psoriasis? No. This chronic health disorder, like many others, develops because of many different causes; some which are known, and some which aren't. Yet, if you're troubled by psoriasis and especially if your history suggests other yeast-related problems, several months course of antifungal medication and a sugar-free special diet could help significantly.

REFERENCES

1. Baker, S.M., "Nystatin for Treatment of Psoriasis." Presented at the *Candida albicans* Conference, Dallas, 1982.
2. Rosenberg, E.W., Belew, P.W., Skinner, R.B. and Crutcher, N., "Response to: Crohn's Disease in Psoriasis," *N. Engl. J. Med.*, 1983; 308:101.

3. Crutcher, N., Rosenberg, E.W., Belew, P.W., et al, "Oral Nystatin in the Treatment of Psoriasis," *Arch. of Dermatol.*, 1984; 120:433.
4. Skinner, R.B., Rosenberg, E.W. and Noah, P.W., "Psoriasis of the Palms and Soles Is Frequently Associated with Oral Pharyngeo *Candida albicans*," *ACTA Derm. Venereol* (Stockh), 1994; Suppl. 186:149–150.

23

Asthma

Based on the research studies of Iwata in the 1960s and 1970s and the clinical observations of Truss and Witkin, superficial yeast infections may adversely affect the immune system. Symptoms that result may adversely affect many different parts of the body. Yet, I'd never thought about the yeast connection to asthma until a physician friend added a note to a Christmas card several years ago, which said:

> "One of my patients with intrinsic asthma showed a marvelous response to Nizoral."

In November 1982, at a medical conference in Colorado, I met a 40-year-old physician (I'll call him Dr. Sam Carroll) who told me that he had suffered from asthma for many years, and had shown a remarkable response to Diflucan.

Subsequently, I received a letter from Dr. Carroll and talked to him briefly on the phone. To learn more about his story, I called him in January 1994 and recorded our conversation. Here's what he had to say.

> "I developed asthma as a child and I've taken bronchodilators off and on as long as I can remember. Also, in between my bouts of asthma, I would develop bronchitis which required repeated courses of antibiotic drugs. Also, from time to time, I took prednisone or other steroids.

"I improved during my teen years and early twenties and required little medication. Then my asthma came back in a much worse form about 15 years ago. I had to take daily theophylline during the late '80s and early '90s. I also took many other therapies, including the Ventolin steroid inhalers. And, when my asthma flared, I'd again take oral prednisone.

"Six or eight years ago, I began to experiment with my diet and I found that when I eliminated milk, sugar and yeasty foods, my asthma improved. At about the same time, I took nystatin and it also helped.

"Then, about two years ago, a pharmaceutical representative gave me samples of Diflucan. After taking 100 mg. a day for three days, and then 100 mg. every other day for a week, my asthma was better than it had been in a long time. I've taken no steroids in the past two years and take only an occasional puff from my Ventolin inhaler when I'm exposed to a lot of dust and smoke.

"During the past year, I've treated three other asthmatics using a yeast-free, sugar-free diet and Diflucan and their response has been remarkable."

Not long after my conversation with Dr. Carroll, I came across an abstract of a study by University of Virginia researchers who described the favorable response of a group of asthmatic patients to antifungal therapy. Here are excerpts from this abstract published in *The Journal of Allergy and Clinical Immunology* in January 1994.

"In a previous study we reported a series of 12 male asthmatic patients with fungal infection of the feet and specific sensitivity of their lungs and noses to *Trichophyton tonsurans (T. tons)*. In that group, some patients had many of the characteristics of intrinsic asthma . . .

"In the current controlled study, ten Trichophyton allergic asthma patients (9 male and 1 female) have been randomized to receive either 22 weeks or 44 weeks of oral fluconazole at 100 mg. daily. After the 10 months of the study, specific bronchial reactivity to *T. tons* had shown a definite decrease in 9/10 patients tested . . . No adverse reactions to fluconazole have been noted in these 10 patients, even in those maintained on fluconazole for up to 2 years."[1]

These investigators also pointed out that fungal infections of the feet in these patients improved. And in 8 patients, there was a progressive reduction in steroid dosage.

A second abstract published in the same issue of the *The Journal of Allergy and Clinical Immunology*, came from Belgian researchers who also described the response of some of their asthmatic patients to a systemic azole antifungal drug. Here are excerpts.

"Ketoconazole (K) is known for its antifungal properties. Since 1986, we observed several cases of asthma improving during treatment with K. The aim of this study was to investigate a possible effect of K in asthma.

"Ten corticosteroid-dependent asthmatic patients, aged 13–62 years, without evidence of fungal infection, entered a double-blind placebo-controlled study."

These observers found that 4 out of 5 of the treated patients improved . . . while 4 out of 5 of the placebo group did not.

These observers found that 4 out of 5 of the treated patients improved after two weeks, while 4 out of 5 of the placebo group did not improve. No side effects of the drug were observed. And they stated:

"We conclude that ketoconazole might be beneficial in some asthmatic patients. Further studies are needed to investigate the mechanism of action and a possible steroid sparing effect of ketoconazole in asthma."[2]

My Comments

I was especially pleased and excited to read the report from Belgium because in this study the asthmatic patients showed no evidence of fungal infections. If an asthmatic does not show evidence of a fungal infection on the skin (as was the case with the 12 male asthmatics in the University of Virginia study), where then would the fungal infection be?

Here are some possibilities. Many patients with chronic asthma have received steroids systemically and/or multiple courses of broad-spectrum antibiotic drugs. Such drugs encourage the proliferation of candida in the digestive tract. Moreover, inhaled steroids (used almost routinely in many patients with chronic asthma) promote localized yeast infections.

Further reports on the relationship of *Candida albicans* to asthma were noted by Itkin and Dennis, from the National Jewish Hospital in Denver almost 30 years ago. In the introduction of their paper, these investigators said:

> "It is the scientific aim of the allergist to reduce the number of patients who must be classified as suffering from 'asthma of unknown origin.' It is the purpose of this paper to describe three years of experience with provocative bronchial challenge by inhalation as a tool in establishing *Candida albicans* as a significant allergen . . . in patients suffering from severe asthma."

In their article, these investigators cited the observations of Liebeskind, who had noted an increase of *C. albicans* cells following antibiotic and corticosteroid treatment (see *Annals of Allergy* 20:394–396, 1962). They also noted that similar results had been reported by a number of other authors, and they said:

> "Candidiasis of the oropharynx and larynx has been observed after the use of dexamethasone aerosol in the minimum effective dose in patients suffering from severe asthma who have been treated with oral corticosteroids for long periods . . .
> "The results of this study provide adequate documentation that *C. albicans* is an atopic allergen capable of evoking an asthmatic response in suitable subjects . . . The acceptance of *C. albicans* as a common atopic allergen may improve the effectiveness of treatment in some cases and could reduce the number of patients who must be classified as suffering from 'asthma of unknown origin.' "[3]

Here's more. In a more recent article in the *Annals of Allergy,* Gumowski and colleagues also noted that iatrogenic candidiasis due to the use of some drugs, such as long-term corticosteroid treatment (and) antibiotics, destroyed acidophilic bacteria of the gut, and they stated:

"Besides specific clinical pictures due to the pathogenicity of Candida albicans in cases of immune deficiencies, this yeast is known as an important causative allergen in bronchial asthma, chronic rhinitis, chronic urticaria, and food intolerance"[4]

In the 1993 *Physicians' Desk Reference,* under the heading "Warnings," appeared the following comments about the corticosteroid inhalant Beclovent:

"Localized infections with *Candida albicans,* or *Aspergillus niger,* have occurred frequently in the mouth and pharynx and occasionally in the larynx. Positive cultures for oral candida may be present in up to 75% of patients. Although the frequency of clinically apparent infection is considerably lower, these infections may require treatment with appropriate antifungal therapy or discontinuation of treatment with Beclovent inhalation aerosol."[5]

I hope that in the not too distant future researchers will follow up on the above cited studies and carry out further investigation of the relationship of *Candida albicans* to intrinsic asthma. Perhaps nasal and pharyngeal candida smears and cultures can be carried out in a group of patients with chronic asthma.

Those patients with laboratory evidence of infections by *Candida albicans* could then be entered into a double-blind, placebo-controlled study, similar to the study carried out by the Belgian researchers. Half of the patients could be given a systemic azole drug and half could be given a placebo. The response of the patients with asthma in each group could be monitored. And at the end of the treatment program, nasal and pharyngeal cultures could be carried out in both groups.

In addition, especially in patients who have received systemic steroids and antibiotics, stool examinations for *Candida albicans* could provide additional information.

REFERENCES

1. Ward, G.W., Hayden, M.L., Rose, G., Call, R.C., Platts-Mills, T.,"Trichophyton Asthma: Reduction of Specific Bronchial Hyperreactivity Following Long Term Antifungal Therapy," *J. Allergy Clin. Immunol.*, January 1994 (abstract).
2. van der Brempt, X., Mairesse, M., and Ledent, C., "Ketoconazole (K) in Asthma: A pilot study," *J. Allergy Clin. Immunol.*, January 1994 (abstract).
3. Itkin, I.H. and Dennis, M., "Bronchial hypersensitivity to extract of *Candida albicans*," *Journal of Allergy*, 1966; 37:187–195.
4. Gumowski, P., "Chronic asthma and rhinitis due to *Candida albicans*, epidermophyton, and tricophyton," *Annals of Allergy*, 1987; 59:48–51.
5. *Physicians' Desk Reference*, 47th Edition, Medical Economics Company, Inc., Montvale, NJ, 1993; p 574.

PART

SIX

Yeast-Related Health Problems in Other Family Members

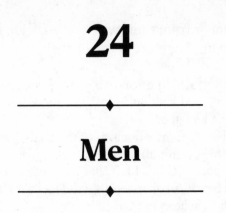

24

Men

Although men are much less apt to develop yeast-related health problems than women, they are not immune. These problems are especially apt to occur in men who:

- have taken repeated or prolonged courses of broad spectrum antibiotic drugs for acne, sinusitis, bronchitis or prostatitis.
- are troubled by persistent "jock itch," athlete's foot or fungus infections of the nails.
- consume lots of breads, sweets, beer and other alcoholic beverages.
- are troubled by fatigue, headache, depression and other nervous system symptoms.
- are bothered by recurrent digestive problems, including constipation, bloating, diarrhea and abdominal pain.
- are bothered by food and chemical sensitivities.
- have been to many different physicians seeking help only to be told "your examination and tests are normal and we cannot find the cause of your symptoms."

Letters I've Received from Men, or from Their Wives or Girlfriends

Within the past decade, 90% of the thousands of letters and phone calls I received came from women who were concerned about their own yeast-related health problems. Yet, I also received hundreds of letters from men, or from their wives or girlfriends, who were concerned about them. Here are some of them.

Mike: "I took tetracycline for two years because of acne. In my early '20s I developed headache, fatigue, abdominal pain and bloating. I just didn't feel good.

"Checkups by my family doctor and by a gastroenterologist who did an endoscopic examination showed no abnormalities. So I began to feel like a hypochondriac. I felt that a 28-year-old guy with a darn good job and a beautiful girlfriend should feel a lot better than I did. But I didn't know where to turn.

> ## Thanks so much. I just wanted you to know that your book had really changed my life.

"Then, in browsing through the book section of a health food store, I came across your book, *The Yeast Connection,* and I was very impressed. I changed my diet, eliminating sugar and most yeast products. I also started taking Mycopryl—a caprylic acid product—and I've noticed a marked improvement in my general health.

"Thanks so much. I just wanted you to know that your book had really changed my life."

David's wife: "This is a letter to say thank you. First for your wonderful book, *The Yeast Connection,* and second for referring me to a doctor who helped us.

"My husband had been ill for 13 years and had been to doctor after doctor. For 10 years they treated him for arthritis with endless new drugs and steroids. Then he started developing sensitivity to tobacco smoke, perfumes and various chemical odors. He was also troubled by headaches and stomach problems. At times we thought he was losing his mind.

"Doctors could not find one thing wrong; yet, David continued to grow weaker and more discouraged. It was then we became aware of your book. Then we got the name of the doctor who lived only a 2-hour drive from home. He told him to start on a sugar-free special diet and he gave him a prescription for nystatin. He made many other suggestions that you know about, including nutritional supplements.

"We've also done some further diet detective work and have found that David is sensitive to milk and wheat.

"We're in the process of writing a book about this nightmare that has completely changed our lives. I'm also compiling a list of recipes. If David and I can be of any help or encouragement to any of your patients, please give them our address and telephone number.

"Thank you again for the book that truly changed our lives."

James: "I'm a 24-year-old male university student. Until 18 months ago, my health was perfect. At that time I began having pains in my lower abdomen and groin. I was diagnosed as having prostatitis and put on a series of broad spectrum antibiotics for 110 days by the university urology clinic. Then I was referred to the university GI clinic.

"They did upper and lower GI x-rays, stool cultures; found nothing and diagnosed me as having irritable bowel syndrome. After that I went to a famous mid-western clinic where they did a chest and kidney x-ray and offered no explanation except that I did not have a serious illness.

"Then I came across *The Yeast Connection* and scored 191 on the test questionnaire. After reading it, I'm convinced that my health problems are candida-related, especially since my original symptoms occurred shortly after a 7-day course of tetracycline for a rash on my lower leg which I thought was a bacterial infection.

"My major problem now is finding a doctor that understands my problem and is willing to prescribe nystatin. The doctors at the university have been unreceptive to your book or my self-diagnosis. I'm desperate to find a physician who is knowledgeable and empathetic. I will be grateful for any help you can provide."

Larry: "I'm 23 years old and have always had a stuffy nose, fungus nails on right foot, jock itch—especially after consuming sugary foods—feeling bad all over for no reason, fatigue, confusion, craving for sugar foods to bring me 'up'—but then I feel 'down.'

"For years I've thought that something was wrong, but did not know what to do. I never drank alcohol because I thought it would flip me out, as I always felt 'drunk' anyway. When driving I feel tipsy sometimes.

"I'm a graphic designer working at a typesetting company. The work is not pressured or anything. There's nothing in my life that could cause the "mental low" or semi-depression that I think my mind and body are in. Everything just seems like slow motion.

"After reading your book, I think my past history gives me a clue. When I was young I always had bronchitis and the doctors loaded me up with antibiotics. Yet, nothing worked. Then I went to an allergist and was given allergy shots which did help end the terrible coughing every spring and fall. But my allergy symptoms still persist.

"I know this sounds like a lot—IT IS! And they're all questions I do not have an answer for.

"When I read your book and read about the Arizona man who was considered to be drunk even though he had never had alcohol, that really hit me. Whenever I drink a 7-Up or other soft drink, I often get hot and sweaty a few minutes afterward. Could this be a reaction of the candida yeast consuming the sugar?

"Thanks for reading this letter. I sure hope you can answer my questions and help me out. It will be a miracle if this is my problem."

Bill: "I would like to thank you for publishing your insights regarding the possible connection between candida and immunological breakdown. For many years I suffered from a wide variety of perplexing and seemingly unrelated symptoms. Yet, I'm thrilled with the progress I've made in recent months under the supervision of Dr. Paula Davey of Ann Arbor, Michigan.

"I hope to continue to improve, although I still have a distance to go before achieving full recovery. Now, however, I can see the light.

"I'll be graduating from the University of Michigan's MBA program next spring and would like to become involved in a business related capacity of what I call alternative forms of health care service. My long search for improved health and now subsequent improvement convinces me that environmental and orthomolecular medicine, and specifically yeast suppression, holds great promise for significantly impacting the health of many individuals.

"I would like to contribute in some way to that process, but I'm not clear where to start looking. I would greatly appreciate your response. Thank you."

Tom: "I'm sure you've read this type of letter hundreds of times, but I hope you'll read through one more. My history reads like many of the examples you cite in your book, *The Yeast Connection.*

"For me it started with a simple urinary tract infection some 3½ years ago. I was treated with an antibiotic for one week and the symptoms cleared. Unfortunately, about a week after finishing the prescription, my symptoms returned. Needless to say, I went back to the doctor who prescribed two more weeks of the drug while commenting, "These things can be quite stubborn."

"This began a vicious cycle (sound familiar!) of antibiotic usage over the next 2½ years (tetracycline, Bactrim, Septra D.S. and at least three more). I was on at least 10 or 12 administrations, many for extended periods. *Each time it was blamed on a virus.*

"My symptoms became more prevalent with each antibiotic and included fatigue, thrush, rectal itching, sinus itching, abdominal pain and bloating. I've seen several doctors, including urologists, who could come up with nothing. I had countless urine tests, a cystoscopy and blood tests which ruled out everything but candida.

"I also noticed my symptoms would be triggered by beer and sweetened foods. My physical symptoms were accompanied by mental ones, including lack of concentration and poor memory. It was all I could manage to read one chapter after being an A and B student my whole life. I still can't believe I managed to graduate.

I asked my family physician to let me try nystatin and he agreed. The improvement is incredible.

"Then I came across Dr. Truss' book and felt like I was reading my autobiography. I couldn't believe how close it followed. I asked my family physician to let me try nystatin and he agreed. The improvement is incredible, most of my symptoms disappeared within a week. Unfortunately, though, that was all that he would allow me to take.

"My symptoms subsided for about 4 months, then they began to return. And recently I've begun experiencing severe headaches, tingling of the extremities, muscle aches and blurred vision. I'm also increasingly sensitive to all chemicals.

"I would appreciate any help you can give me. I'm willing to travel 1000 miles to see you if it means any chance of relief. Or perhaps you could contact my family doctor and provide him with more information about anti-yeast medications other than nystatin."

Ronald: "I'm 50 years old and have suffered for more than 20 years from all the maladies so vividly described in *The Yeast Connection*.

"After reading your book, I began on the diet and convinced my doctor to give me a prescription for nystatin. *Literally, within hours, I felt a substantial improvement in my overall general physical condition.* Here's what I'm talking about.

1. I don't feel any internal ear pressure, nor do I suffer any longer from the general feeling of malaise that accompanied these attacks.
2. My stomach, which had been diagnosed on various occasions as being 'nervous,' 'pre-ulcerated,' 'hiatal hernia'—immediately settled down.
3. I found myself in a state of general well-being.
4. My athlete's foot and jock itch, which has been a part of my life for 30 years, has started to clear up.

"Let me extend my best wishes and thanks to Dr. Truss and to you. I don't really know what the hell is going on, but I'm glad to feel 'normal' for the first time in many years."

A Sugar-Free Special Diet and Antifungal Doesn't Solve Every Problem

In *The Yeast Connection,* and in various parts of this book, I've compared the chronic health problems which many people struggle with to an overloaded camel. And I've said in effect:

"To get your health and life back on track, you'll need to unload many bundles of straw. Moreover, the bundles which are weighing you down may differ from those which overload others."

Here's a man's story which illustrates what I'm talking about.

Edgar: An anesthesiologist practicing in a major industrial city gave a history of repeated antibiotics. In his late thirties and early forties he developed headache, fatigue and other symptoms. He noted that his symptoms were aggravated in the hospital when he was exposed to chemical odors of various sorts.

Although he improved after making dietary changes, taking anti-fungal medication and controlling chemical exposures in his home, his symptoms continued to a disabling degree.

Because chemicals played such a major role in causing his symptoms, he left his practice and went to a dry, arid area in the west, away from almost every form of civilization. There, he felt great! But when he returned to his home city, his symptoms returned, even though he did not go back into the hospital. So he gave up his practice and moved to a pollution free home in Santa Fe, New Mexico.

In the summer of 1992, Edgar said:

"My general health is great and my chemical sensitivity is a lot less than it was 7 to 8 years ago. I was even able to return to my former home for a week's visit without developing significant symptoms. Yet, I feel that if I remained there, and breathed the chemical fumes on the freeway, or in the hospital, my health problems would return again.

"I value my health more than anything else and I have little desire to go back."

In *The Yeast Connection,*[1] I included the story of Paul, a 40-year-old factory worker who came to see me in the early '80s. On a comprehensive program of management, including a yeast-free, sugar-free diet, nystatin and nutritional supplements, including 2000 or 3000 mg. of vitamin C a day, Paul steadily improved. And at a follow-up visit a few months later, he said:

"I'm much better. Now my bad days are as good as my good days were before I started treatment. My stomach no longer hurts; I don't need to take Tagamet and my tolerance to tobacco and other chemicals has improved."

During the decade of the '80s, I saw Paul for occasional checkups and at each visit he said:

"I'm doing well, but I still experience symptoms when I'm exposed to chemical fumes and odors at work. Yet, they're better now that they've changed the place I work in the plant."

Then in 1993, Paul called and reported he was experiencing some of his old problems. During our conversations, I learned that he was still working in the factory and was exposed to chemicals. He also was a part-time farmer and sprayed chemicals on his crops. Yet, he said:

"In spite of these symptoms, I'm still much, much better than I was ten years ago before I started on the diet, nystatin and supplements."

I told Paul that I felt that the chemical exposure was probably the main cause of his recurring symptoms. I was especially worried about the work he was doing with agricultural chemicals, so I advised him to have someone else do that part of the job. And I said:

"I know from what you've told me that you need to make a living from your factory work and your farm work. Yet, if you continue to experience symptoms, you may have to make a living doing something that doesn't make you sick."

REFERENCE

1. Crook, W.G., *The Yeast Connection*, Third Edition, Professional Books, Jackson, TN and Vintage Books, New York, 1986; pp 187–188.

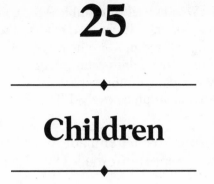

25

Children

Should a chapter on children be included in a book which focuses on the health problems of women? I asked myself this question from time to time as I gathered information for this book.

Because of the many letters I received from women who told me of yeast-related health problems in their children, I began to feel that such a chapter would be appropriate. One reason is, of course, that women are usually the main caretaker for their children. But, if I had any doubts about my decision, I put them aside after receiving a letter from Ellen Blake in August 1994. Here are excerpts.

> "I'm writing you this letter on an impulse. I have candida-related health problems and have been successfully treated by my gynecologist. Now I'm reading your book, *The Yeast Connection,* to learn all that I can, so that I can treat my children as well. They've both been troubled by chronic ear infections and my older daughter has some symptoms of candida; my younger child does not, but I would like to prevent them.
>
> "As you well know, many physicians don't even consider candida in their diagnosis and treatment. It infuriates me! My question is this: How can I, and all the other believers, including mothers, get the AMA (or whoever) to require nystatin when antibiotics are prescribed for children and adults? Why hasn't this occurred to them yet?
>
> "I'm extremely interested in 'crusading' for this. I'm one of those who was told by many doctors, 'It's a woman's thing. Live with it.'

I thank God that Dr. Michael Burnhill had the courage to try something new for his patients. He changed my life. I would like to bring this relief to everyone and prevent the problems in our children.

"Thank you for your kindness and taking the time to review my letter. My address and phone number are listed below if you'd like to get in touch with me. Appreciatively, Ellen."

As you might guess, that letter made my day, and here now is my discussion of yeast-related disorders in children.

My first significant experience with a yeast-related disorder in a child came many years ago. It was some 9½ months after I returned to the USA from France at the end of WWII. At the age of only a few days, Elizabeth, my first born daughter, developed white patches in her mouth.

At first my wife, Betsy, and I thought they were fragments of milk. But when we couldn't wipe them away with a soft cloth, I realized that Elizabeth had *thrush*, a mild infection caused by *Candida albicans*.

We painted Elizabeth's mouth with a bright purple solution (gentian violet) several times a day for three days. The mouth rash disappeared and Elizabeth seemed no worse for the experience.

During my many years of pediatric practice, I saw other infants—and occasionally an older child—with thrush. And in the 1960s, I read an article in a pediatric journal which said in effect:

> "At least half of the chronic diaper rashes experienced by young infants are caused, in part, by *Candida albicans*. And to handle them properly, anticandida agents should be a part of the treatment program."

Yet, it wasn't until 1979 that I first learned from Dr. Truss that superficial and seemingly innocent yeast infections could play a part in causing symptoms in distant organs in people of all ages—and both sexes—including children.

The Observations of Orian Truss

In his article, "The Role of *Candida albicans* in Human Illness," Dr. Truss dealt mainly with adults. Yet, he also commented about children's health problems. And in summarizing the categories of illness in which the relationship of yeast is well established, as well as those in which the evidence is strongly suggestive, he listed six different categories including infants, children and teenagers. And in discussing problems in this age group, he said:

"Infants and children with frequent infections and much antibiotic. Bowel disturbances, oral thrush, diaper rash, and respiratory allergy are common. Chronic irritability and hyperactivity, and even one case of stuttering, have been seen in children, many of whom carry the diagnosis of 'learning disabled.'

"The manifestations of candidiasis after puberty . . . interference with sex hormone physiology is added to the manifestations of the childhood years, often with devastating effect on mood and on intellectual functions. It is vital to recognize this problem in early adolescence . . ."[1]

In his book *The Missing Diagnosis*, in the chapter on infants and children, Truss commented:

"The problem of chronic candidiasis in infants and children is especially important, not only as it relates to their health at this period of their lives, but also as it may relate to problems with yeast later in life."

Truss pointed out that antibiotics are frequently given to an infant for a respiratory infection such as a cold, bronchitis or otitis. And he said:

"After the use of antibiotic has been discontinued, the previous state of health may not return . . . Restlessness, discontent and irritability often accompany the runny nose."

And he presented in detail the story of a 16-month-old boy who gave a history of almost constant health problems beginning at the age of 2½ months. During that time, the infant was given his first antibiotic for a cold. *During the ensuing months, he was given antibiotics repeatedly for ear and other infections. And at the age of 10 months, tubes were put into both ears.*

In spite of the antibiotics and the tubes, the child's respiratory problems continued. At the time of the child's first visit, Dr. Truss prescribed oral nystatin. After one week, the mother reported that the child felt better all over and was "running around and clapping his hands."

During the ensuing ten weeks, the child was essentially asymptomatic. At that point, Dr. Truss decided to stop the nystatin to see if it was no longer needed. But when the loose stools returned, he was again placed on nystatin and it was continued during the next four months. Dr. Truss commented:

"The month was October when it was discontinued. The next time I heard from his mother was the following April. She said he might be having a little hay fever from the pollen, but he had a good winter.

"Once again illness that had turned into a nightmare was suddenly reversed by thinking of and treating chronic candidiasis. The abruptness of the reversal of so many symptoms once nystatin was started leaves little doubt that the yeast problem had underlain the vicious cycle . . ."

In his continuing discussion of this child's symptoms which included crying, irritability, inability to sleep, constant diarrhea, cough and chronic discomfort in both ears, Truss said:

"In my opinion, this is not an isolated problem. In fact, it is probably very common. Antibiotics save countless lives, but as with most forms of medical treatment, some individuals are left with residual problems related to their use.

"Perhaps a single most fascinating and potentially important aspect of this case was the abrupt cessation of the ear infections. *This suggests that Candida albicans was actually causing this problem and makes one wonder about the possible relationship of this yeast to what seems almost a national epidemic of otitis and 'tubes in the ears.'"*

Truss also discusses other health problems in children, including learning disabilities and depression. He said:

"At any age, but particularly in young children who experience difficulty with school, this condition [meaning candidiasis] is worth considering."[2]

Observations and Experiences in My Own Practice

Although I didn't know that systemic and nervous symptoms in my pediatric patients could be yeast related, beginning in the late 1950s I learned that such symptoms were often caused by food sensitivities. Common troublemakers included especially milk, wheat, corn, chocolate and egg.

Yet, it wasn't until the early '70s that I learned that the ingestion of cane, beet or corn sugar were important causes of hyperactivity—even though I didn't understand the mechanism. Here are typical comments of parents excerpted from my office records.

CRS, 2¹/₂-year-old girl: "As little as one teaspoon of sugar will cause constant crying, irritability and tantrums. Since taken off sugar, I feel as though someone has given me a different child."

WO, 6-year-old boy: "Even a few bites of sugar, corn or eggs cause hyperactivity, nervousness, stuffy nose, hoarseness and other symptoms. Last year when W. was in kindergarten, he had continued problems with discipline, paying attention to the teacher and being still in class. This year he is learning very fast and is in the top group in all of his classes."

P, 9-year-old boy: "Peter's worst troublemakers are sugar and corn. However, wheat, potato, milk and egg also cause problems. During the elimination diet, I found that it was plain old sugar out of the sugar bowl that caused the severe hyperactivity and we suffered for three days. He's doing beautifully now because we constantly watch his diet and give him food extract injections every 4 or 5 days."

JRW, 8-year-old boy: "Table sugar is our worst offender. Other sugars cause trouble to some extent. Hot dogs also cause a terrific reaction."

In the 1970s, at the suggestion of the late Dr. Amos Christie (my pediatric chief at Vanderbilt), I kept a record of every new patient who came to see me because of complaints of hyperactivity, attention deficits and other behavior and learning problems.

During a five-year period (January 1, 1973—December 31, 1977), I saw 182 children with these complaints. They ranged in age from 18 months to ten years. However, most were between four and eight.

Each child was given a comprehensive workup which included a carefully planned and executed seven-day elimination diet. Permitted foods included any meat but bacon, sausage, hot dogs and luncheon meat; any vegetable but corn; any fruit but citrus; any grain but wheat and corn. Here are the dietary ingredients which were eliminated: beet and cane sugar, milk, wheat, corn, egg, chocolate, yeast, citrus and food coloring and additives. *If and when the child's symptoms improved (as they usually did), the eliminated foods were returned to the diet one food per day and reactions were noted.* At the end of a five-year period, through questionnaires and personal and telephone interviews, I obtained the following information:

Seventy percent (128) of the parents were absolutely certain that their child's hyperactivity was related to specific foods in the diet. In addition, eight parents (4.7%) noted clear-cut improvement in their child's symptoms on the diet. However, the cause and effect relationship to specific foods was not clearly identified.

The foods causing hyperactivity in 136 children included sugar, 77; colors, additives and flavors (especially red food coloring), 48; milk, 38; corn, 30; chocolate, 28; and wheat, 15. However, many other foods were reported as causing trouble. I published my observations in the *Journal of Learning Disabilities* in 1980.[3]

The Controversy Over Sugar and Hyperactivity

My observations on the relationship of sugar to hyperactivity led the Sugar Association to invite me to a fancy golfing resort in Florida in 1981. I was "wined and dined" and I played golf with the president of the association the first two days of the meeting.

The night of the second day, I gave my talk and they naturally didn't like what I had to say. The following morning, I called my office in Tennessee and said jokingly, "If I don't get home, come down and look in the alligator ponds."

The Sugar Association then began to fund studies by a number of investigators, including Dr. Mark Wolraich and associates at the University of Iowa.

In the early 1990s, Dr. Wolraich moved to Vanderbilt University and in February 1994 he published still another study[4] which appeared to give sugar a clean bill of health as a cause of hyperactivity. Yet, a number of people expressed a different point of view.

Stephen J. Schoenthaler, Ph.D., California State University, in a letter to the editor in the *New England Journal of Medicine* said:

> "Wolraich et al (February 3rd issue), concluded that neither dietary sucrose nor aspartame affects children's behavior or cognitive function, even when intake exceeds typical dietary levels. This conclusion is not justified."[5]

In my letter published in the same issue of *NEJM*, I summarized my experiences in studying children with hyperactivity and other nervous system symptoms, and I noted that several other observers had published studies showing that some children are sensitive to sugar. In my commentary, I said:

> "What is the explanation for these sharply differing results? Although I do not claim to have all the answers, here is one of them:

Sensitivity to a dietary ingredient can best be determined by an elimination/challenge diet."[6]

Another professional who disagreed with the Wolraich findings, Michael F. Jacobson, Ph.D., Executive Director, Center for Science in the Public Interest, in a letter to the editor of the *New York Times* said:

> "The sugar industry must be pleased that a new study is being pointed to as proof that sugar does not cause hyperactivity in children. The study, conducted by Dr. Mark Wolraich, of Vanderbilt University . . . shows only that a small number of children whose parents believed they were sugar sensitive, did not react to table sugar (corn sugar, a widely used sweetener was not used).
>
> "Several previous studies, as well as numerous reports from pediatricians and allergists, found that sugar indeed causes some children to become more active, or to engage in inappropriate behavior. The effects of sugar could well be exacerbated by the effects of dyes or other food ingredients, commonly found in sugary foods.
>
> "The message to parents is not affected by the new study: *If you think your child is sensitive to sugary foods, remove them from your child's diet for a week. If you see improved behavior, restore foods one by one until you find one or more that trigger a reaction* [emphasis added]."[7]

Here's more. Further support for the relationship of sugar to hyperactivity in children came from a nationally syndicated radio commentator and columnist, Paul Harvey. In an article, "You May Crave What's Bad For You," Harvey said:

> "It is a cruel irony that people who are sensitive to some specific food and drink are likely to crave it. Responsible studies demonstrate that hyperactivity in children often develops because of sensitivity to common foods—including sugar.
>
> "Yeast infections in women most often result from repeated courses of antibiotic drugs and are aggravated by diets loaded with sugar.
>
> "Quite understandably, these studies were not sponsored by

sugar merchants. Instead, they represent recent research studies, as well as careful clinical observations over a period of 40 years, along with an ever-improving understanding of nutrition medicine."

Harvey cited my observations and those of others who had found that sensitivity to common foods plays an important part in causing behavioral changes. And he said:

"Dr. William Crook has invested 40 years in assembling empirical and clinical evidence relating to diet.

"As long ago as 1958, he reported to the Allergy Section of the American Academy of Pediatrics on Children 'whose behavior improved when food such as milk, egg, corn and wheat, were eliminated from the diet.' "

In his continuing discussion, Harvey emphasized the importance of withholding suspected foods from the child for one week, then returning them to the diet one at a time and noting reactions. And he said:

"Why do sweets often cause trouble for a child? In 1993 studies from St. Jude Hospital found that sugar promoted yeast overgrowth in the intestinal tract of mice.

"For intestinal or vaginal yeast infections, stay away from sugar!

"Again, people sensitive to some dietary ingredient may crave it. Your appetite is not a reliable measure of what's good—or bad—for you."[8]

Why and How Does Sugar Cause Hyperactivity and Other Nervous Symptoms in Children?

There are several different mechanisms. One of them was pointed out by Schoenthaler, who said:

"The study (by Wolraich) ignored the fact that high sugar diets, with sucrose ranging from 25 to 60% of caloric intake, may be displacing essential minerals, vitamins and amino acids necessary for brain function."[5]

Here's another possibility: One of my mentors and heroes, pioneer food allergist, Theron Randolph, M.D., of Chicago many years ago noted that sensitivity to sugar depends, in part at least, on the botanical source of the sugar.[9]

In my own practice, I also found that some of my patients reacted to cane sugar who did not react to beet sugar and vice versa. I also found that corn sugar or corn syrup caused reactions in other of my patients. Yet, some of these children did not seem to be bothered by cane sugar.

But 15 years ago, after learning about Dr. Truss' observations, I began to ask myself, *Is it possible that my sugar-craving children who show hyperactive behavior when they eat sweets are developing these nervous symptoms because sugar feeds their candida? And is this the answer rather than sugar allergy?*

Today I think this is certainly a part of the answer and I now feel that sugar-sensitive-hyperactive children (especially those who have taken repeated courses of antibiotic drugs) react to sugar because the sugar promotes the proliferation of candida.

Moreover, research studies, that I first read about and heard about in the late '80s and early '90s, suggest that disturbances in the normal content of microorganisms in the intestinal tract create what has been called a "leaky gut." Such disturbances lead to the absorption of toxins of various types and food antigens that normally exist in the intestine.

The attention deficit/hyperactivity disorder (ADHD) and other behavior and learning problems affect millions of American children. Moreover, the number of children with these disorders seem to be increasing. In my experience, the causes of these disorders resemble a jigsaw puzzle.

The important pieces include food sensitivities, nutritional deficits, genetic factors, lead, cadmium and other toxic minerals, psychological and other factors.

Yet, in my experience, if a hyperactive, learning disabled child gives a history of recurrent ear and other infections, and his hyperactive behavior is triggered by sugar, I feel that a sugar-free special diet and antiyeast medication should be important parts of his overall management.

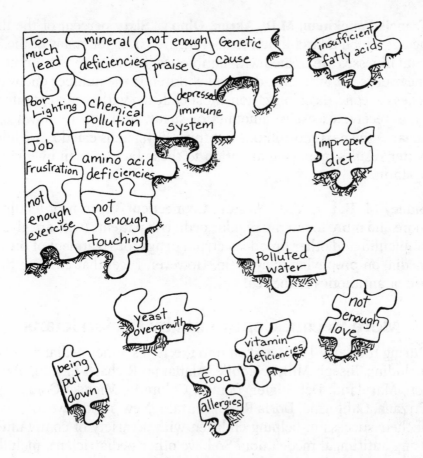

Comments of Physicians

At a conference in Dallas in the early '80s, several pediatricians told of their experiences in treating children with a low sugar diet and nystatin.

Aubrey Worrell, M.D., Pine Bluff, Arkansas   "Over the years I've seen kids who are sick one week out of a month and each time they seem to require antibiotics. A year and a half ago, I began to use small doses of nystatin three times a day for 4 to 6 weeks. My patients seemed to do better. I think it works."

Francis Waickman, M.D., Akron, Ohio "Sixty percent of the illnesses which take children to doctors are viral. Yet, many of these viral illnesses are treated with antibiotics. In my opinion, stopping the overuse of antibiotic drugs in children is the number one way to lessen candida colonization. Most children with recurrent infections receive excessive amounts of sugar. And cutting down on sugar is the next most important thing physicians can do. I've had better results by paying attention to these factors than by giving nystatin."

Sidney M. Baker, M.D., Weston, Connecticut "I'm now tending more and more to put my regular pediatric patients (who are given ampicillin and other broad-spectrum drugs for treatment of otitis media) on prophylactic nystatin. However, I feel that curbing the use of antibiotics is the real key."

More Recent Comments by Pediatricians

During the early 1980s and on into the 1990s, other pediatricians, including Joseph Miller, Mobile, Alabama; Richard Layton, Towson, Maryland; Del Stigler, Denver, Colorado; Michael Goldberg, Tarzana, California; Doris Rapp, Buffalo, New York, have told me of their success in helping children with a variety of complaints using antifungal medication. So have other pediatricians, including:

Allan Lieberman, M.D., North Charleston, South Carolina "I treat almost every patient I see, including children with hyperactivity, behavior and learning problems, using a therapeutic trial of the anticandida program. The dramatic results I've obtained in so many children encourage me to continue this approach. I've found that young children with recurrent respiratory and ear infections seem to really benefit. So do children, especially teenagers, with chronic depression."

Gary Oberg, M.D., Crystal Lake, Illinois "Children with learning and behavioral problems often have many causes contributing to their difficulties. Effective management requires identifying and treating all contributing factors. In the group that has received repeated courses of broad-spectrum antibiotics, treatment with nystatin and sugar elimination will often result in improvement of many of their symptoms."

Morton Teich, M.D., New York, New York "I've treated quite a number of hyperactive children and have done quite well with them, using the anticandida approach. One of our most significant findings in studying hyperactive patients was the history of sugar craving. This relationship is so striking that I've come to feel if the patient doesn't have some form of sugar and yeast craving, I tend to question the diagnosis."

Comments of Other Physicians

Physicians in other specialties have also made similar observations. Included among these physicians are, Harold Hedges, Little Rock; Nick Nonas and William Wilson, Denver; George E. Shambaugh, Jr., Hinsdale, Illinois; Sherry Rogers, Syracuse; Stephen Edelson, Atlanta, Robert Payne, Salt Lake City; John Curlin, Jackson, Tennessee and Young Shin, Atlanta.

In a recent letter to me, Dr. Edelson said:

"Today I'm taking care of several children, ranging in age from 5 to 12, who have attention deficits and hyperactivity. All of them are being treated with a comprehensive program which includes anticandida therapy, environmental controls, nutritional counseling and EPD immunotherapy. I've had wonderful results in several and good results in others."

In the third edition of *The Yeast Connection*, I included the fascinating story of a Utah child with yeast-related health problems. Here are excerpts from Dr. Payne's summary of her story.

"Susie (not her name) developed pneumonia at the age of 10 days. She received massive doses of antibiotics. Subsequently, she developed severe asthma and sleep apnea syndrome. She failed to thrive and weighed only about 15 lbs. at the age of one year . . . She was very unresponsive, sort of like a glob of clay. She also experienced continual respiratory infections and repeated asthma attacks."[10]

On a special diet and nystatin, this child showed a dramatic improvement both physically and developmentally.

To obtain a follow up on Susie, I called Dr. Payne in May 1994. Here are excerpts of his report.

"I talked to Susie's mother recently. She's doing well, has had rare, if any, infections, is vigorous, alert and does well in school. She's a perfectly normal child. It's certainly been gratifying for me to be able to watch her progress after all the problems she had the first year of life.

"I've seen a lot of other children with yeast-related problems who respond to diet and nystatin. These include children with learning disabilities, depression and emotional and affective disorders. Also, children with immune dysfunction and recurring infections.

"I usually keep these children on nystatin for a year and a half, along with a good diet and nutritional supplements. In regard to Ritalin, which is such a popular medication in Utah, I despise having my patients on this medication and I have gotten almost all of them off it by now."

In *The Yeast Connection* I cited Dr. Curlin's observations. He said in effect:

"During her teen years one of my daughters was an especially well-coordinated gymnast. Yet, ever since infancy she had shown periods of moodiness, depression and fatigue. Then at the age of about 12 she noticed periodic changes in her ability to concentrate and coordinate her movements.

"Because of these symptoms I put her on nystatin and an anticandida diet. On this program she did extremely well. However, if she did not follow her diet or take the nystatin, her moodiness and fatigue returned. Also, interestingly, she'd show a lack of physical coordination in her gymnastics.

"Our youngest son was fed only breast milk during his first six months of life and was continued on breast milk plus other foods until the age of one year. Nevertheless, he was constantly irritable and suffered from a chronic rhinitis. *Almost within 24 hours after I began giving him small doses of nystatin powder, his rhinitis cleared and he showed a noticeable change in personality. His irritability subsided and he became much more pleasant.*

"This was so impressive that his six older siblings could recognize when his daily doses of nystatin had been forgotten by the sudden changes in his behavior. Then when he received his nystatin, he settled down."[11]

Dr. Curlin's comments about his young son led me to speculate about some of the hundreds of crabby, irritable and colicky infants I've seen. Many of these babies experienced persistent abdominal pain and discomfort, regardless of formula changes or other treatment measures I prescribed. Moreover, I've seen many colicky or crabby infants who were totally breastfed.

Would a therapeutic trial of nystatin be appropriate for such infants? And would it be safe?

Again, my answer is "Yes."

Abdominal discomfort and other digestive problems occur so commonly in adults with candida-related health problems, it seems reasonable to anticipate that similar abdominal problems also trouble infants.

As already noted, candida-related health problems, including colic, should especially be suspected in infants who have received antibiotics, who have been troubled by persistent diaper rashes, and/or thrush, or whose mothers have experienced candida-related health problems.

Ear Problems in Children and the Yeast Connection

During over 40 years of pediatric and allergy practice, thousands of children with otitis media sought help from me and my pediatric associates. Problems in some of these children were difficult for us to manage and frustrating for the parents and the children. Yet, I can recall only a rare child who developed mastoid infections, or other complications.

Antibiotics save lives. No doubt about it. Yet, during recent years I've begun to feel that antibiotics may be causing unexpected, untoward effects. And they seem especially apt to cause problems in children who take repeated or long term courses of these medications for ear infections. My concern about today's management of middle ear problems is shared by other professionals, and in a guest editorial in the *Annals of Allergy*, Raoul Wientzen, M.D., a Georgetown University Infectious Disease specialist, said:

> "Seventy percent of children by three years of age will have suffered from a single bout of OME (Otitis media with effusion) and 33% of children will have experienced repetitive bouts of OME. *Fully half of acute care visits to pediatricians in this country in some way involve the diagnosis, treatment and follow up management of OME* [emphasis added]."

In his continuing discussion, Wientzen said that much had been learned about the causes, the diagnosis and the treatment of these problems, but he also said, "Much has not!"[12]

Wientzen also said that more than one million tympanostomy (ear) tubes are placed in children's ears each year in the U.S.; yet, by contrast, European physicians have not felt that this procedure significantly improves the prognosis of middle ear fluid over the long run.

In 1987, Kenneth Grundfast, M.D., Chairman of the Department of Otolaryngology of Children's Hospital National Medical Center in Washington, DC and Cynthia J. Carney, a health writer and a former contributor to the *Washington Post* health section, published a book entitled, *Ear Infections in Your Child*. I was especially interested in the two-page comments by Carney, *"From a parent's point of view."* She told of . . .

> "A blur of sleepless nights, visits to doctors, struggles with administering antibiotics and days of holding and comforting my lethargic and feverish child."

In her continuing discussion, Carney pointed out that even though she has co-authored a book about childhood ear infections, she does not have all the answers to her son's illness. And she said:

"Neither myself nor my physician understand why Brandon has had continual ear infections since he was eight months old, and my husband and I have finally accepted that we will never know the reasons."

And in his preface, *From A Doctor's Point of View*, Dr. Grundfast said:

"I've come to realize that many parents want to know more about the causes and treatment of their children's ear infections—the more information parents have, the more secure they feel in making decisions about care for their children . . . If you are a parent of a child who has been troubled by ear infection, and you want to play a more active role in the management of your child's ear infections, I hope that this book will enable you to achieve an understanding of a problem that has seemed frustrating and bewildering to you."[13]

I was pleased to see that the authors of this book pointed out that allergies to milk and other foods, and the frequent and/or indiscriminate use of antibiotics may contribute to recurrent problems. And I was even more pleased—even excited—to read their brief comments about fungal infections in children who had been treated with prophylactic antibiotics and to see their reference to *The Yeast Connection*.

In that book, I told of the observations of Dr. Truss, as well as those of George E. Shambaugh, Jr., M.D., Emeritus Professor of Otolaryngology, Northwestern University and a former president of the American Academy of Otolaryngology. I pointed out that Dr. Shambaugh urged pediatricians, otolaryngologists, allergists and other physicians to take a look at the allergic aspects of ear problems in children.

I also provided readers with a detailed report of the story of

Wesley, a youngster born in 1979. Like many American children, this child was troubled by repeated ear infections during the first two years of life. Although he was given repeated courses of broad-spectrum antibiotics, the infections continued to recur.

Wesley was referred to me for consultation in August 1982. A review of his history at that time showed, in addition to his ear problems, he was troubled by nervous system symptoms. At the time of one of his visits, the referring physician made these notes in Wesley's medical record.

"Having temper tantrums, beats his head and carries on for at least an hour. Bites his sister. Nothing seems to help. Attacks not brought on by frustration or being upset. Sleeps poorly. Mother worn out!"

Because of these problems, Wesley was referred to a clinical psychologist who advised a behavior modification. Yet, it didn't work and the hyperactivity continued. So did the bouts of ear infections.

At the time of my first visit, Wesley's mother told me that sweets of any kind triggered behavioral symptoms and corn was a major troublemaker.

Because of these symptoms, and the history of multiple courses of antibiotics, I put Wesley on nystatin and a sugar-free, corn-free special diet. In one month, Wesley was "like an entirely different child"; yet, when he was challenged with sugar and junk food, the hyperactivity and irritability returned.

Wesley continued the diet and nystatin on a regular basis for two years. Then he was able to relax just a little bit on the diet. Yet, major infractions would always cause problems.

In the fall of 1993, I called Wesley's mother to find out how he was getting along. She told me he was doing fine and she wrote me a letter to put in his chart. Here are excerpts.

"My son Wesley had repeated ear infections and took many, many antibiotics. We never spent a day that he hadn't cried. He never slept the whole night through. His outbursts were such that we were afraid he was going to hurt himself or someone in the family.

"When we took him to a physician we were told to send him to a mental health doctor. Yet, we found on our own that sugar made a big difference.

"Then after our visit with you we put him on a low sugar diet, nystatin, magnesium and vitamins. *The results were amazing.* Within a three to four week period a different child emerged.

"We now had a calm easy going child who was actually sitting on the floor, feet in the front, looking at the book. We had to take his picture because we had never seen him slow down enough to do this before.

"Wesley is now 14 years old and he still follows a good diet and takes a good supply of vitamins, magnesium and nystatin to control yeast in his body. He never had to take Ritalin or other drugs. He's doing well in self-esteem and in his school work."

More About Ear Problems
in Infancy and Later Hyperactivity

In a May 1987 report published in *Clinical Pediatrics*, Randi J. Hagerman, M.D., and Alice R. Falkenstein, M.A., M.S.W., from the Child Development Unit, The Children's Hospital and Department of Pediatrics, University of Colorado Health Sciences Center, Denver, Colorado, and Yeshiva University, Psychology Department, New York, New York, published the results of their study which showed that infants who had repeated bouts of ear problems were prone to develop later hyperactivity. Here's their abstract of the article.

"An association between the frequency of otitis media in early childhood, and later hyperactivity, is reported in this study. The subjects were 67 children referred to a child development clinic for evaluation of school failure. Ranging from 6 to 13 years old, all the children demonstrated specific learning problems, and 27 were considered hyperactive by two or more raters.

"Sixteen of the hyperactive children were treated with central nervous system stimulant medication. In retrospect, there was positive correlation between an increasing number of otitis media infections in early childhood and the presence and severity of hyperactive behavior.

"Ninety-four percent of children medicated for hyperactivity had three or more otitis infections, and 69% had greater than 10 ear infections. In comparison, 50% of nonhyperactive school failure patients had three or more infections and 20% had greater than 10 infections. Twenty-two of 28 children (79%), known to have more than 10 infections, experienced recurrent otitis before one year of age."[14]

In the discussion section of their article, these authors pointed out that not all hyperactive children have a history of early otitis and not all patients with recurrent otitis become hyperactive. They speculated on possible reasons for this association, and they said:

"Further investigation is necessary to evaluate etiologic aspects of this association."

In my opinion, repeated antibiotics given for ear infections set up a vicious cycle which includes recurrent infections and nervous symptoms of various types. Here's a chart which summarizes what I feel is happening.

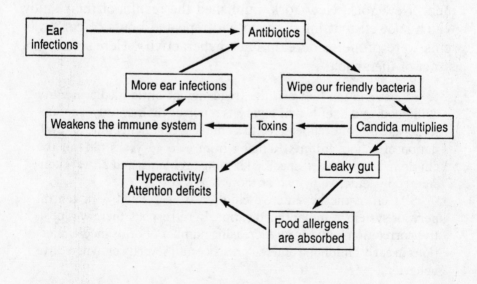

Suggestions for Research on Ear Problems in Infants and Young Children

In the third edition of *The Yeast Connection* published in the fall of 1986, I said in effect:

> "I hope the observations of Drs. Truss, Teich, Curlin and my own anecdotal report will stimulate physicians, both in practice and academic centers, to carry out studies to document the relationship of candida to—health problems which are troubling children and their parents and perplexing their physicians."[15]

Yet, few physicians were interested. In the late '80s and early '90s, I continued to receive reports from parents who were frustrated by their children's repeated ear infections. Here's a typical letter.

> "My son has had a history of chronic ear infections and I feel that antibiotics aren't the answer. In addition, I feel they may be causing the problem. Everywhere I go I hear other mothers frantically discussing the ear problems their own children are experiencing. Almost without exception, all these children have taken many different antibiotics, many times with no good results.
>
> "Nearly always the next subject mentioned is the yeast connection, which develops in these children. Many mothers tell of the extreme redness of the genitals and the diaper rashes. Tell me why the physicians are not required to advise every mother that yeast infections will occur unless precautions are taken. These include giving acidophilus and keeping the child off of sugary foods. Something must be done for these innocent children. I am outraged."

Public Meeting to Discuss the Diagnosis and Treatment of Otitis Media

In the spring of 1992, I received a notice from the U.S. Federal Register that a "public meeting on the clinical practice guidelines for diagnosis and treatment of otitis media" would be held on Monday, May 19, 1992, in Bethesda, Maryland.

According to the notice:

"Representatives of the organizations and other individuals are invited to provide relevant written comments and information and to make a brief oral statement to the panel. A consortium of three nonprofit organizations was awarded a contract to develop guidelines for *Diagnosis and Treatment of Otitis Media in Children*.

"The organizations are the American Academy of Pediatrics, the American Academy of Family Physicians and the American Academy of Otolaryngology—Head and Neck Surgery . . . Registration should be made with and written material submitted to the . . . American Academy of Pediatrics."

After receiving this notice, I wrote to the American Academy of Pediatrics and was invited to make a five-minute presentation and to submit written comments.

In my presentation, I emphasized the disturbances in the intestinal tract caused by broad-spectrum antibiotic drugs, including overgrowth of candida yeasts. And I cited the published reports of the Japanese researcher, Iwata[16,17,18], which showed that candida may act as an immunosuppressant. I also cited the observations of Steven S. Witkin,[19] a Cornell Medical School researcher who also noted that *Candida albicans* infections which develop following the use of antibiotics "may cause defects in cellular immunity."

I then cited the observations of other researchers, including W. Allan Walker[20] of Harvard and John Hunter[21] of England, who have reported that alterations in the bacterial content of the colon may lead to the absorption of food antigens (allergens). I also referred to the observations of the Georgetown Medical School researcher, Talal Nsouli* and his associates, who reported that food allergies contribute

---

*In September 1994 these researchers published the findings of a study which examine the prevalence of food allergy in patients with recurrent serous otitis media. They found that 81/104 patients showed a significant statistical association between food allergy and recurrent otitis media. The elimination diet led to a significant amelioration of serous otitis media in 70/81 patients.

significantly to ear problems in young children. These investigators stated:

> "The possibility of food allergy should be considered in all pediatric patients with recurrent serous otitis media. . . ."[22]

I also cited the research studies carried out at St. Jude Hospital in Memphis[23] which showed that sugar ingestion increased the growth of candida in the digestive tract. Finally, I pointed out that a handful of physicians, including C. Orian Truss and ear specialist, George E. Shambaugh, Jr.,[24] have found that the administration of oral nystatin (in sugar-free powder), and a low-sugar diet, interrupted the cycle of recurrent ear infections in a number of their patients.

Based on these observations, I urged the Consortium of professional organizations and the AHCPR to investigate the relationship of *Candida albicans* in the gut to recurrent otitis media in children.

Although I was given a courteous hearing, my comments and suggestions were not included in the 1994 report on otitis media by the American Academy of Pediatrics.

In my continuing efforts to bring the relationship of yeast overgrowth to ear infections into the medical mainstream, I wrote a letter to the editor of the *Ear, Nose and Throat Journal* which was published in the May 1992 issue. In that letter, I cited the observations and comments of Grundfast and Carney who pointed out a number of drawbacks to antibiotic therapy, including the development of fungal infections in children who have been treated with prophylactic antibiotics. And I said:

> *"Could these antibiotic induced fungal infections in the gut contribute to the epidemic of ear problems in American children? In my opinion the answer is YES!"*

In my continuing discussion, I said:

> "Based on the observations of Truss and my own observations, I'm writing to suggest a simple non-blinded study of healthy infants

in the hope it will provide information that may help interrupt the vicious cycle of ear infections. Here's a brief outline of the study.

- Infants would be enrolled at birth and divided into two groups.
- Infants in group A who experience an ear infection would be treated in the usual manner.
- Infants in group B would be treated in a similar manner. *In addition, infants in this group would also be given oral nystatin powder* three times a day during the time they were receiving broad-spectrum antibiotic drugs, and for one week after the antibiotic was discontinued.*
- Infants in group B would also be placed on preparations of *Lactobacillus acidophilus* three times a day for four months.
- Infants in group B who experienced a second ear infection would be placed on nystatin, 100,000 units three times a day for 4 months."[25]

During the two years since this letter was published, I've discussed the possibility of this study with several pediatricians, yet none of them have been interested.

If you know a pediatrician or family physician who would like to carry out this simple study, ask him/her to call or write me. Funds **may** *be available from the International Health Foundation, Inc., to help cover a part of their cost in carrying out this simple research project.*

Comments of Otolaryngologist
George E. Shambaugh, Jr.

In an August 1994 letter to me, Dr. Shambaugh said:

"I've seen a number of children in my practice who are troubled by repeated bouts of otitis media and related respiratory infections. Almost without exception, all of these children have been given repeated rounds of antibiotic drugs.

---

*I do not recommend Nilstat suspension (Lederle) or Mycostatin suspension (Squibb). Here's why: *They are loaded with sugar.* Instead you can obtain pure sugar-free nystatin powder (on prescription) from a number of pharmacies. You'll find additional information in Part Seven.

"In managing these children, I give them tiny amounts of nystatin powder, three or four times a day. My results have been quite good. The liquid nystatin has so much sugar in it that it certainly is not as good as the plain powder. Lacking powder, or when the patient refuses to take the powder, the tablets are useful.

"I think it is quite important for both children and adults to take acidophilus and nystatin during any antibiotic treatment and to continue it for a month after to prevent a flare up in the yeast problem."

Concluding Comments

Candida isn't "the" cause of ear disorders in infants and children. Yet, the response of Wesley and other of my pediatric patients, along with reports from Drs. Truss, Shambaugh and other physicians, suggest that a low-sugar diet and oral powdered nystatin could relieve much suffering and lessen the cost of managing ear problems in young children.

Other measures which may help include: the avoidance of tobacco smoke (and other indoor chemical pollutants); the use of elimination/challenge diets to identify sensitivities to milk and other foods; nutritional supplements, including soluble vitamin C powder, 100 to 250 mg., three to four times daily (If loose stools or other digestive symptoms develop, the amount of vitamin C can be reduced); Kyolic odor-free liquid garlic extract, five to ten drops, three times daily; zinc sulfate liquid, 5 mg., once daily.

The Yeast Connection to Autism

In *The Yeast Connection,* I told the story of Rusty, a 5-year-old child who had been troubled with recurrent ear infections and hyperactivity during the first two years of life.[26] Yet, his developmental milestones were normal until the age of 2½ at which time specialists at a university center made a diagnosis of "pervasive developmental disorder with symptoms of autism."

On a comprehensive treatment program which included nystatin, a special diet and the avoidance of chemical pollutants, the child improved significantly—even dramatically—although he continued to experience developmental problems.

I also told the story of Duffy Mayo, a California child with autistic-type behavior who improved on anticandida therapy. Duffy's story was described in the *Los Angeles Times,* and subsequently he was featured on Charles Kuralt's TV program, "American Parade."

Other Reports of Yeast-Connected Autism

On a number of occasions beginning in the early-80s, Bernard Rimland, Ph.D., head of the Autism Research Institute, San Diego, California, told me of reports he had received of other autistic children who had improved following anticandida therapy.

During the late 1980s, I saw several more children in my practice with autistic-like symptoms who improved on a sugar-free, special diet and nystatin. And during the early '90s, I received dozens of phone calls and letters from parents of autistic children.

Almost without exception, autistic symptoms in these children first appeared during the second year of life following repeated ear and other infections. I heard many similar reports at national conferences on autism (Indianapolis, 1991; Albuquerque, 1992; Stamford, Connecticut, 1993; and St. Louis, 1994).

I realize that autism, like many other chronic and often devastating disorders, may develop from many different causes. Yet, I feel that autism which first appears during the second year of life is, in many children, yeast connected. Here's a report I received from Elizabeth Smith (not her name) on November 16, 1993, which is typical of the stories I've heard from many parents.

"My 6½-year-old daughter, Melissa, was a normal healthy child during her first year of life. She was bright, alert and she passed all of her developmental milestones with flying colors. Yet, she was troubled by a series of ear infections. All were treated with amoxicillin and other broad-spectrum antibiotic drugs. Her autistic symptoms began to appear at the age of 16 months.

"I recently heard and read that a number of parents of children with late-onset autism improved following the use of a sugar-free special diet and the antiyeast medications nystatin or Diflucan. I'd like further information."

In responding to Elizabeth, I told her that based on the reports I'd received from many sources, late-onset autism was often yeast related. In our continuing discussion, I asked:

"Is your physician kind and caring—even though skeptical of the yeast connection? If your answer is 'yes,' I'll send you a packet of information which you can share with the physician. Then ask him/her if he/she will work with you and Melissa."

On December 23, 1993, I received a letter from Elizabeth. Here are excerpts.

"Dear Dr. Crook, I want to thank you for all of your help. It's made a big difference in our lives. Melissa is doing fine. We upped the Diflucan to 50 mg. a day and give her acidophilus three times a day as you suggested.

"When we first started the Diflucan, she told us through facilitated communication that her mind started clearing up. For about three days, she talked about it getting clearer. At that time, she said it was very clear.

"A week later she had an ear infection and was put on an antibiotic, Augmentin. Her mind immediately started 'fogging up.' Melissa was very upset, but improved when we upped the dose of Diflucan. Here are some of the changes we've seen since we started the Diflucan:

"She now sleeps through most nights and she's calmer. Her Dad and I are really enjoying that. Comments from teachers have also noted these changes.

"She's also told us, *Things don't move around when I try to look at them.* Her coloring has improved and her desire to color has increased. And she loves to color. As a matter of fact, for the first time, my walls, countertops and anything close has been colored on. Yet, it's hard to complain because it's so great to have her coloring.

"She has also increased her eye contact. She tells me that since my face isn't moving around, it isn't as scary. So she says, 'I like to look at your face now.'"

In her long letter, Elizabeth included comments about Melissa's reactions to various foods.

> "Sensitivity to common dietary ingredients bother her, especially sugar, orange juice, popcorn and carbonated drinks. Also, peanuts and fresh yeast bread. These foods make her feel bad, even agitated."

> "She now seems to be able to experience pain—she didn't in the past. Her eardrums would burst and she never complained of pain, now she knows if her ears hurt."

More Support for the Yeast Connection to Autism

During the 1960s, Bernard Rimland, Ph.D., published a book on autism. The purpose of the book was to show that this devastating disorder is not caused by the failure of the parents to provide the infant and young child with loving care. Instead, he pointed out that autism develops because of biological disturbances which affect the child's nervous system.

In the 1970s, Rimland established the Autism Research Institute (formerly the Institute for Child Behavior Research), 4182 Adams Ave., San Diego, California 92116. Through this institute he has provided information about the biological causes of autism to professionals and nonprofessionals, including parents all over the world. He also publishes a newsletter and collects and disseminates information packets and books.

In the October 1994 issue of *Autism Research Review International,* he included a 2-page review, "Parent Ratings of the Effectiveness of Drugs and Nutrients." Here are excerpts from this report.

> "The parents of autistic children represent a vastly important reservoir of information on the benefits and adverse effects . . . of the large variety of drugs and other interventions that have been tried with their children . . . The data presented in this paper have been

collected from the more than 8700 parents who have filled out questionnaires designed to collect such information . . .

"The 31 drugs listed first were prescribed by the child's physician in each case. Note that Ritalin, the drug most often prescribed, is near the bottom of the list. Only 26% of the parents reported improvement, while 46% said the child got worse on Ritalin."[27]

I studied the graphic charts in the report and I was delighted to see that nystatin (or ketoconazole) ranked higher than any other prescription drug. Of the 208 children who were given one of these medications, 49% found that the child was "better" on the medication and only 4% said that the child was "worse." The better/worse ratio was over 12 to 1.

By contrast, none of the other drugs showed a better/worse ratio of more than 2.7 to 1 and many prescription medications, including Ritalin, which was given to 1,661 children, showed a better/worse ratio of 0.5 to 1. (This means that twice as many children were made worse by Ritalin as those who were helped.)

The ratio for Cylert, which was given to 294 children and Dexedrine, which was given to 629 children, was also less than 0.5 to 1.

My Comment

This study does not "prove" that the manifestations in all autistic children are yeast-related and/or that antifungal medications provide a "quick fix." Yet, based on the reports I've received, as well as the research data gathered by Dr. Rimland, I feel that all autistic children should be given prescription antifungal medication and a sugar-free diet as an integral part of their management program—especially those children:

- whose developmental status was normal during the first 6 to 12 months of life,
- who were treated with broad-spectrum antibiotics for ear or other infections,
- whose autistic symptoms developed during the second or third year of life.

Rimland's data also showed that nutritional supplements, especially high doses of vitamin B_6 and magnesium, provided significant help to many autistic children.

Why Autism May Be Yeast Connected

There appear to be several mechanisms. One of these appears to be the direct effect of candida toxins. In a report describing his studies on candida toxin in mice, Kazuo Iwata, a Japanese mycologist, commented:

"Canditoxins produced unique clinical symptoms. Immediately after... intravenous injection (of toxin) animals exhibited ruffled fur and unsettled behavior. Toxicity was so acute and severe that the majority of treated animals succumbed... within 48 hours. Within 10 minutes after being given a dose of toxin, the animals became unsettled and irritable; had congestion of the conjunctiva, ears and other parts of the body and finally developed paralysis of the extremities."[16]

In a paper published in another journal describing his research studies on mice, Iwata commented:

"When injected into uninfected mice, Canditoxin exerted toxic manifestation in spleen lymphoid cells... This indicates the possibility that... the toxin produced in the invaded tissues may act as an immunosuppressant to impair host defense mechanisms involving cellular immunity."[17]

A second way candida may be related to autism is through the disturbance of the normal balance of microorganisms in the intestinal tract. When this occurs, the protective membrane lining the intestines is weakened. As a result, food allergens are absorbed which may cause adverse reactions in the nervous system.*

---

*See also the references on page 292 to the observations of Walker and Hunter in the discussion of ear problems in infants and young children.

REFERENCES

1. Truss, C.O., "The Role of *Candida albicans* in Human Illness," in *The Missing Diagnosis*, 1986, p 173.
2. Truss, C.O., *The Missing Diagnosis*, Second Edition, P.O. Box 26508, Birmingham, AL 35226, 1986; pp 77–82.
3. Crook, W.G., "Can What a Child Eats Make Him Dull, Stupid or Hyperactive?" *Journal of Learning Disabilities*, 1980; 13:53–58.
4. Wolraich, M.L., et al, "Effects of Diets High in Sucrose or Aspartame on the Behavior and Cognitive Performance of Children," *N. Engl. J. Med.*, 1994; 330:301–307.
5. Schoenthaler, S.J., "Sugar and Children's Behavior," *N. Engl. J. Med.*, 1994; 330:1901.
6. Crook, W.G., "Sugar and Children's Behavior," *N. Engl. J. Med.*, 1994, 330:1901–1902
7. Jacobson, M.F., "Sugar *Is* to Blame for Little Monsters," *New York Times*, February 24, 1994 (Letters).
8. Harvey, P., "You May Crave What's Bad for You," *Conservative Chronicle*, March 16, 1994; Vol. 9 No. 11.
9. Randolph, T.G., "Corn Sugar as an Allergen," *Annals of Allergy*, 1949; 7:651–661.
10. Crook, W.G., *The Yeast Connection*, Third Edition, Professional Books, Jackson, TN and Vintage Books, New York, 1986; pp 376–377.
11. Curlin, J., In *The Yeast Connection*, Third Edition, Professional Books, Jackson, TN and Vintage Books, 1986; p 196.
12. Wientzen, R.L., "Otitis Media with Effusion: More than a pain in the ear," *Annals of Allergy*, 1984; 53:369.
13. Grundfast, K. and Carney, C.J., *Ear Infections in Your Child*, Warner Books, New York, 1987.
14. Hagerman, R.J. and Falkenstein, M.A., "An Association Between Recurrent Otitis Media in Infancy and Later Hyperactivity," *Clinical Pediatrics*, 1987; Vol. 26 No. 5.
15. Crook, W.G., *The Yeast Connection*, Third Edition, Professional Books, Jackson, TN and Vintage Books, New York, 1986; p 201.
16. Iwata, K., In *Recent Advances in Medical and Veterinary Mycology*, University of Tokyo Press, 1977.
17. Iwata K. and Uchida, K., "Cellular Immunity in Experimental Fungus Infections in Mice: The influence of infections in treatment with a canditoxin on spleen lymphoid cells," *Mykosen Suppl.* 1, 1978; pp 72–81.
18. Iwata K. and Yamamoto, Y., "Glycoproteins Produced by *Candida albicans*." Proceedings of the 4th International Conference on the Mycoses, June 1977. PAHO, Scientific Publication No. 356.

19. Witkin, S.S., "Defective Immune Responses in Patients with Recurrent Candidiasis," *Infections in Medicine*, May/June 1985. p 129.
20. Walker, W.A., "Role of the Mucosal Barrier in Antigen Handling by the Gut" in Brostoff, J. and Challacombe, S.J., *Food Allergy and Intolerance*, London, Balliére Tindall, 1987; pp 209–222.
21. Hunter, J.O., *The Lancet*, 1991; 338:495–496.
22. Nsouli, T.M. et al, "The Role of Food Allergy in Serous Otitis Media: A Challenge for the Allergists," Poster presentations, American College of Allergy and Immunology. *Immunology and Allergy Practice*, 1991; 8:37. *Annals of Allergy*, 1991; 66:91.
23. Vargas, S.L., Patrick, C.C., Ayers, G.D. and Hughes, W.T., "Modulating Effect of Dietary Carbohydrate Supplementation on *Candida albicans* Colonization and Invasion in a Neutropenic Mouse Model," *Infection and Immunity*, 1993; 61:619–626.
24. Shambaugh, G.E., Jr., Personal communication, January 1992.
25. Crook, W.G., Letters to the editor, *Ear, Nose and Throat Journal*, 1992; 71:206–207.
26. Crook, W.G., *The Yeast Connection*, Third Edition, Professional Books, Jackson, TN and Vintage Books, New York, 1986; pp 189–191.
27. Rimland, B., "Parent Rating of the Effectiveness of Drugs and Nutrients," *Autism Research Review International*, Autism Research Institute, 4182 Adams Ave., San Diego, CA 92116, October, 1994.

PART

SEVEN

More About

26

Diet

Whether you're sick or well—or somewhere in between—you've read countless articles, commentaries and books which focus on diet. You've also seen and heard short and long TV programs which discuss foods of different types.

Those which tell you about contaminated beef, chicken and fish may have prompted you to eat more vegetables, fruits and grains, and fewer animal products. So have programs and advertisements which tell you that high fat diets promote all sorts of health problems ranging from heart disease to cancer.

Like you, and most other Americans, until about 25 years ago I ate the typical American diet, including meat three times a day. Bacon for breakfast, a hamburger for lunch and fried chicken or a pork chop for supper. I also liked ice cream cones, cokes and candy. Although I ate a few vegetables and fruits, high-protein and high-fat animal foods were major parts of my diet.

Pritikin—A Nutrition Pioneer

I first learned about the importance of high-complex-carbohydrate diets from the late Nathan Pritikin—a business man who had developed a crusading interest in preventing chronic illnesses through dietary changes and exercise. In his books, television appearances, lectures and in his programs at the Longevity Research Institute in California, Pritikin urged people to use less protein and fat and more complex carbohydrates.

Pritikin found that such diets helped individuals with serious vascular diseases (including high blood pressure and blocked arteries) regain their health without drugs or surgery. He also found that many people with adult-onset diabetes were able to throw away their insulin syringes and pill bottles when they changed their diets.

In the early 1970s, I was invited to give a presentation on food sensitivities at a conference in Florida which focused on preventive 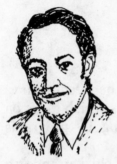 medicine. At a dinner on the last night of the conference, I, by chance, sat at the same table with Pritikin. The plates of everyone at the table, except for Pritikin and his wife, Naomi, contained a large serving of roast beef. By contrast, the Pritikins' plates were loaded with vegetables.

In the weeks and months following this conference, Pritikin and I began to correspond, and at some point he invited me to serve as a member of the Advisory Board of his Longevity Research Institute (LRI).

On two different occasions in the 1970s, I attended LRI conferences in California. At one of those conferences, I met Dr. James Anderson, a Professor of Medicine at the University of Kentucky, who for many years had recommended diets high in complex carbohydrates. I also met and sat at the dinner table with Senator George McGovern. And everyone at the conference was eating lots and lots of vegetables, fruits and whole grains—many times a day.

At one of these conferences, *a scientific study was presented that should interest you—especially if you've been bothered by memory and concentration problems.*

Here's a brief summary of this study.

Intellectual tests were given to people who came to the LRI before they started on a treatment program which featured a high-complex-carbohydrate diet and exercise. The tests were repeated after the same people had been following the program for four weeks. *Their findings: significant improvement in performance and test scores.*

In the third edition of *The Yeast Connection*, I told the story of my good friend and neighbor, Turner Bridges, who, at the age of 69, was found to have diabetes and an elevated blood cholesterol

(260). On a modified Pritikin diet, Turner's diabetes vanished and his cholesterol dropped to 165. Today, at the age of 85, Turner plays golf, exercises on his rowing machine, works on his home computer and enjoys better health than many men half his age.

During the '80s and on into the '90s, the importance of diets containing fewer animal products and more vegetables, fruits and grains has been emphasized by increasing numbers of professionals and nonprofessionals.

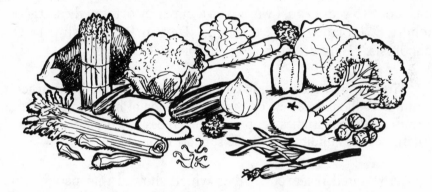

Proteins—You May Be Eating More Than You Need

To meet your nutritional requirements, you need to eat a variety of foods. And one of these food groups we call *proteins*. They're an essential part of your diet. You need them to build and maintain your muscles, hair, nails, skin, eyes and internal organs, including your heart muscle and your brain. Yet, according to the October 1994 issue of the *Mayo Clinic Newsletter*, Americans are eating twice as much protein as they need.

In discussing proteins in his beautifully written, comprehensive book, *Staying Healthy With Nutrition*, Elson M. Haas, M.D., commented:

"Our immune defense system requires protein, especially for the formation of antibodies that help fight infections. Hemoglobin, our oxygen-carrying, red-blood-cell molecule is a protein, as are many hormones that regulate our metabolism, such as thyroid and insulin. Protein is needed for growth and the maintenance of body tissues; it is vitally important during childhood or pregnancy and lactation. *However, we can eat too much protein.*"[1]

High-Protein Diets Play a Part in Causing Osteoporosis

While attending a Pritikin conference in Santa Monica, California, about 15 years ago, I was given a paper by orthopedic surgeon, Robert E. Morrow, M.D., entitled, "Diet in Relationship to Osteoporosis." Here are some of Dr. Morrow's comments:

"Traditionally the building blocks underlying a solid bone structure were thought to rest on the consumption of high protein food sources. Recent studies . . . proved this to be inaccurate . . . even a detriment to building firm bone support in our bodies."

Morrow cited research studies which showed that people who consumed a lower-protein diet were able to maintain a "positive calcium balance." He said that protein foods produce an acid urine and calcium is released from the bones to neutralize it. By contrast, vegetables and fruit produce an alkaline urine. So the bottom line is that people who eat adequate—but lower—amounts of protein lose less calcium in the urine.

In his 1993 book, *Food For Life*, Neal Barnard, M.D., in a section entitled, "Keeping Strong Bones," talked about how changes in diet and lifestyle may prevent this disorder which disables countless women—especially after menopause. He focused his attention especially on the dairy industry, and he said that in countries where dairy products are commonly used, there is actually *more* osteoporosis than in other countries.

In documenting his statement, he cited studies which showed that high calcium diets did not lead to stronger bones in a group of premenopausal women. And he said that although milk contains calcium, that, "for the vast majority of people, the answer is not boosting calcium intake, but, limiting calcium loss. As surprising as it sounds, one major culprit in osteoporosis may be protein—especially animal protein."[2]

In citing the reasons why animal protein may cause bone loss, he pointed out that animal protein has high phosphorus to calcium ratios (over 14:1). By comparison, the ratio in fruits and vegetables is more on the order of 1.5:1 to 2:1 and broccoli (President George Bush's nemesis) has about the best ratio of all (0.4:.1).

In his 1994 book, *Preventing and Reversing Osteoporosis,* nutrition authority Alan R. Gaby, M.D., said:

> "The American diet tends to contain too much, rather than too little, protein. Studies have shown that excessive dietary protein may promote bone loss. . . . The effect of dietary protein in osteoporosis might be explained in part by the phosphorous content of many high protein foods. Of course, phosphorous does appear to have an adverse effect on bone health."[3]

Can You Get Enough Protein from Vegetables?

From all that I read and hear, my answer to this question is "yes"—and the job isn't too complicated. In his book, *Choose to Live,* Joseph D. Weissman, M.D., commented:

> "Amino acids are the building blocks of protein . . . We must obtain these from food, but not necessarily from meat. In fact, we're able to use the amino acids obtained from vegetable sources very efficiently. It is virtually impossible to develop a protein deficiency on a vegetarian diet . . .
>
> "Another misconception is that it is very difficult to obtain *complete* protein on a vegetarian diet . . . The Seventh Day Adventists, many of them total vegetarians, have followed their own form of the low toxin diet and have an outstanding health history . . . A reluctance to change to a vegetarian diet may have social and psychological causes, but it has no nutritional foundation."[4]

During the past decade, I've also received a lot of information about the benefits of vegetarian diets from Drs. Calvin and Agatha

Thrash of the Uchee Pines Institute.* In their newsletters, books and lectures, and in their program at the Institute which helps sick people get well, they, of course, feature vegetarian diets which are lower in protein.

Sadja Greenwood, M.D., an Assistant Clinical Professor at the University of California Medical Center in San Francisco, in her 1992 book, *Menopause Naturally*, urges women to use meat as a flavoring for grains rather than as a centerpiece of the meal. And she said:

> "You can eliminate milk, eggs and all animal protein from your diet and still be healthy in your adult years. Complete vegetarians, known as vegans, get their calcium from broccoli, kale, collards and other plant foods (and all the protein they need in beans and whole grains)."[5]

Comments from the *Nutrition Action Healthletter*

This authoritative, delightfully illustrated newsletter**, has played an important role in teaching me things about nutrition that I didn't know before. Moreover, Michael F. Jacobson, Ph.D., head of CSPI and executive editor of this newsletter, and I have been friends for many years.

As is the case with friends (even with your spouse) or other family members, you sometimes disagree. And Mike and I took different positions on the importance of nutritional supplements. Yet, he has strongly supported me (and my friends in the health food industry) on other issues, including the role certain food ingredients contribute to hyperactivity, attention deficits and related disorders in children.

But back now to a discussion of protein. In the April 1987 issue of the *Nutrition Action Healthletter*, Elaine Blume said:

---

*Uchee Pines Institute, 30 Uchee Pines Rd. #15, Seale, AL 36875.
**Published ten times a year by the Center for Science in the Public Interest, Suite 300, 1875 Connecticut Ave., N.W., Washington, DC 20009–5728.

"Long seen as the epitome of nutritional goodness, protein is beginning to lose its glow ... Evidence is growing that consuming large amounts of protein can contribute to osteoporosis, heart disease and certain cancers. A high protein intake is also harmful to individuals who suffer from kidney disease."

> **Long seen as the epitome of nutritional goodness, protein is beginning to lose its glow.**

In the June 1993 issue of this same newsletter, associate nutritionist David Schardt, in an article entitled, "The Problem With Protein," cast some doubt about the relationship of high protein diets to cancer, brittle bones and worn out kidneys. Yet, he said:

"If you have high cholesterol, switching from animal protein to plant protein could help lower it. In some cases, dramatically. But the connection between protein and cancer, osteoporosis and kidney disease is less clear ... especially in healthy Americans.

> **If you think the more protein you eat the better, you're wrong.**

"Even so, one thing is certain—if you think the more protein you eat the better, you're wrong.

"The average American gets ⅔ of his or her protein from meat, fish, dairy, poultry and eggs. Only ⅓ comes from plants (beans, legumes and grains mostly). Unfortunately, most animal protein carries a hefty price tag—artery-clogging, saturated fat and cholesterol.

"But what if you restrict yourself to fish, low fat dairy and the leanest cuts of meats? Is there something wrong with eating that kind of animal protein? For some people, yes ... You don't need any animal protein to be healthy."

Fats

Fats are an important constituent of foods and are found in just about every part of your body. Like carbohydrates, they are sources of metabolic energy. They help move the fat-soluble vitamins across the walls of your intestines into your bloodstream.

Although fats are present in foods of all kinds, they're found especially in animal products, including meat, dairy products and eggs. So to reduce your fat intake, sharply limit or avoid these foods.

How's Your Diet?—Take the CSPI Nutrition Quiz

The cover story of the March 1992 issue of the *Nutrition Action Healthletter* was entitled, "How's Your Diet?—Take the CSPI nutrition quiz." Forty multiple choice questions were listed. Readers were given four or five choices with scores ranging from +3 to −3. *The higher your score, the more apt you were to be ranked as a "nutrition superstar."*

Here are a few of the questions which focused especially on your fat intake.

How many times a week do you eat unprocessed red meat (steak, roast beef, lamb or pork chops, burgers, etc.)?

a. Never		+3
b. One or less		+2
c. 2–3		0
d. 4–5		−1
e. 6 or more		−3

How many times per week do you eat deep fried foods (fish, chicken, vegetables, potatoes, etc)?

a. None		+3
b. 1–2		0
c. 3–4		−1
d. 5 or more		−3

How many times per week do you eat processed meats (hot dogs, bacon, sausage, bologna, luncheon meats, etc.)?

a. None	+3
b. less than 1	+2
c. 1—2	0
d. 3–4	−1

Many other questions on this quiz dealt with other dietary ingredients, including fruits and vegetables. And as you might guess, you'd make a high score if you consumed a lot more of these foods. Yet, you'd end up with a low (or even a "minus") score if you loaded up on fats, processed foods or sugar.

Why High Fat Diets Lead to Health Problems

Why are you more apt to experience health problems if you consume a high fat diet? Here are a few of the reasons.

1. Such diets cause you to put on extra pounds. And people who are overweight are more apt to develop diabetes, high blood pressure and other health problems. Fats are rich in calories (270 calories per ounce, as compared to 120 calories per ounce in carbohydrates and proteins). So if you want to control your weight, cutting down on your fat intake should rank high on your list of priorities.
2. Most fats, especially those found in animal products, contain relatively few vitamins, minerals or fiber. So the calories in these foods are often labeled "empty."
3. High fat diets make you more apt to develop heart disease and cancer. In discussing this relationship in their book, *World Medicine,* Tom Monte and the editors of East/West Natural Health, cited the 1979 recommendations of the U.S. Surgeon General, which urged Americans to reduce the overall fat intake to reduce their risk of cancer and heart disease.

They also cited a 1990 report in the *New England Journal of Medicine* which studied the relationship between diet and colon cancer. In this six year study, researchers followed 88,751 women between the ages of 34 and 59, according to dietary habits and health patterns. And they said:

> "The results showed that as fat intake and red meat consumption rose, so too did the rates of colon cancer. Those eating the most animal fat were twice as likely to develop colon cancer as those eating the least. These findings were consistent with an enormous body of evidence that has been showing for decades that dietary fat causes colon cancer."[6]

In his book, *Staying Healthy with Nutrition,*[7] Elson M. Haas, M.D., pointed out that there's also an association between excessive dietary fat intake and cancers of the breast, uterus and ovaries.

Why do high fat diets cause cancer? I'm sure there may be many reasons, including some that I know about and some that I do not. I first learned one of these reasons from Dr. Joseph Weissman, and I again cite comments from his book, *Choose to Live*.

He pointed out that man-made chemicals of many kinds pollute our water, air and soil. These include petrochemicals, coal tar derivatives and industrial byproducts and wastes of many types. These pollutants make their way into the air we breathe, the water we drink and the food we eat. And he said:

> "All foods are affected: fruits, vegetables, grain, fish, poultry, eggs, dairy products. Some foods store more toxins than others for some are *bioconcentrators* and *biomagnifiers*."[8]

This means that when an animal consumes a toxic substance (for example DDT), it is concentrated and stored in the fat. Moreover, even lean meat, chicken and fish contain high concentrations of these xenobiotic chemicals. Dr. Weissman feels that these chemicals have been responsible for "the appearance of new man-made diseases."

Sources of Pesticide Residues in the U.S. Diet

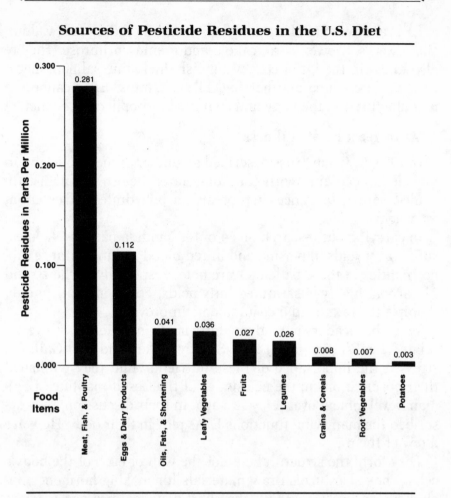

Source: Modified from data in G. Q. LIpscomb and R. E. Duggan, "Dietary Intake of Pesticide Chemicals in the U.S.," *Pesticides Monitoring Journal* 2 (1969): 162–69; and P. E. Cornelliussen, "Pesticide Residues in Total Diet Samples," *Pesticides Monitoring Journal* 2: (1969) 140–52, 5: (1872) 313–30.

More About Fats—Especially the Good Fats

Everywhere you turn, someone is bashing fats. And rightly so. But let's not throw out the baby with the bath water. *You should not avoid all fats because there are good ones, as well as bad ones. The good ones are called essential fatty acids (EFAs). You need them to enjoy good health.*

EFAs are found in plants and their seeds, including flax, walnut, sunflower, safflower, corn, canola and evening primrose. They're also found in the fat of cold water fish, including salmon, mackerel, sardines, tuna and herring. Like vitamins, EFAs cannot be manufactured in the body and so must be supplied in the diet.

EFAs in Yeast-Related Illness

In 1984, C. Orian Truss described a number of metabolic abnormalities in patients with candida-related health problems. Included were disturbances in proteins, carbohydrates and essential fatty acids.

In carrying out research on 24 of his candida patients, he measured fatty acids in plasma and in red blood cell membranes. Abnormalities in these patients were noted, especially in the 20 and 22 carbon, highly-unsaturated fatty acids. Following anticandida therapy, the fatty acid measurements improved.[9]

Two other leaders in studying fatty acids in patients with yeast-related health problems, Drs. Sidney Baker and Leo Galland, stressed the importance of these nutrients. And they published their observations in the newsletter of the Gesell Institute of Human Development over ten years ago. In their discussion, they described the many vital functions EFAs play in their body. Here are a few of them.

They form the structural core of the wall of each of the body's cells. They also furnish raw materials for making hormones, including the *prostaglandins*, the short-distance message carriers that are made by all of the cells of the body.

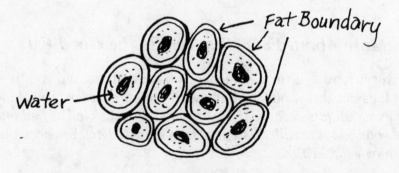

In his continuing discussion of the importance of EFAs, Baker points out that our bodies are composed of billions of cells of various sizes, shapes and functions. Each cell has around it a waterproof boundary that is made of oils. Numerous membranes inside the cell where the cell's "business" takes place are also made of oils. Baker has calculated that all the cell membranes of an adult human, if they were laid out on a flat surface, could cover about ten football fields.

Flexibility of these membranes, which is critical to their proper functioning, is imparted by the content of the EFAs. Essential fatty acids come directly and only from our foods. In no other way is the expression "you are what you eat" more accurate.

Because of their many diverse functions, EFAs are important in preventing health problems of many types, including eczema and other skin disorders, arthritis, heart disease and PMS.

There are two general classes of EFAs—the Omega 3 fatty acids and the Omega 6 fatty acids. Here's how they get their names. Each long chain of fatty acids begins with a carbon atom that has three hydrogens hitched on to it. This is called the CH3, or Omega, end of the molecule. Omega 3 fatty acids have the first double bond on the third carbon atom from the CH end of the molecule; the Omega 6 fatty acids have the first double bond on the sixth carbon.

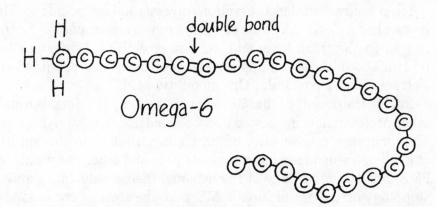

During the past decade, almost without exception, physicians treating patients with yeast-related health problems have used EFA supplements as a part of their treatment program. In the spring of 1994, in responding to my question about the EFA supplements he recommends for his patients, Dr. Galland said:

> "The majority of people are getting more than enough Omega 6 oils in their diet. What's lacking in the American diet are Omega 3s. I like to use flax seed oil as a source. Yet, I will use fish oils as well."

The usual dose of flax oil is one to two tbs. a day. It can be mixed with lemon juice and used as a salad dressing, or can be taken straight. Because flax oil can become rancid, it should be dispensed in dark glass bottles and kept refrigerated. Moreover, the bottles should be dated, as it has a short shelf life; three to four months at most.

Omega 3 oils can also be purchased in capsules; they, too, can get rancid after a time. In discussing the capsules with Galland, he said that the capsules which appear to have the least amount of contamination or peroxidation are MaxEPA and SuperEPA.

Along with the flax oil supplement, patients are instructed to eat more vegetables and to avoid sugar, alcohol and the bad fats (hydrogenated vegetable oils and saturated fats).

The Observations of David Horrobin, Ph.D.

I first read about the observations on essential fatty acids of this researcher in 1981. A couple of years later, while attending a conference in Montreal, I met and had dinner with Dr. Horrobin who told me about his fascinating work with oil of evening primrose—a rich source of a particular Omega 6 fatty acid.

During the decade of the '80s, I read reports by Dr. Horrobin and other professionals interested and knowledgeable in studying evening primrose oil. Benefits of supplementation with this oil included: relieving premenstrual breast pain and other symptoms of PMS; preventing atrophy of the lacrimal (tear producing) glands; stopping nerve deterioration in MS; and, improving certain kinds of eczema.

In 1990, Horrobin edited a book on the essential fatty acids which included articles by a number of different professionals, including two Scottish researchers, Peter O. Behan and Wilhelmina M.H. Behan of the Departments of Neurology and Pathology, Glasgow University, Glasgow, G12, Scotland.

These researchers used a special EFA preparation which contained both Omega 3 and Omega 6 fatty acids in treating polysymptomatic patients with the post-viral fatigue syndrome. Patients receiving EFAs improved significantly as compared to a control group of patients who received placebo capsules containing only olive oil. *Symptoms that showed improvement included dizziness, vertigo, depression, memory loss, exhaustion, muscle weakness, aches and pains and lack of concentration.*

In summarizing their observations, the Behans said:

> "There were no adverse events. We conclude that essential fatty acids provide a rational, safe and effective treatment for patients with the Post Viral Fatigue Syndrome."[10]

The Observations of Edward N. Siguel, M.D., Ph.D.

I first heard about the observations of this Boston University researcher from a presentation he made in 1994 on Dr. Jeffrey Bland's *Preventive Medicine Update*™[11] audio-tape. I learned more about Dr. Siguel's observations from an abstract of a presentation he made on April 2, 1994, at the International Symposium on Functional Medicine, Rancho Mirage, California. Here are excerpts.

> "The concept of Essential Fatty Acid Deficiency (EFAD) is well known . . . We believe that EFAD is associated with significant disease states and may underlie many of the chronic diseases prevalent in western societies . . . Individuals who maintain normal or low body weight by eating low calorie, low fat, processed foods . . . are at higher risk for Essential Fatty Acid Insufficiency (EFAI).
>
> "The huge social pressure for women to be slim, combined with their lower metabolic rates (and potential greater EFA needs with pregnancy) lead many women to diets very low in EFAs. The problem of EFA caused by diets low in EFAs is increased by the use of hydrogenated oils leading to elevated levels of circulating *trans* fatty acids. . . ."[12]

In September 1994, at the Natural Products Expo East Conference in Baltimore, I attended Dr. Siguel's lecture and took many notes. I also bought a copy of his new book, *Essential Fatty Acids in Health and Disease*,[13] and picked up a number of his handouts. Included were copies of articles published in the August 24, 1994, issues of the *New York Times* and the *Chicago Tribune* and excerpts from an article published in the scientific journal, *Metabolism*. Here's a summary of several of Dr. Siguel's recommendations.

- EFAs are good for you. They help to prevent and treat high cholesterol, high blood pressure and cardiovascular disease.
- Balance is the key to healthy nutrition. Linolenic acid (Omega 3) and Linoleic (Omega 6) are Essential Fatty Acids (EFAs). A balance of oils and foods rich in these EFAs helps prevent and treat disease.
- Very low-fat diets can be harmful and should not be used by people trying to lose weight.
- The cholesterol content of food has relatively little impact on cholesterol levels. Rather, it is excess saturated fat and calories which cause your body to make more cholesterol.

A New Book on Fats

At the conclusion of Dr. Siguel's lecture, I had a brief visit with a Canadian friend, Udo Erasmus. Later in the day, while visiting the Nutri-Books booth, I obtained a copy of Erasmus' new book, *Fats That Heal, Fats That Kill*. I can't claim I've read all of it. Yet, I read enough to say this book is fantastic! Moreover, it's written by an internationally recognized authority with impressive credentials. These include two years of post graduate study in genetics and biochemistry and a Ph.D. in nutrition.

This book, as the title implies, literally "covers the waterfront." It provides professionals and nonprofessionals with comprehensive, yet clearly written, information on subjects we all need to know about.

In his discussion of the good oils, he includes a discussion of flax which is one of the world's oldest known cultivated plants. He also points out that it's the richest source of the Omega 3 oils and is beneficial in the treatment of PMS and all major degenerative diseases. These include MS, cancer, heart disease and arthritis.

Erasmus also includes a comprehensive discussion of evening primrose, borage and black currant oils—the Omega 6 oils. And he points out that when these oils are taken, they must be combined with Omega 3 oils, including flax oil or fish oil.

In discussing the bad fats, he talks about frying, and he said:

> "Frying and deep frying are two of the most popular methods of (fast) food preparation, but they are also the most damaging to health. . . . Frying with oils will not kill us, and so seems harmless. Our body copes with the toxic substances. But over 10, 20 or 30 years, our cells accumulate altered and toxic products . . . (which) interfere with our body's life chemistry, our 'biochemistry.' Cells then degenerate, and these degenerative processes manifest as degenerative diseases.

Frying and deep frying are the most damaging to health.

> "Frying is not recommended, because safe frying is a contradiction in terms. Frying temperatures are too high. When foods turn brown, they have been burned. The nutrients in the brown material have been destroyed . . . Although frying cannot be recommended for health, some oils and some frying methods are safer than others. Knowing them can be helpful to those who will not give up this destructive practice."[14]

The Observations of Ann Louise Gittleman, M.S.

In 1980, this academically-educated certified nutrition specialist became the director of nutrition of the Pritikin Longevity Center in Santa Monica. In the foreword to her 1988 book, *Beyond Pritikin,** she said:

---

*To be updated in 1995.

"The Pritikin Center proved to be a refreshing professional and personal change. After three years in the public health field, I was growing frustrated with apathy toward change regarding the high saturated fat, high sugar and low fiber content of the hospital and federal food programs."

She said that Nathan Pritikin was always gracious and helpful to her. Yet, in 1982, she resigned her position as director of nutrition to pursue a wider field of clinical and research interests regarding the underlying causes of degenerative diseases. And she said:

"There was a whole new world of research findings which were coming to light about essential fatty acids, food allergies and *Candida albicans* . . . that raised nutritional concerns not covered by the Pritikin prescription."

Gittleman's book points out that the heart of the Pritikin diet is its extremely low-fat content. Yet, she said that his diets fail to stress the importance of the essential fats. She also cited a March 1986 article in the *New England Journal of Medicine* which indicated that oils, like olive, are just as effective in lowering cholesterol levels as a low-fat, high-carbohydrate diet. And she said:

"The Greek island of Crete has the highest olive oil consumption in the world and also the lowest mortality rate due to cardiovascular disease. Olive oil has been a staple in the Mediterranean country for 5000 years."[15]

The Observations of Joe D. Goldstrich, M.D.*

For a number of years this board certified cardiologist served as medical director at the Pritikin Longevity Center in California. Like other Pritikin disciples and supporters, he advocated a very low-fat-vegetarian diet for preventing and reversing coronary heart disease. Yet, he has now modified his approach.

---

*See also Dr. Goldstrich's comments on the importance of nutritional supplements in Chapter 28.

In the preface to his 1994 book, *The Cardiologist's Painless Prescription for a Healthy Heart and a Longer Life*, Goldstrich said:

"Diet is extremely important. If I had coronary heart disease, I would become a vegetarian overnight. However, most people can't, or won't, make all the sacrifices that are necessary to maximize diet therapy."

In his book, Dr. Goldstrich points out that people in the Mediterranean countries of Europe show little heart disease, even though they eat red meat. And he feels that a part of the reason is their consumption of olive oil. He especially recommends extra virgin olive oil or virgin olive oil, and he says:

"Olive oil smokes at 390 degrees. The better the olive oil, the lower the smoke point. Smoking oil is oxidized oil. *Never eat food cooked in oil that has been heated to the smoke point.* That oil is rancid/oxidized/spoiled. You have to be careful when you cook with olive oil not to get it too hot."

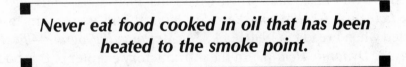

Never eat food cooked in oil that has been heated to the smoke point.

Goldstrich points out that fat is a necessary nutrient for health and that our bodies require the essential fatty acids in order to maintain a number of important and vital body functions. He also includes a brief discussion of flax seed oil and he said:

"Flax seed oil . . . is a rich source of the polyunsaturated essential fatty acid, linolenic acid. Flax seed oil is the richest source known for linolenic acid . . . It is the only major source of Omega 3 fatty acids for vegetarians."

In his continuing discussion of fats, he isn't nearly as enthusiastic about flax oil as I am, yet he points out that it can be used as a supplement or as an ingredient in salad dressing. He also said that vitamin C, B_3, B_6, zinc and magnesium are required if a person is to fully utilize and enjoy the benefits of flax seed oil.

In making a further recommendation about olive oil, he said:

> "It is best not to use either butter or margarine. If you need to put some fat on your bread or vegetables, try a little olive oil like the Italians and Greeks, who have the lowest coronary heart disease risk."[16]

Complex Carbohydrates

As I have repeatedly emphasized in many places in this book, complex carbohydrates, especially vegetables, play a critically important role in enabling you to enjoy good health.

The Observations of John A. McDougall, M.D.

While in the "green room" of a TV station in the late 1980s, I first heard about John A. McDougall, a California physician, who, like Pritikin, emphasized the importance of vegetarian diets.

And I was fascinated when I read his 1985 book, *McDougall's Medicine—A Challenging Second Opinion* and even more fascinated when I read his 1990 book, *The McDougall Program—Twelve Days to Dynamic Health.*[17] In the introductory chapter of this book, he told how and why he became interested in diets which feature plant foods. Here are a few of the highlights.

McDougall was reared in the 1950s on the traditional diet of eggs and sausage for breakfast, roast beef, ham, hamburgers, hot dogs, pork chops, fried chicken and other foods which were "washed down with big glasses of creamy whole milk." He kept eating these foods when he went off to college.

While in college, he suffered a stroke which caused a complete paralysis of the left side of his body. This experience played a major role in his decision to become a physician.

After finishing medical school and a year of surgical residency, McDougall took a job on a sugar cane plantation. There he saw patients with diabetes, heart disease and other chronic health disorders who, rather than improving, went slowly downhill.

Then, in 1973, in what he labeled as the turning point of his life, a friend who came in for a chat suggested the possibility that his patients' diets had something to do with their health problems.

> **McDougall began to ask every patient who walked into his office what he or she ate.**

So, in the months that followed, McDougall began to ask every patient who walked into his office what he or she ate. He noted that most of his older Chinese, Japanese and Filipino patients were in excellent health. He said that they were trim, hard working, felt good and functioned well even in their seventh, eight and ninth decades of life.

By contrast, the younger generation who had been eating a typical American diet were fat, and an increasing number of them were plagued with diabetes, colon cancer, heart disease and other chronic health disorders.

This experience led McDougall to become even more convinced of the importance of diet. And, like Pritikin, he began to write books to tell people what he had learned. He also established a hospital and health center in northern California. There he put together a 12-day program that has enabled many people to change their lives for the better.

In commenting on the adequacy of diets he recommends, McDougall pointed out that plant foods contain enough calories to meet the energy requirements of the active person. He also said that they contain plenty of protein (including all the essential amino acids), essential fats, fibers and minerals required to meet people's daily dietary needs.

Observations by Other Physicians

In the early 1990s, other physicians began to write and talk about the importance of diets containing less fat and more complex carbohydrates. One of these physicians, Dean Ornish, M.D., said:

"Vegetarian foods in their natural form are primarily complex carbohydrates. For example, grains, beans, vegetables, fruits and so on. Complex carbohydrates are very filling. In contrast, simple carbohydrates are 'empty calories'—that is, calories without any nutritional value. So it's easier to eat a lot of calories without being aware of it . . . Besides being more filling than simple sugars . . . complex carbohydrates are hard for your body to convert into fat."[18]

Simple carbohydrates are 'empty calories'—that is, calories without any nutritional value.

As you probably know, the Ornish program, like the Pritikin program, was designed primarily to treat and prevent heart disease. And *studies published in major medical journals in the 1990s show that heart disease in women occurs much more often than had been previously written about or talked about.*

So a high-complex-carbohydrate diet will not only help you feel better and improve your present health, it will also lessen your chances of developing heart disease as you grow older.

On the NBC "Today" program on Saturday morning, November 22, 1993, Jackie Nespral highlighted Dean Ornish and his diet designed to prevent heart disease. She also included comments of heart specialists who said that the value of such diets was "unproven." Yet, Nespral said that Ornish had attracted the attention of people all over the country, including Bill and Hillary Clinton, who invited him to the White House.

Neal D. Barnard, M.D., and Joe S. McIlhaney, Jr., M.D, have also recently emphasized the importance of complex carbohydrates. In his 1993 book, *Food For Life*, Barnard urged readers to eat more grains, legumes, vegetables and fruits in order to lessen their chances of developing heart disease, cancer, overweight, diabetes and other diet-related illnesses. And he said:

"The high fat content of the customary diets of western countries causes an artificial elevation of estrogen, the female sex hormone. Reducing the fat content of the diet not only reduces cancer risks, but also makes menstrual periods much more comfortable."[19]

And in his comprehensive book, *1250 Health Care Questions Women Ask,* McIlhaney outlined five basic principles, including reducing the intake of fat, sugar, salt and cholesterol. Here's his first principle.

"Increase the amount of carbohydrates consumed to where you've doubled the amount of calories you get from carbohydrate foods, especially those rich in fiber and low in refined sugar. To do this, eat more fruits, vegetables, legumes and whole grains. . . ."[20]

In discussing diets, Dr. McIlhaney cited the classic observations of the British physician, the late Dennis Burkitt, who worked for 20 years as a surgeon in Africa. For some years Burkitt was a member of the Advisory Board of the Pritikin Longevity Research Institute, and I met him at a conference in Santa Barbara in the 1970s.

During our conversations, Burkitt told me that heart attacks, gallstones, diverticulitis, appendicitis, hemorrhoids, cancer, diabetes and obesity affect people in the U.S. and other western countries in almost epidemic proportions. Yet, he said these diseases were unknown or rare in Africans who ate their native diets.

Such diets consisted mainly of vegetables, whole grains and fruits. Yet, when Africans began to eat the "typical American diet," they developed heart disease, diabetes, cancer and the other diseases which occur so commonly in the so-called "civilized" western world.

I was so fascinated by Burkitt's observations that I invited him to come to Tennessee, and he accepted my invitation. He gave the feature address at the annual "Ladies' Night" meeting of the Consolidated Medical Assembly of West Tennessee.

In his presentation he showed a dozen slides of vegetables, fruits and grains. He showed an equal number of slides of loose stools which resembled those passed by a cow! And Burkitt, said in effect:

"If you want to be healthy, you should consume a lot more fiber. It promotes a 'rapid transit time' through the intestinal tract. As a result, the healthy person will pass two to three loose BM's a day."

> **The healthy person will pass two to three loose BM's a day.**

Burkitt pointed out that most Americans—even those who aren't constipated—feel that their stools should be formed and shaped like a banana. Yet, he said:

"If you want to remain healthy, let the waste pass through you promptly so that your stools will resemble those of the healthy Africans."

Comments from the Lay Literature

During the past several years, many articles in magazines and newspapers have emphasized the importance of complex carbohydrates. One such article, in the March 10, 1992, *New York Times* by Natalie Angier, emphasized the nutritional value of plant foods. In her discussion she pointed out that some scientists propose that our forebears evolved largely as vegetarians and that people ate foods that were most easily available—plant foods.

> **You don't have to give up meat entirely to enjoy the disease-fighting rewards of plant foods.**

And in her 1991 book, *The Food Pharmacy to Good Eating*,[21] syndicated columnist Jean Carper, in a chapter entitled "The Vegetarian Advantage," urged readers to eat fruits and vegetables with abandon. She pointed out that vegetarians have a definite health advantage and that we should eat at least five servings a day. And she said you don't have to give up meat entirely to enjoy the disease-fighting rewards of plant foods.

In her 1993 book, *Food—Your Miracle Medicine—How Food Can Prevent and Cure Over 100 Symptoms and Problems,*[22] Jean Carper again emphasized the importance of foods, including the cruciferous vegetables (such as cabbage, broccoli and collard greens), garlic, soybeans, onions, carrots, tomatoes and all green and yellow vegetables, and fruits, especially citrus.

In April 1994 the cover stories of two important publications, CSPI's *Nutrition Action Healthletter* and *Newsweek,* featured *phytochemicals.*

What are phytochemicals? According to CSPI reporter David Schardt, they're:

> "...not vitamins or minerals. They're not fiber or complex carbohydrates. Yet, they could explain—at least in part—why eating more broccoli or soybeans or citrus fruits may help prevent cancer.
>
> "These are the hundreds—perhaps thousands—of *phytochemicals* found in plant foods. You've probably heard some of them mentioned in the news: *genistein* in soybeans, *flavones* in dried beans, *indoles* and *isothiocyanates* in broccoli."

In his *Nutrition Action Healthletter* report, Schardt interviewed epidemiologist John Potter of the University of Minnesota who had been studying the relationship between diet and cancer for more than 15 years. Here are excerpts from that interview.

Schardt: How many vegetables and fruits should we be eating?
Potter: More is better, but I don't know how much more. It's extraordinary how little we eat, though, and how many people don't eat any at all.

(In the late 1980s, the average American was eating about 1½ servings of vegetables, less than one serving of fruit, and less than ⅓ of a serving of legumes or nuts a day. That comes to about 2½ servings a day, not counting potatoes. And a serving is pretty tiny—only half a cup.)

Schardt: Can you eat too many vegetables and fruits?

Potter: I doubt it. The National Cancer Institute and other authorities advocate five servings a day. But for the last year, my research group has been studying a few hundred people who've been told to eat up to eight servings a day.[23]

In his continuing comments, Potter pointed out that initially people who increase their consumption of fruits and vegetables may suffer from considerable inconvenience, including more bloating and gas. Yet, he also said that their preliminary data strongly suggest that people eventually tolerate these diets, like them and feel better while consuming them.

Sharon Bagely, in her *Newsweek* article (which was put together with the support of Karen Springer in Chicago and Mary Hager in Washington), also quoted the observations of Dr. Potter. She pointed out that phytochemicals seem able to throw a biochemical wrench into one or more of the mechanisms leading to a tumor. "At almost every one of the steps along the pathway leading to cancer, there are one or more compounds in vegetables or fruits that will slow up or reverse the process."[24]

More recently, in an article, "The Live Longer Diet," in the May 1994 issue of *Longevity* Magazine, Peter Radetsky told about the findings of Cornell University nutritional biochemist T. Collin Campbell, Ph.D.

Campbell, in collaboration with scientists from Cornell, Oxford University, the Chinese Academy of Preventive Medicine and the Academy of Medical Sciences in Beijing, studied the diet and lifestyles of 6500 adults from 130 villages and 65 counties of rural China. According to Radetsky, the Campbell study was:

"... the most comprehensive study ever undertaken on the relationship between diet and disease ... the answers are chilling. Better cut way down, Campbell is saying, to every meat and dairy eating American, or suffer possible life-threatening consequences."[25]

Here are a few of Campbell's findings.

- The incidence of heart disease, cancer and diabetes in the Chinese was a small fraction of what it is in the U.S.
- Plant foods contain lots of antioxidant nutrients which protect people against free radical build up.
- Diets containing lots of animal protein cause girls to menstruate sooner. This, in turn, generates higher levels of circulating estrogen, making them ultimately more liable to develop breast cancer.

In an accompanying article in *Longevity*, "Re-inventing the Pyramid," registered dietician, Janis Jibrin, recommends a change in the USDA Food Guide Pyramid. The older four food groups were meat, dairy, grains and fruits/vegetables. Jibrin suggests replacing it with a pyramid which puts much less emphasis on meat and dairy products.

Here are her recommendations for the foods we should eat every day.

- 8 or more servings of whole grains, including whole wheat bread, pasta, cereals and brown rice.
- 6 or more servings of vegetables, including dark green and leafy vegetables, sweet potatoes, squash, cabbage and brussel sprouts.
- 4 or more servings of fruits, including citrus fruits, papaya, strawberries, mango, apricot and cantaloupe.
- 2 or 3 servings of dried beans and tofu.
- 2 or 3 servings of calcium-rich foods such as collard greens, kale, seaweed and non-fat milk or yogurt.
- Up to 4 tsp. of monosaturated oils, such as canola and olive.

And she said:

"Follow our guidelines and you can't go wrong; load up on the foods highlighted in each group, as special health gold mines, and you'll go even further towards the healthiest and longest life possible."[26]

Evidence is piling up at a fast pace, confirming that fruits and vegetables are full of exotic health-promoting compounds that boost bodily defenses against disease in all sorts of ways. There's no doubt about it. The message is clear. *Vegetarians, and even meat eaters who eat lots of plant foods, enjoy impressive health advantages.* Here is a summary of the health benefits of complex carbohydrates.

- They promote friendly intestinal bacteria which may counteract candida overgrowth.
- They provide vitamins, minerals and antioxidants.
- They provide fiber, promoting normal elimination, lessening your chances of absorbing food allergens and other toxins.
- They promote the absorption and retention of calcium lessening your chances of developing osteoporosis.
- They promote the release of glucose to meet your energy needs.

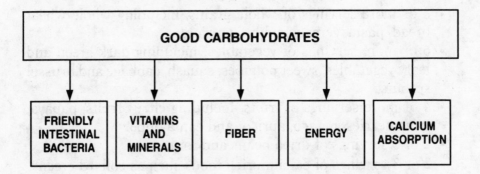

Are High-Complex-Carbohydrate Diets Always O.K.?

Like every other person, you are unique. Your diet requirements may not be the same as those of other people with candida-related health problems. Also, not all physicians agree on the diet that may be most appropriate for you—especially during the early weeks of the diet.

Candida pioneer C. Orian Truss emphasizes the importance of a diet low in foods with high yeast or mold content and also low in all carbohydrates during the early weeks of treatment. Then, as his patients improve, he tells them to increase the complex carbohydrates. In discussing diets, he pointed out that yeasts thrive on carbohydrates. And he said:

> "Limiting the intake of sweets and starches deprives candida of the nutrient that allows its maximum multiplication . . . Additional benefits may derive from carbohydrate restriction. Many patients are allergic to the cereal grains . . . Carbohydrate restriction may eliminate such food allergens from the diet."[27]

Candida clinicians who also favor a lower complex carbohydrate diet during the early weeks include Geraldine Donaldson, M.D., of Livermore, California, and Ken Gerdes of Denver.

In February 1994, I asked Dr. Gerdes to tell me about the diets he recommends for his patients with yeast-related problems. He said:

> "Basically I haven't changed much in the last five years. I still put people on a diet containing no sugar, no fruit and 80 grams of starch during the early weeks. Then, as they improve, I gradually increase the amount of starches and I bring back the fruit, one piece at a time, depending on what the person can tolerate."

In the mid-1980s, I interviewed John W. Rippon, Ph.D., author of a comprehensive text on yeast and mold infections, and a former member of the faculty of the University of Chicago. In discussing the dietary ingredients which promote the growth of yeasts in the digestive tract, he said:

> "Yeasts thrive on the simple carbohydrates. These include cane sugar, beet sugar, honey, corn syrup, maple syrup and molasses. *In addition, eating fruits promotes yeast growth.* Here's why. Fruits are loaded with fructose; in spite of their fiber content, fruits are readily converted to fructose and other simple sugars in the intestinal tract, thereby encouraging the growth of *Candida albicans*."

> **Yeasts thrive on the simple carbohydrates.**
> **These include cane sugar, beet sugar,**
> **honey, corn syrup, maple syrup**
> **and molasses.**

In his continuing discussion, Dr. Rippon said that in his opinion, peas and beans don't usually cause trouble because they don't contain a large percentage of utilizable carbohydrates. He also said that he felt that potatoes, grains and other high carbohydrate vegetables rarely, if ever, cause problems. And he said:

> "The whole grains are difficult to digest and whole wheat, brown rice and other whole grains are digested only slowly. Accordingly, they don't seem to be broken down to the point where yeasts can easily ferment them.
> "There really isn't any experimental evidence I can find on the subject except grains, by themselves, aren't utilizable by yeast. So it would seem to me that whole grains would be against the metabolism of yeast, in contrast to the fruits."[28]

Other Comments About Diets by Professionals

To gain more information about diet, in 1993 and 1994 I interviewed a number of physicians interested and experienced in treating patients with yeast-related health problems. Here are some of their comments.

Leo Galland, M.D., New York, New York: "The intestinal tract is one of the most important parts of the body as far as whether one is sick or well. I'm not talking just about food allergies, but the reason we're seeing an increasing prevalence of food intolerance is because of an unhealthy and imbalanced gut flora. The problem may be with the diet itself, or it may be from antibiotics or parasitic infestation.

"I use low-sugar and low-yeast and dairy-free diets to begin with. But I allow complex carbohydrates. Then if a patient isn't getting better, I'll put them on a very low-carbohydrate diet for 2 to 3 weeks. Then, most people can increase their complex carbohydrates without problems."

Harold Hedges, M.D., Little Rock, Arkansas:　"The symptoms in some patients with possible yeast-related disorders are caused by adverse food reactions. These patients clear on a seven-day elimination diet.* Those who show little or no response are treated with the full candida protocol, i.e., nystatin, nutritional supplements, etc."

Marcelle Pick, R.N.C, NP, Yarmouth, Maine:　"Sugar is the most difficult issue and 97% of the women I see have issues with this food. I think we have to be really careful when we introduce a restrictive diet to them because some of them go bonkers; it pushes them to their limits.

"I allow people to eat what they want as long as it's grains and other complex carbohydrates. I even allow them to eat fruit, although I keep them off prunes and raisins because of their high sugar content."

Walter Ward, M.D., Winston-Salem, North Carolina:　"I recommend a high fiber, high complex carbohydrate, low fat, moderate protein, organic food diet, including *Lactobacillus acidophilus* every day. On this diet I ask patients to eliminate wheat, oat, cheeses, fruits, coffee and tea. Sugar and mushrooms should be eliminated forever."

Food Yeasts Often Cause Problems

If your health problems are related to the common yeast, *Candida albicans*, consuming foods and beverages which are loaded with yeast may trigger your symptoms. Here's a summary of other things I learned from Dr. Rippon.

- People with candida-related health problems are often sensitive or allergic to foods that contain yeast. Yet, eating yeast-containing foods doesn't make candida organisms multiply.

*See Chapter 36.

- The yeast cell is composed of cytoplasm and cell walls. The cell wall is usually the most reactive part of the yeast organism. Some people may be allergic to cell wall and show no reactions whatsoever to the cytoplasm.
- There are hundreds of families of yeasts. The one we deal with in most foods and beverages are the Saccharomyces. They're found in beer, wine and breads, as well as brewer's yeast and baker's yeast.
- In beer and wine you have yeast protein, but you don't have yeast cell wall.
- All yeasts are not the same and nutritional yeast is an excellent source of enzymes, B vitamins and amino acids. So every person with a yeast-related health problem may not need to avoid yeasty foods.

> **All yeasts are not the same and food yeasts are an excellent source of nutrients.**

What I Learned About Yeast from Dr. Sidney M. Baker

In his delightful booklet, *Notes on the Yeast Problem,** Dr. Baker said:

"Yeast is a kind of a fungus. Mildew, mold, mushrooms, monilia and candida are all names that describe distant relatives of the yeast that inhabit ones body. Yeast also lives on the surfaces of all living things. It leavens breads, brews wine and beer . . .

"Yeast itself is nutritious; it manufactures (and smells like) many of the B vitamins, as well as other essential nutrients . . . The small amounts of yeast that give bread its good yeasty taste are not enough to add much directly to the nutritional value of the bread. Instead, yeast's contribution comes from its ability to release minerals present in the wheat. Zinc, for example, is easier for our intestines to assimilate if the wheat is 'treated' with yeast."

---

*Out of print.

In his continuing discussion, Dr. Baker talked about the diets he recommended for his patients. And he said:

"Truly yeast-free diets are impossible to come by. Yeast and other molds are ubiquitous on the surfaces of fruits, vegetables and grains and they can only be avoided completely by eating only fresh dairy, meat, fish and peeled fruits and vegetables. *So from a practical standpoint, the complete avoidance of yeasts and molds in ones diet is really not feasible* [emphasis added]."

According to Dr. Baker, the main sources of yeast in the diet include leavened foods (breads, bagels, pastries, pretzels, crackers, pizza dough and rolls), fermented and aged products, including alcohol, cheeses, commercially prepared juices (including any but home, fresh-squeezed citrus juices), dried fruits, condiments, sauces and mushrooms. In his continuing discussion of yeast problems, Dr. Baker said:

"Doing a five-day avoidance of yeast is one of the simplest and most reliable ways to find out if such a factor may play a role in a person's health. After strict adherence to the five-day yeast avoidance, a person may choose to 'challenge' themselves with a heavier load of yeast to see if it provokes symptoms. The challenge should be avoided if the response to being off yeast is so clear cut that no question remains as to the relationship between yeast and the diet and symptoms . . .

"The five-day yeast avoidance and challenge is usually done when nothing else is being changed and symptoms are observed from a few minutes to 2–3 days following restarting yeast in the diet . . . *Remember that once you have already decided that you are sensitive to yeast, you will need to be your own judge as to how much you tolerate various foods that may contain some yeasts or molds."*

You will need to be your own judge as to how much you tolerate various foods that may contain some yeasts or molds.

Reactivity to Candida Albicans and Sensitivity to Baker's Yeast

In a spring 1994 article, Betsy B. Jorgensen, M.S., described her research studies on yeast sensitivity. Here are excerpts from the abstract of her study.

"We evaluated the clinical records of 487 patients who had been allergy tested with the modified RAST (Radioallergosorbent) enzyme test for both *Candida albicans* and baker's yeast. There were 343 females and 144 males in the study sample—a Chi-Square statistical analysis of the data demonstrated a highly significant relationship between RAST responses to *Candida albicans* and baker's yeast.

" . . . Recommendations were made to eliminate yeast and yeast foods and products from a *Candida albicans* positive patient's diet for at least 3–4 months, rather than the usual 4–6 weeks. Reintroduction of yeast and yeast foods and products should be carefully monitored and be very gradual."[29]

As I've said elsewhere in this book, you're unique. And the diet which is suitable for you may differ in many ways from the diet of other people with yeast-related health problems. And if your health problems are candida-related, my recommendation is to "take it easy when it comes to loading up on yeast-containing foods."

Sugar Makes Yeast Multiply— No Doubt About It

Between 1992 and 1994, to learn more about yeast-related health problems, I "picked the brain" of dozens of people, including some 20 physicians. One of these physicians, C. Richard Mabray, a gynecologist from Victoria, Texas, told me about his reactions when he first heard Dr. Truss talk about the relationship of candida vaginitis to chronic fatigue, PMS and other symptoms, and he said:

"As a gynecologist, I found these stories difficult to believe because candida vaginitis was one of the most common problems I saw. Moreover, I was using nystatin orally and vaginally. And I did not see any of the dramatic results that were being described."

Then he said he learned to put his patients on a diet low in sugar and other simple carbohydrates, along with the nystatin. And he said:

> *"I was absolutely astounded. Within two weeks I had several people calling to tell me what a genius I was because for the first time in a long time they felt really good* [emphasis added]."

> ### Within two weeks I had several people calling to tell me what a genius I was.

Another of my consultants, gynecologist Philip K. Nelson, said:

> *"I've been amazed at the number of patients who reported an improved sense of well being by restricting sugar."*

Scientific Reports Confirm the Role of Sugar in Promoting the Growth of Candida

During the past decade, researchers have published studies which showed that the ingestion of sugar and other carbohydrates played a part in causing recurrent vaginitis. Even more impressive is a 1993 research study of mice with weakened immune systems. The animals who consumed sugar (dextrose) developed a tremendous increase in the growth of *Candida albicans* in the digestive tract.*

What Can I Eat? What Must I Avoid?

Thousands of people have written and called me during the past five years asking about diets. Here's an excerpt from a letter from Belinda which is typical of many I have received.

---

*See also Chapter 9.

"Dr. Crook, I've read and heard so many things about candida diets I'm confused. Please tell me what I should eat and what I must avoid."

Another letter came from John, who said:

"I know that sugar makes yeasts grow, and I've read that red meats, bacon, sausage and lamb chops are loaded with fat and aren't good for me. I also saw on TV that most chickens are now contaminated with salmonella bacteria and fish may be loaded with chemicals. And you're telling me that I may be allergic to dairy products, wheat, corn and yeasty foods. And that fruit and sugar make yeast multiply . . . *What's left for me to eat and drink?!"*

In replying to Belinda and John, I told them that I could understand their confusion and frustration. I also admitted that I had, at times, been confused by the different messages I've heard. Moreover, I've changed my advice on several occasions.

For example, the first edition of *The Yeast Connection*, published over 10 years ago, included three different diets. I also listed in grams the carbohydrate content of most common foods and I asked my patients and readers to carefully count the grams.

In subsequent editions, including the 1986 paperback edition, I urged readers to eat lots of low-carbohydrate vegetables, along with some high-carbohydrate vegetables. I also recommended meats for every meal. Because I wasn't satisfied with my recommendations, in 1988 I sent a questionnaire to physicians, nurses and patients to obtain more information about diets. Here are a few of the questions I asked.

- Do potatoes, yams, peas, beans and other high carbohydrate vegetables promote the growth of candida?
- Do you feel that grams of carbohydrate need to be counted?
- Does everyone with a candida-related health problem need to avoid all yeast-containing foods?
- How often do you find food allergies and sensitivities in your candida patients?
- Do these sensitivities improve following anticandida therapy?

The responses I received were interesting and varied. Yet, the great majority recommended:

- Avoiding sugar and refined carbohydrates.
- Eating more complex carbohydrates.
- Eliminating yeasty foods during the first couple of weeks of the diet, then experimenting to see if they really cause trouble.

I received different answers about fruit. One of my consultants said:

"The diet is already hard enough, and fruits are nutritious foods. So I don't eliminate them initially unless the patient isn't improving."

Another physician commented:

"Fruits are important troublemakers and I always eliminate them the first two to three weeks of the diet, then I tell people to experiment."

All respondents, without exception, commented on the sensitivities to common foods which were always present in individuals with candida-related health disorders. Major offenders included yeast, wheat, dairy products and corn.
Several of the people who wrote me, including professionals and nonprofessionals, wanted more information, including recipes which contained less meat and other fatty foods and more vegetables. And many wanted recipes and menus that would be tasty and would suit everyone in the family. One consultant asked, "Why don't you write a nutrition guide and cookbook?"

Since I didn't spend much time talking about nutrition in *The Yeast Connection*, I agreed that such a book was needed and I decided to tackle the task. In preparing my material, I reviewed many articles, books and other references. I also sought the help of Nell Sellers, a nurse associate and allergy technician, who had worked with me for many years. Nell and I reviewed and modified many recipes we obtained from various sources, including her own kitchen.

Yet, in spite of our hard work, I wasn't pleased with our recipe section. So I sought the help and consultation of Marjorie Hurt Jones, R.N., a professional cook, author and editor whose publications I had long admired. As many readers of this book know, Marge "took over" and together we co-authored and published *The Yeast Connection Cookbook* in 1989. Features of this book included recipes and menus which:

- featured more complex carbohydrates and less protein and fat,
- contained no sugar or other quick acting carbohydrates,
- featured vegetables of all sorts, including some most people know little about,
- included important information about the grain alternatives, amaranth, quinoa and buckwheat,
- provided kitchen and family tested recipes for breakfast—perhaps the most difficult meal of the day,
- provided recipes for readers with sensitivities to yeast, dairy products, wheat, corn and other common foods.

A Special Word About Grains

Over 60 years ago, Albert Rowe, M.D., of Oakland, California, began to write and talk about the favorable response of many of his patients to cereal-free, milk-free diets. Then in the 1940s, Theron Randolph, M.D., of Chicago, reported on the favorable response of many of his patients to dietary changes, and corn ranked high on the list of troublemakers. After learning about the Rowe and Randolph observations, I put many of my patients on elimination diets and was pleased by their response.

During the past decade, I've received reports from both physicians and nonphysicians who have found that wheat may play a part in causing their symptoms. One such report came from Edward Leyton, M.D., of Kingston, Ontario, who, in responding to my article on interstitial cystitis in the IHF newsletter, *Healthline*, said:

> "I'm writing to report that I've had success in treating interstitial cystitis with a yeast-free diet and a wheat-free diet in combination with nystatin."

In 1992 Dr. A. V. Costantini, an American who worked with the World Health Organization and now lives in Germany, talked to physicians at a conference in Dallas and again at a meeting of the American Academy of Environmental Medicine[30] in Sparks, Nevada, in October 1993. Although what Dr. Costantini had to say was rejected by some, others became "believers." Costantini especially emphasized the troublemaking effect of toxins which form in grains before they're ingested.

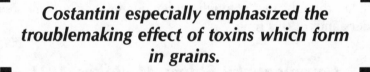

Costantini especially emphasized the troublemaking effect of toxins which form in grains.

In discussing reactions in her patients to wheat, Barbara Solomon, M.D., of Baltimore commented:

> "The gluten in the wheat is certainly a factor. Yet, another thing I've been thinking about is what happens in the stored grains. I wonder how much yeast the grain has in it when it's sent to the bakery.
> "Some people react to some forms of wheat and not to others. It seems to me it could be the mold the food had before it got to the bakery. So I thought Dr. Costantini's observations were fascinating."

Dr. Richard Mabray commented:

> "Hearing Dr. Costantini speak about fungal toxins prompted me to realize that as important as candida is, it is only one of the really important things.
> "When we encourage people to do a candida diet, we automati-

cally are affecting other fungal toxins as well. I suspect that is why sometimes things work so well. Dr. Costantini recommends that patients stay away from beer, bread, sugar, chicken fat, yeast products and grains, especially corn and wheat."

A "crusading" friend of mine, Elizabeth Naugle, College Station, Texas, has strongly supported the observations of Costantini. So has another friend, Maggie Burston of Kleinburg, Ontario. To obtain more information about his observations, I consulted Dr. Sidney Baker who commmented:

"Although I don't agree with everything he has to say, especially about uric acid, his review of the literature, including references to the fungal infections in poultry, is intriguing and I think he should be listened to.

"He's certainly making a point that must be true—that the interaction between human beings and fungal toxins, although complicated, probably has a much wider scope than anyone really understands at this time."

Comments by Sidney M. Baker, M.D.

As readers of *The Yeast Connection* and several of my other books know, I've cited the observations of Dr. Baker many times. Moreover, I included a number of his concepts, drawings and charts in Section C of *The Yeast Connection*. So to get his current thoughts about diet, I interviewed him again in early 1994. Here are excerpts from his comments:

"I try to emphasize to people the difference between a *diagnostic* diet and a *treatment* diet. A diagnostic diet is maybe three weeks. After that it really depends on what a person can tolerate. *I encourage people to experiment.*"

In our continuing discussion, Baker pointed out that some people, even those who are yeast, dairy and fruit sensitive, can take a little of these foods if they don't take too much, too often. And he said:

"Some of the people I'm seeing have been on a very strict yeast-free diet which has no fruits, no dairy products, no nothing. Sometimes they've been on these quite extravagant diets for a year and they haven't been doing any good, and they're still on it . . .

"If we're trying to promote good health, we should not be putting people on low carbohydrate diets with the idea that we're starving the yeast. Eating a diet rich in complex carbohydrates is the best way to promote normal bowel flora in the person who has some immune dysfunction . . . *We shouldn't be putting people on an unhealthy diet in our efforts to make them healthy* [emphasis added]!"

A Special Word About Animal Products

In the third edition of *The Yeast Connection* published in 1986, I included meal suggestions for the early weeks and more meal suggestions after the first few weeks. And I provided you and other readers with a dozen pages of illustrated menus for breakfasts, lunches and main meals. There were recipes which featured steak, meat loaf, sauteed liver slivers and a pork chop casserole. *This book contains no such recipes.* Here's why.

Based on scientific reports and observations of growing numbers of reliable observers, I am now convinced that people who consume varied diets, which avoid or sharply limit animal products, are much more apt to enjoy better health.

> **People who consume varied diets, which avoid or limit animal products . . . enjoy better health.**

You'll find dozens of superb, tasty vegetarian recipes in the books by Barnard, McDougall, Ornish and many others, including John Robbins' fantastically informative book, *Diet For A New World.* (An Avon paperback book which you can find in most health food stores and some bookstores.)

You may not be ready to become a vegetarian, but if you eat

meats, select them carefully. And in some areas, organically-raised animals are becoming available.

If you eat fish (which a decade or two ago were considered to be safe and health promoting), try to get ocean fish. They are less apt to be contaminated with chemicals and toxins of various sorts. Be especially cautious about eating raw oysters.

Also, as you probably know from reports you've seen on television, chicken, which today is usually produced on assembly lines, is often contaminated with salmonella and other bacteria. So are eggs. So if you eat these foods, *select and store them carefully and cook them thoroughly.*

Here are still other reasons for avoiding (or limiting your consumption of) animal products. Many animals are given antibiotics. When you consume these antibiotic-laden foods, they may cause alterations in the balance of the normal bacteria in your intestinal tract. Along with these alterations, *Candida albicans* may proliferate.

Farm animals are often injected with hormones. When their flesh or milk is consumed, these hormones enter our body. Finally, as noted by Weissman (and mentioned earlier in this chapter), animals consume insecticides and other toxic chemicals and concentrate them in their fat tissues. So when we eat animal products, we take on a bigger load of substances which Weissman calls "xenobiotics."

My Diet Recommendations for the Mid- to Late-1990s

Outlining my diet recommendations for this book hasn't been easy. There are so many factors which must be considered, including individual likes and dislikes, availability of desirable foods and preferences of other family members. Added to these are concerns about pesticides and other contaminants found in many foods.

I'm increasingly an advocate of vegetarian diets. Such diets can be balanced and tasty and provide all of the essential nutrients. *Vegetarians are healthier than meat-eaters. No doubt about it.* But in spite of the increasing interest and acceptance of diets containing few (if any) animal products, most people (including many of my consultants) like and eat some low fat animal foods.

> ## Food sensitivities are present in almost every person with candida-related health problems.

Food sensitivities are present in almost every person with candida-related health problems. They play a major role in causing symptoms, so they must be indentified and properly managed. You'll find a cornucopia of information in Chapter 35 and detailed instructions for carrying out an elimination/challenge diet in Chapter 36.

What's more, a Canadian physician, Ronald B. Greenberg, several years ago published a fascinating, comprehensively documented paper, "Is The Yeast Syndrome Food Allergy?"[31] In his report, which includes 87 references to the medical literature, Greenberg describes his experiences in studying 33 consecutive patients who felt that their symptoms were yeast related. Thirty-one of the patients were allergy tested and placed on elimination diets. Twenty-four (77.4%, p < .001) had a good or partial response, and seven had no response to the elimination of dietary allergens.

Why do individuals with yeast problems develop food sensitivities? Recent studies by both practicing physicians and researchers suggest that candida overgrowth in the gut may harm the mucosal barrier. This may lead to the absorption of incompletely digested food molecules which cause sensitivity reactions. It's what a number of clinicians call "the leaky gut syndrome."

Frequent food offenders, in addition to those already listed, include eggs, citrus and the legumes. *However, any food may cause an adverse reaction.*

Now, having said all those things, here are my recommendations.

- *Clean up your diet:* Avoid "junk" foods—foods which are refined, overly processed and loaded with sugar, salt, food coloring, additives and hardened (hydrogenated or partially hydrogenated) vegetable oil and other hidden ingredients.
- *Avoid all simple sugars:* These include cane sugar, beet sugar, fructose, corn syrup, maple syrup, honey and molasses. The candida "critters," like baby birds looking for worms, thrive on these simple carbohydrates. Sugar promotes the multiplication of *Candida albicans,* just as it does the tooth decay germs.
- *Feature nutritious foods from a variety of sources:* Eat more vegetables. Add to your diet once a week (or more often) kamut, spelt or teff and one of the grain alternatives, amaranth, quinoa, or buckwheat.
- *Divide your diet into two parts:* The first part, *the more difficult diagnostic diet,* lasts about three to four weeks. The second part, the long-term treatment diet, will be easier.

On the diagnostic diet you avoid all sugars and fruits and the yeast-containing foods, including breads, bagels, pastries, pretzels, crackers, pizza, rolls, fermented and aged products, alcohol, cheeses, commercially prepared juices, dried fruits, condiments, sauces and mushrooms.

Then, try the yeast challenge as recommended by Dr. Sidney Baker. If you pass this challenge, you can relax a bit and, in the days and weeks ahead, you can experiment further and decide how much of the yeast-containing foods you can tolerate.

If you pass the yeast challenge, you can add fresh, frozen or unprocessed nuts and seeds to your diet. I especially recommend walnuts, almonds, pecans, cashews and sunflower and pumpkin seeds. For now, avoid peanuts and pistachios as they are much more apt to contain molds.

During the diagnostic part of your diet avoid fruits. Here's why. Although they contain complex carbohydrates and furnish many excellent nutrients, they're readily converted into simple sugars in the intestinal tract.

After you've been on your diet for about two or three weeks, do a fruit challenge. Here's how: Take a small bite of banana. Ten minutes later eat a second bite. If no reaction occurs in the next hour, eat the whole banana.

If you tolerate the banana without developing symptoms, try strawberries, pineapple or apple the next day. If you show no symptoms following these fruit challenges, chances are you can eat fruit in moderate amounts. *But feel your way along and don't overdo it.*

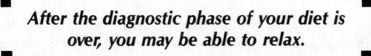

After the diagnostic phase of your diet is over, you may be able to relax.

After the diagnostic phase of your diet is over, you may be able to relax and go along with what I call the long-term treatment diet. Such a diet should feature nutritious foods from a variety of sources with a particular emphasis on vegetables of all sorts.

Food Allergies and Sensitivities

If after a month or two of a sugar-free diet, antifungal medication and other therapies you're still experiencing problems, you'll need to track down your hidden food allergies.

Here's a brief outline of the steps you'll need to take.

- You can eat and drink the following:
  —any vegetable but corn
  —any fruit but citrus
  —any meat but bacon, sausage, hot dogs or luncheon meats
  —rice, oats and the grain alternatives amaranth, quinoa and buckwheat
  —unprocessed nuts that are fresh, refrigerated or frozen
  —water, preferably bottled or filtered
- You'll need to avoid the following:

  milk   chocolate   sugar   citrus   corn
  yeast   soft drinks   punches   wheat
  processed and packaged foods   food coloring and additives

- Pick a convenient time for the diet; don't try it during a holiday or when you're visiting; before beginning the diet keep a symptom and food diary for three days; continue the diary while you're eliminating foods and while you're eating them again; if you're away from home, take your food with you.
- The elimination part of the diet lasts about a week, or until you show convincing improvement in your symptoms.
- The second week, eat the foods you've eliminated, one food per day, and see if your symptoms return.

If you identify one or more food troublemakers and are still having problems, you'll need to try the Cave Man Diet, since apple, chicken, potatoes or other foods may cause symptoms. On this diet you avoid any and every food you eat more than once a week.

- *Diversify or rotate your diet:* Even if you aren't able to carry out a carefully designed and executed elimination diet, by rotating your diet you may be able to identify foods that may be disagreeing with you and causing your symptoms.

In rotating your diet, you eat a food only once every 4 to 7 days. For example, in rotating fruits, you'd eat oranges on Monday, bananas on Tuesday, apples on Wednesday and pineapple on Thursday. Then on Friday you could start over again with oranges. The same system can be used with other food groups, including meats, vegetables and grains.

You'll find a further discussion of rotation diets in Part Nine.

What You Can Drink

Water Everyone needs to drink water. Yet this vital fluid, like the proverbial old gray mare, "ain't what she used to be." No longer can we turn on the water in our homes and offices and be sure that what flows out is free of lead and other contaminants. You'll find suggestions for obtaining safer water in Chapter 52.

Fruit Juices Whether frozen, bottled or canned, they're prepared from fruits that have been allowed to stand in bins, barrels and other containers for hours or days. All juices are loaded with yeast and molds, except for fresh squeezed orange juice or other freshly prepared juices.

Coffee and Tea   These popular beverages, including herbal teas, are prepared from plant products and are subject to mold contamination. How much mold is uncertain. If you aren't allergic to yeast, you can drink these beverages and experience no problems. If yeasty foods bother you and you can't get along without your coffee or tea, you'll have to experiment and see what happens.

Diet Drinks   *I do not recommend them.* They have no nutritional value and they usually contain aspartame and many contain caffeine, food coloring and other ingredients which may disagree with you. However, since they do not contain mold, you may tolerate them in limited quantities. If you use them, don't go overboard. (Read also my comments about aspartame in Chapter 27).

Alcoholic Beverages   All alcoholic beverages are loaded with yeast. If you're allergic to yeast, avoid them. There are other reasons you should avoid or limit your intake. They contain large amounts of quick acting carbohydrates which make yeast "go crazy."

Suggestions for Breakfast and Eating on the Run

Breakfast is your most difficult meal, especially on the diagnostic diet. In the recipe section of *The Yeast Connection Cookbook,* my collaborator and co-author, Marge Jones, commented:

> "What can I eat for breakfast? Time and time again I hear this and it is a valid concern for people on a diet to control Candida.
> "If you strip breakfast of yeast, you'll eliminate toast, French toast, bagels, sweet rolls, even sourdough bread. If you also omit wheat, milk, corn, sugar, soy and egg, you end up with a gaping void in your menus where breakfast used to be."

Marge then gives you lots of breakfast suggestions, including pancakes or flat bread that you can make a few days ahead, package and freeze. Then when you're ready, you can put them in your toaster oven.

"Eat these versatile little treasures with your fingers, like dainty pieces of toast, or top them with your favorite filling or bean dip for open-faced mini-sandwiches. They go brown bagging easily and travel well on trips too."

Marge is a real authority on the non-grain alternatives, amaranth, buckwheat and quinoa. These nutritious foods are rich in carbohydrates and help fill you up. They're also useful for people who are sensitive to wheat and corn.

She also tells you how to fix breakfast "pudding." Ingredients in this recipe include foods which you may not think of as breakfast foods, such as sweet potatoes, and/or other vegetables. Another suggestion, especially during the diagnostic phase of your diet, is a big bowl of oatmeal plus chopped nuts or well-cooked eggs with lean meat.

When eating on the run, plan ahead. Don't wait until you're rushing off to work. Make sure that you can fill your "brown bag" with nutritious foods, including raw vegetables, nuts and rice cakes. You may also get some of the nutritious vegetable-based burgers from your health food store (see Chapter 52).

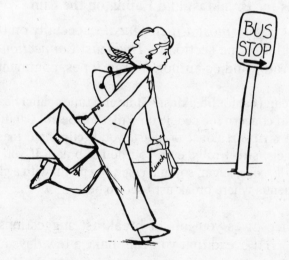

REFERENCES

1. Haas, E.M., *Staying Healthy with Nutrition*, Celestial Arts, Berkeley, CA, 1992; pp 39–63.
2. Barnard, N., *Food for Life*, Harmony Books, New York, 1993; pp 19–20.
3. Gaby, A.R., *Preventing and Reversing Osteoporosis*, Prima Publishing, Rockland, CA, 1994; p 15.
4. Weissman, J.D., *Choose to Live*, Grove Press, New York, 1988; pp 11–21.
5. Greenwood, S., *Menopause Naturally*, Volcano Press, Volcano, CA, 1992; pp 162–164.
6. Monte, T., and editors of East West Natural Health, *World Medicine*, Jeremy P. Tarcher, Putnam, New York, 1993; pp 96–97.
7. Haas, E.M., *Staying Healthy with Nutrition*, Celestial Arts, Berkeley, CA, 1992; p 76.
8. Weissman, J.D., *Choose to Live*, Grove Press, New York, 1988; p 18.
9. Truss, C.O., "Metabolic Abnormalities in Patients with Chronic Candidiasis," *J. of Ortho. Psych.*, 1984; 13:66–93.
10. Horrobin, D.F., *Omega 6 Essential Fatty Acids—Pathophysiology and Roles in Clinical Medicine*, Alan R. Liss, Inc., New York, 1990.
11. Bland, J., *Preventive Medicine Update*, P.O. Box 1729, Gig Harbor, WA 98335.
12. Siguel, E.N. in Bland, J., Second International Symposium on Functional Medicine, 1994. Rancho Mirage, California. HealthComm, P.O. Box 1729, Gig Harbor, WA 98335.
13. Siguel, E.N., *Essential Fatty Acids in Health and Disease*, NuTrek Press, Brookline, MA, 1994.
14. Erasmus, U., *Fats That Heal, Fats That Kill*, Alive Books, Burnaby, B.C., Canada, 1993; pp 125–126, 269–274 and 279–287.
15. Gittleman, A.L., *Beyond Pritikin*, Bantam Books, New York, 1988.
16. Goldstrich, J.D., *The Cardiologist's Painless Prescription for a Healthy Heart*, 9-Hart-9 Publishing, Dallas, TX, 1994.
17. McDougall, J.A., *The McDougall Program—Twelve Days to Dynamic Health*, Plume/Penguin, New York, 1990; pp 15–28.
18. Ornish, D., *Dr. Dean Ornish's Program for Reversing Heart Disease*, Ballentine Books, New York, 1990; p 257.
19. Barnard, N., *Food For Life*, Harmony Books, New York, 1993.
20. McIlhaney, J.S., Jr., with Nethery, S., *1250 Health Care Questions Women Ask*, Focus on the Family Publishing, Colorado Springs, CO, 1992; pp 808–813.
21. Carper, J., *The Food Pharmacy to Good Eating*, Bantam Books, New York, 1991; pp 9–13.

22. Carper, J., *Food—Your Miracle Medicine*, HarperCollins, New York, 1993.
23. Schardt, D., "Phytochemicals: Plants against cancer," *Nutrition Action Healthletter*, Center for Science in the Public Interest, Washington, DC, 1994; 21:1, 9–11.
24. Bagely, S., "Better than Vitamins," *Newsweek*, April 25, 1994; pp 45–49.
25. *Longevity*, "The Live Longer Diet," May 1994; pp 40, 42, 44, 78 and 80.
26. *Longevity*, "Re-inventing the Pyramid," May 1944; pp 40–41.
27. Truss, C.O., *The Missing Diagnosis*, P.O. Box 26508, Birmingham, AL 35226, pp 152–153.
28. Crook, W.G., *The Yeast Connection*, Third Edition, Professional Books, Jackson, TN and Vintage Books, New York, 1986; pp 71–72.
29. Jorgenson, B., "Baker's Yeast Allergy in Candidiasis Patients," *J. of Advan. in Med.*, 1994; 7:43–49.
30. Costantini, A.V., "The Fungal Etiology of Autoimmune Diseases, Malignancies, Arteriosclerosis and Hyperlipidemia. Presented at the American Academy of Environmental Medicine, 28th Annual Meeting, October 9–12, 1993, Sparks, New York.
31. Greenberg, R.B., "Is the Yeast Syndrome Food Allergy?" *Clinical Ecology*, 1989; 7(2):27–33.

27

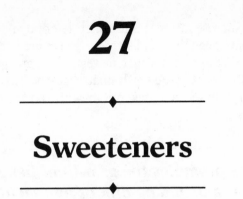

Sweeteners

Every week I receive phone calls and letters from people who say, "If I can't use sugar, what can I use?" Sometimes I say something like this, "Everybody likes sweets, certainly I do. Even young infants will smile if you put something sweet in their mouths. Yet, during the early stages of your diet, avoiding sugar, corn syrup, honey, molasses, maple syrup and other simple carbohydrates is an essential part of any candida treatment program. But diets are not forever and after a few weeks (or months) you can experiment."

Also, I tell people that if they tolerate fruits they can use them in some of their recipes. Or they can put a banana, peach or other sweet fruit in a blender with a little water and make a "slurry" to pour on cereal or add to other foods.

But, I also have some good news about a relatively new sweetener with a big name, fructooligosaccharides (FOS), and about one of the artificial sweeteners, pure liquid saccharin.

FOS: A Healthful Sweetener

About two years ago, while thumbing through a copy of one of my favorite health food magazines, *Let's Live,* I came across an article by Betty Kamen, Ph.D., entitled, "FOS: A Healthful Sweetener (No kidding!)." In this article Kamen told me for the first time about FOS, a sweetener which was (and is) used in hundreds of foods in Japan. Here are excerpts from this article.

"FOS are sucrose molecules to which 1, 2 or 3 additional fructose molecules have been linked in sequence. FOS are widely distributed in a variety of edible plants such as vegetables and grains and some fruits. They're not absorbed by human digestive enzymes in the gastrointestinal tract or pancreas, but are utilized by your friendly intestinal bacteria.

> ## FOS promotes the growth of beneficial bacteria including bifidus and lactobacilli.

"FOS promotes the growth of beneficial bacteria including bifidus and lactobacilli. And in doing so they interfere with the growth of disease-causing organisms."

In her article, Kamen cited numerous scientific studies which validate the use of FOS, and in her concluding comments she said:

"In Japan, FOS are considered food, not an ingredient or additive. We all know how difficult it is to give up that sweet tooth. Since FOS functions similarly to sucrose in a wide variety of food applications, it could effectively replace all or part of the sucrose in processed foods . . . More than that, it is a health enhancer. FOS—watch for it."[1]

Comments By Marjorie Hurt Jones

I received additional information about FOS in Jones' newsletter, *Mastering Food Allergies*. In an article, "FOS, A 'Good For You' Sweetener!," she said:

"Here comes a new sweetener galloping into our consciousness . . . and it wears a white hat! Fructo-oligo-saccharides or FOS for short . . . may reportedly nourish the 'good guys' of the gut selectively . . . but can NOT be utilized by candida and other yeasts, or by salmonella and certain other harmful bacteria . . .

"FOS occur in small amounts in nature, in onion, garlic, burdock and other vegetables, in bananas and a few other fruits, and in wheat, rye, barley and oats. Commercially produced FOS appear to be identical to those from natural sources."

In her continuing discussion, one "downside" Marge pointed out was cost. And she said:

"With supplies in this country still quite limited, supplement companies have jumped in and are selling 60–100 grams of FOS for $10–$12. (100 grams equals ½ cup.) If you want to use 1–2 teaspoons a day, therapeutically, that may be okay. But if you want to bake cookies—you will need $20–$40 worth of FOS for one batch! Ouch!"[2]

I received still more information from a Colorado friend, Nicolette M. Dumke, author of several excellent books about allergy cooking, and she said, "Dr. Crook, I'm excited about the efficacy of FOS. I think you'll like it." She even dumped ¼ of a teaspoon of FOS in the envelope. I touched it to my tongue and it tasted like sugar.

The next chapter in my FOS "saga" came during an interview with Charles Resseger, D.O., in December 1993. In our conversation we talked about many things, including the antifungal medications Diflucan and Sporanox. And he said:

"I'm really enthusiastic about FOS. It's a polysaccharide—very sweet. It is so complex that yeast cannot utilize it at all, yet bacteria can. If you put it into the digestive tract with the friendly bacteria, the good acidophilus just grows like crazy.

> **If you put it into the digestive tract . . . the good acidophilus just grows like crazy.**

"That makes sense because what we're really trying to do is to repopulate the colon with good bacteria. And my results are phenomenal. My patients who are taking it say that the stuff really tastes good.

"This makes so much sense I can't believe that somebody hasn't thought of it sooner. I'm giving it to all of my yeast patients along with good acidophilus bacteria."

To get further information about FOS, I wrote to Beatrice Trum Hunter, food editor of *Consumers' Research*, who has written and published over a dozen books on food issues. In early February 1994, she sent me an article in a peer-reviewed journal which documented the safety and benefits of FOS. Here are excerpts from this comprehensive, scientific article.

"*Fructooligosaccharides can have beneficial effects as food ingredients* . . . In Japan, FOS are considered food, not food ingredients, and are found in more than 500 food products, resulting in significant daily consumption . . . Numerous in-vitro and in-vivo studies have been conducted to evaluate the potential toxicity of FOS to animals and man . . . *Results provided no evidence that FOS possessed any genotoxic potential* . . . [emphasis added]."

Numerous clinical studies in Japan revealed that FOS was selectively utilized by bifidobacteria; the authors found that this activity improved intestinal flora, relieved constipation, improved blood lipids and suppressed the production of putrefactive substances.

The article pointed out that FOS are found naturally in many foods, especially fruits and vegetables. The authors focused their report on the addition of FOS to plain unsweetened yogurt to improve its taste. In discussing possible side effects, they pointed out that none were noted in animals who took FOS over long periods of time, and they said:

"The only effect noted was the occurrence of soft stools or diarrhea after ingestion of large quantities of FOS (more than 5%)."

In other animal studies these researchers cited findings in chicks, piglets, dogs and cats. And they said:

"Numerous feed efficiency studies . . . reveal no adverse effects related to feed supplementation of FOS, and feed efficiency was enhanced. These results are consistent with studies in other species where FOS have a positive effect on the gut flora and health outcomes.

> **Numerous feed efficiency studies . . . reveal no adverse effects related to FOS.**

"FOS . . . are resistant to digestion . . . therefore, are nondigestible by humans but can be utilized by select gram positive organisms, such as bifidobacteria . . . [they] may possess some dietary fiber-like function."[3]

Later, Beatrice Trum Hunter sent me another peer-reviewed article which described other health benefits of FOS.

- proliferation of bifidobacteria and reduction of detrimental bacteria
- reduction of toxic metabolites and detrimental enzymes
- prevention of pathogenic and autogenic diarrhea
- prevention of constipation
- protection of liver function
- reduction of serum cholesterol
- anticancer effect
- production of nutrients

After receiving all of these reports, I ordered a bottle of FOS and sprinkled some on my cereal. It tasted just like sugar. To obtain still further information, I called culinary authority, Marge Jones. Here are excerpts from our conversation.

Crook: Marge, if you're counseling a client who has just purchased a bottle of FOS, what do you tell her?

Jones: I have her start very cautiously, perhaps ¼ tsp. twice a day. She can sprinkle it on her food or drop it in her tea.

Crook: How does FOS compare to sugar?

Jones: It's perhaps half as sweet.

Crook: Are there side effects?

Jones: Some people may develop a few digestive symptoms, including abdominal pain, gas and even diarrhea. These symptoms occur because FOS isn't digestible. It's too large a molecule. Although few, if any, problems have been reported in people using FOS, it's a good idea for them to use it cautiously until they determine their own tolerance.

Crook: Marge, I can recall that you've been interested in another natural sweetener, stevia, for some years. What do you think of it now?

Jones: I like it. I think the secret of getting satisfactory results with stevia is to play around with it until you learn the least amount that will produce sufficient sweetness to satisfy you. If you put too much in, you may pick up bitterness as an aftertaste.

Crook: Do you use it on any kind of a regular basis?

Jones: Yes, I go through these sweeteners cyclically, based in part on what I'm going to write about or what I'm curious about. When I go on a kick of being interested in stevia, I use it two or three times a week.

Crook: Can you use it in cooking—and preparing a recipe?

Jones: Yes, you can and Nicolette Dumke has developed an even greater experience, which she describes in her latest book, *Allergy Cooking With Ease*."[4]

Another Source of FOS

In October 1994, Dr. Susan Busse, a family physician, told me about Jerusalem artichoke flour. According to Busse, this flour can be sprinkled on cold or hot cereal as a topping, or used in a bread muffin or cookie recipe as a partial flour replacement (up to 10%). More information about this flour can be obtained from HealthCo International, P.O. Box 544, Bloomingdale, IL 60108 (800-477-3949).

Saccharin

U.S. laws require that products containing saccharin carry this label: *Use of this product may be hazardous to your health. This product contains saccharin, which has been determined to cause cancer in laboratory animals.*

Yet, in the third edition of *The Yeast Connection*,[5] I cited a report in *Pediatric News* which said that saccharin has shown no evidence of carcinogenic potential in 20 human studies and 14 single-generation animal studies. The report also stated that while saccharin has been associated with the development of bladder cancer in rats after exposure at high levels in utero and throughout life, the manner in which this occurs is not known.

In 1994, to obtain current information about saccharin, I called Linda Farmer and Becky Parks at the Learning Center at the Jackson Madison County General Hospital. Here are excerpts from a report they sent me. The first one came from South Dakota State University.

"Almost from its discovery in 1879, the use of saccharin as an artificial, non-nutritive sweetener has been the center of several controversies regarding potential toxic effects, most recently focusing on the urinary bladder carcinogenicity of sodium saccharin in rats when fed at high doses in two-generation studies.

"No carcinogenic effect has been observed in mice, hamsters or monkeys, and numerous epidemiological studies provide no clear or consistent evidence to support the assertion that sodium saccharin increases the risk of bladder cancer in the human population."[6]

Another report from the National Cancer Institute entitled "Epidemiology of Bladder Cancer" stated:

"Approximately 49,000 people in the United States develop bladder cancer each year, and about 9700 die of it . . . Smoking accounts for about half of bladder cancer diagnosed among men and about one-third of that among women. Moderate to heavy smokers typically show a two to five fold risk of bladder cancer compared with persons who never smoked . . .

"Clear evidence of bladder cancer risk also is apparent for a small number of occupational groups: dye workers, rubber workers, leather workers, painters, truck drivers and aluminum workers."

> ### *Artificial sweeteners confer little or no excessive bladder cancer risk.*

In the continuing discussion, the article pointed out that coffee drinking was probably not a factor and consumption of fruits, vegetables and foods high in vitamin A are possible protective factors. And they said, "Artificial sweeteners confer little or no excessive bladder cancer risk."[7]

Clear liquid saccharin is available in most any drugstore or grocery store. Brand names include Fasweet (Schering-Plough) and Sweeta (Squibb). I, personally, use small amounts of saccharin to sweeten occasional cups of coffee and tea. And I do not worry about increasing my risk of bladder cancer. I also prefer saccharin to NutraSweet.

Aspartame

Over twenty years ago at a medical conference in Florida, I met H. J. Roberts, M.D., a West Palm Beach board certified internist who shared my interest in nutrition. Over the years we have corresponded and in the June 1991 issue of the IHF newsletter, *Healthline*, I cited a report by Roberts. Here are excerpts.

"A 47-year-old female patient had unexplained confusion, significant memory loss, intense headaches, impaired hearing, light-headedness, severe 'nervousness,' muscle cramps and depression with suicidal thoughts. She also complained of severe dryness of the eyes, requiring one bottle of artificial tears a week . . .

"All symptoms markedly improved after she stopped using aspartame and then disappeared. She no longer required artificial tears and was able to accompany a church group doing relief work abroad two weeks later."

Roberts has published two books dealing with aspartame reactions, including *Sweet'ner Dearest: Bittersweet Vignettes About Aspartame (NutraSweet)*[8] and *ASPARTAME (NutraSweet*), Is It Safe?*.** In the introductory chapter of the latter book, he said:

"Aspartame is responsible for many distressing medical problems, ranging from headaches and memory loss to hyperactivity in children and seizure disorders.

> ### *Aspartame is responsible for many distressing medical problems.*

"Aspartame . . . is now consumed by more than 100 million persons in the United States . . . The consumption of aspartame has increased at an astonishing rate since 1981, when this man-made sweetener was first introduced. By 1985, 800 million pounds of aspartame were used per year in the United States.

"Equally important, the public, increasingly concerned in recent years about all food additives, has been reassured that aspartame is entirely safe and can be used without worry."

He then quotes the safety endorsement of FDA officials in 1981, 1985 and 1987, as well as the recommendations of the American Dietetic Association and the American Diabetes Association. And he said:

"All this sounds very convincing, doesn't it? Why, then, would I, a busy and established internist, take on the formidable task of presenting an opposing point of view . . . arguing that aspartame is by no means as safe as we have been led to believe?"

---

*A registered trademark of the NutraSweet Company.
**Roberts book, *ASPARTAME (NutraSweet), Is It Safe?*, can be ordered from the Charles Press Publishers, P.O. Box 15715, Philadelphia, PA 19103.

He then points out that, based on his experience, products that contain aspartame are capable of producing a wide range of frightening symptoms. And he acknowledges that people may ask up front, "What information does this doctor have to justify stirring up anxiety about aspartame when the American Medical Association and dozens of regulatory agencies have already vouched that the additive is safe?" His answer, "Read the book, weigh the evidence and judge for yourself."[9]

How often does aspartame cause reactions? In my own practice, I've heard about them only occasionally. Yet, the highly reputable *Brain/Mind Bulletin* published a letter to the editor by Gerrard Gormley, Manchester-by-the-Sea, Massachusetts, who talked about depression. Here are excerpts from his letter.

"In March 1986 I quit smoking cold turkey. I didn't miss cigarettes, but I did start consuming a lot of chewing gum and soda containing NutraSweet.

"Within a week or two I slipped into a depression of black hole proportions. With it came total writer's block. I felt as though my brain had been scooped out, blended in a food processor and poured back into my skull.

"For well over a year, I suffered the worst depression of my life. My mood and mental acuity were so severely degraded that I even gave up a lucrative consulting business of 25 years standing . . .

"In August 1987, I stumbled onto a chemical link that made all the difference. I came across a *Science News* article citing MIT lab tests showing that aspartame, the principle ingredient in NutraSweet, destroys neurotransmitters, the chemicals that convey messages between neurons in the brain . . .

> **Within a week or two I was back to normal, writing productively every day.**

"I decided I could live without aspartame and eliminated it from my diet. Within a week or two I was back to normal, writing productively every day. Once again, I was decisive, mentally sharp and more energetic than I had felt in 18 months. I generally got my life back on an even keel.

"It seems clear that aspartame was the major factor causing and/or aggravating my depression."[10]

I don't really know what percentage of people experience adverse reactions to aspartame. Maybe concern about it isn't all that important unless you happen to be a person like Gerrard Gormley.

Another physician who agrees with Dr. Roberts' observations, Dennis W. Remington, in collaboration with Barbara W. Higa, R.D., published an informative 234-page book, *The Bitter Truth About Artificial Sweeteners*,[11] and like Dr. Roberts, he focused especially on the adverse effects of aspartame.*

He presented data to show that artificial sweeteners may interfere with obtaining adequate nutrients essential for good health and rather than helping people lose weight, may promote weight gain!

REFERENCES

1. Kamen, B., "FOS: A Healthful Sweetener (No kidding!)," *Let's Live*, October 1992; pp 32–34.
2. Jones, M., "FOS—A 'Good for You' Sweetener!" *Mastering Food Allergies*, November 1992; Vol. 7 No. 10, MAST Enterprises, Inc., 2615 N. 4th St., #616, Coeur d'Alene, ID 83814.
3. Spiegel, J.E., et al, "Safety and Benefits of Fructooligosaccharides as Food Ingredients," *Food Technology*, January 1994; pp 85–89.
4. Dumke, N., *Allergy Cooking with Ease*, Starburst Publishers, P.O. Box 4123, Lancaster, PA 17604, 1993.
5. Crook, W.G., *The Yeast Connection*, Third Edition, Professional Books, Jackson, TN and Vintage Books, New York, 1986; p 392.
6. Ellwein, L.B., Cohen, S.M., "The Health Risks of Saccharin Revisited," *Critical Reviews in Toxicology*, 1990; 20(5): 311–326
7. Silverman, D., Hartge, P., Morrison, A. and Devesa, S., "Epidemiology of Bladder Cancer," *Hematology/Oncology Clinics of North America*, February, 1992; 6(1):1–30.

---

*Unfortunately, Dr. Remington's book is now out of print.

8. Roberts, H.J., *Sweet'ner Dearest: Bittersweet Vignettes About Aspartame (NutraSweet)*, Sunshine Sentinel Press, P.O. Box 8697, West Palm Beach, FL, 33407, 1992.

9. Roberts, H.J., *ASPARTAME (NutraSweet), Is It Safe?* Charles Press Publishers, P.O. Box 15715, Philadelphia, PA 19103.

10. *Brain/Mind and Common Sense*, Interface Press, Box 42211, 4717 N. Figueroa St., Los Angeles, CA 90042, April 1991.

11. Remington, D.W. and Higa, B.W., *The Bitter Truth About Artificial Sweeteners*, Vitality House International, Provo, UT, 1987.

28

Vitamins and Other Nutritional Supplements

Today, over half of all Americans take vitamin supplements. Increasing numbers of physicians (including some who were once skeptical of their value) are taking them too. Moreover, they're recommending vitamins and other nutritional supplements to others.

Here's an example of what I'm talking about. For many years, beginning in the 1970s, I saw and heard Dr. Art Ulene on the "Today Show." His presentations on a variety of medical topics were always thorough and informative. About 15 years ago we began to correspond and in the late '80s and early '90s I visited him in his office on two occasions. And we exchanged phone calls and many more letters.

Like most physicians, Art's point of view could be described as "conservative," so I was surprised—even startled—to learn that Art had written a book, *The Vitamin Strategy*, which recommends vitamin and mineral supplements. I found this book, co-authored by Art and his daughter, Dr. Val Ulene, at the Nutri Books booth at the Natural Products Expo East Convention in Baltimore. Here are excerpts from Art's foreword.

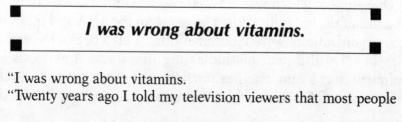

I was wrong about vitamins.

"I was wrong about vitamins.
"Twenty years ago I told my television viewers that most people

didn't need vitamin supplements. If you were eating well, I said, buying and consuming vitamin pills was a waste of money.

"I certainly wasn't alone in this belief. At that time few people in the medical community supported vitamin supplementation. Even today, most physicians, and perhaps most registered dieticians and nutritionists, insist that people in the United States get all the vitamins they need from their diet alone. It's not surprising that health professionals feel this way. After all, that's what we were taught in medical school . . .

"I now know that many of the pronouncements I heard about the uselessness of vitamins simply aren't true. No matter what your age, no matter what your health status, according to new research, optimal doses of vitamins and minerals can improve the state of your health and reduce your chances of developing many diseases and disorders once considered almost unavoidable."[1]

Like Dr. Ulene, until the early 1970s, I was one of those conservative physicians. But gradually I began to change my mind based on articles I read in health food magazines. (My mother, an organic gardener, faithfully read these magazines and passed relevant articles on to me.) I also began to receive favorable reports from my patients who were taking vitamins, minerals and other nutritional supplements, including many of my patients with food and chemical sensitivities.

Then, in the mid-1970s, one of my patients brought me a copy of *Executive Health*,[2] a monthly periodical which I had seen advertised in the *New York Times* and the *Wall Street Journal*. Consultants listed on the front page of this newsletter included two Nobel Prize winners, Linus Pauling, Ph.D., and Albert Szent-Györgyi, Ph.D. There were also other consultants with impressive credentials, including the late Alton Ochsner, M.D., founder of the world famous Ochsner Clinic in New Orleans.

One subject which was covered was the importance of vitamins and minerals, including doses larger than the AMA and other medical organizations were recommending. I also began to read articles in scientific journals indicating that many Americans were deficient in calcium, magnesium, zinc and other nutrients and micronutrients. By the early '80s, our most conservative medical journals began to talk about osteoporosis and the need for calcium supplements.

Then, in 1981, Mary Ware, who at that time was president of the Southwestern Health Organization (SWHO), invited me to talk on food allergies at a conference in San Antonio. I was impressed by the integrity, dedication, sincerity, knowledge and expertise possessed by many of the people I met there.

> ## I was impressed by the integrity . . . and expertise possessed by many of the people I met there.

Those I met and visited with included Frank Ford,* head of a Texas company specializing in organically grown grains. Among other things, Frank explained to me the advantages of "expeller pressed" vegetable oils—oils which were not subjected to high temperatures during processing.

I also learned for the first time something about the virtues of garlic from Vera Weido, a San Antonio health food store owner. Vera gave me a package of Kyolic-Aged Garlic Extract, saying, "Dr. Crook, you may wish to give this product to your patients. I've read research reports which show that it helps control candida. You ought to be taking it yourself."

About the same time, I became reacquainted with Elmer Cranton, M.D., a graduate of Harvard Medical School and a pioneer in preventive and holistic medicine. Dr. Cranton and I had served on the Advisory Board of the Pritikin Research Foundation in California, but I hadn't seen or talked to him in several years.

Dr. Cranton had co-authored with Richard Passwater, Ph.D., a book on minerals, trace elements, hair analysis and nutrition.[3] He had also written several papers about the importance of antioxidants and other nutrients in combating free radical pathology.

---

*In 1987 Ford became a member of the Advisory Board of the National Health Foundation.

In the early '80s, after corresponding with Dr. Cranton and reading his book, I began to prescribe nutritional supplements for my patients, my family and I began to take them myself. These included products which contained 20–100 mg. of the different B vitamins, 1000–1500 mg. of vitamin C, 50–200 mcg. of selenium, 1000–1500 mg. of calcium, 500–800 mg. of magnesium, 15–30 mg. of zinc, plus a number of other nutrients and micronutrients.

Then, after learning about the importance of the essential fatty acids from David Horrobin, Ph.D., Donald Rudin, Ph.D., Sidney Baker, M.D., Leo Galland, M.D., and Orian Truss, M.D., I began to prescribe and take supplemental Omega 3 and Omega 6 fatty acids, including flax seed oil, fish oils and evening primrose oil.

Controversy Over Vitamins

For the past decade, several self-appointed vocal spokesmen, including Stephen Barrett, M.D., of Allentown, Pennsylvania, and Victor Herbert, M.D., of New York, have vigorously and bitterly challenged those who favor nutritional supplements. And they say, in effect, "Taking vitamins, minerals and other nutritional supplements is 'quack' medicine."

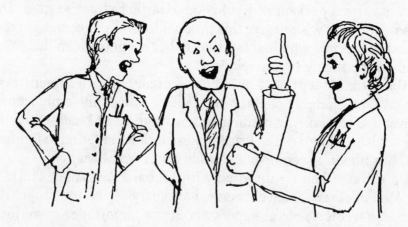

An opposite point of view has been expressed by a number of scientists with impeccable academic credentials. The late Roger Williams, Ph.D., of the University of Texas and the late Linus Pauling, Ph.D., a double Nobel Prize winner, were among those who supported the use of many of the vitamins, including vitamin C and vitamin B complex.

Support for the use of nutritional supplements was also expressed by Robert A. Good, M.D., Ph.D., Chairman of the Department of Pediatrics, University of South Florida, Tampa, who commented:

> "An explosion of new information shows that the proper combination of nutrients, combined with the reduction of caloric intake will fortify the body's immune system and aid in fighting disease."[4]

During the late 1980s and early 1990s, the controversy has continued. Yet, the importance of nutritional supplements, in addition to a good diet, has been reported in a number of major publications.

Support for Nutritional Supplements

In the March 10, 1992, issue of the *New York Times*, in an article titled, "Vitamins Win Support As Potent Agents of Health," reporter Natalie Angier said:

> "Long consigned to the fringes of medicine and accorded scarcely more credibility than crystal rubbing or homeopathy, the study of how vitamins affect the body and help prevent chronic diseases is now winning broad attention and respect among mainstream medical researchers."

> *Scientists are gathering . . . evidence that vitamins influence the health . . . of nearly every organ.*

In her discussion, Angier pointed out that scientists are gathering provocative evidence that vitamins influence the health and vibrancy of nearly every organ. And she said that they may help forestall or even reverse many diseases including cancer, heart disease, osteoporosis, a weakening of the immune system, nerve degeneration and other chronic disorders.

A group of nutritional supplements called "free radical scavengers," received special emphasis, especially vitamins E, C and beta-carotene. These compounds, also known as "antioxidants," may battle cardiovascular disease by preventing the body from turning otherwise harmless cholesterol into a form that can plug up the arteries.

Angier quoted a number of authorities, including Dr. Simin N. Meydani of the Human Nutrition Research Center on Aging at Tufts University in Boston, who said:

"We used to think about vitamins strictly in terms of what you needed to prevent short-term deficiencies. Now, we're starting to think about what is the optimal level of vitamins for lifelong health and to prevent age-associated diseases."

Angier also cited a number of other researchers, some of whom made presentations at a recent conference in Arlington, Virginia, sponsored by the New York Academy of Sciences.

Vitamins: A *Time* Cover Story

In the April 6, 1992, issue of *Time,* the introduction of this cover story read, "The New Scoop On Vitamins—*They May Be Much More Important Than Doctors Thought At Warding Off Cancer, Heart Disease and the Ravages of Aging—and no—you may not be getting enough of these crucial nutrients in your diet.*"

In her comprehensive report, the author of the article, Anastasia Toufexis, said:

"It's raining. Flooding to be precise. But business is as brisk as ever at Ms. Gooch's Natural Foods Market in West Los Angeles . . . Inside, crowds jam the supplement section . . . Maryanne Latimer is among the faithful . . . she has been plagued by chronic fatigue syndrome and has therefore expanded her usual menu of vitamins and minerals.

"But, for every true believer in the power of vitamins . . . there is an agnostic, a skeptic who insists that vitamins are the opiate of the people."

In her continuing discussion, Toufexis points out that more and more scientists are finding evidence that suggests that nutrients play a much more complex role in assuring vitality and optimal health than was previously thought. And she quotes Dr. Jeffrey Blumberg, Associate Director of the Human Nutrition Research Center on Aging at Tufts University, who said:

We are now entering the second wave of vitamin research.

"We are now entering the second wave of vitamin research. The first wave was the discovery of vitamins in a role in combating nutritional deficiencies such as rickets and beriberi. Now we're on the second wave. *You don't need to take vitamin C to prevent scurvy in this country today, but you could need it for optimal health and the prevention of some diseases* [emphasis added]."

Vitamins Enter the Medical Mainstream

During the late '80s and early '90s, more and more physicians have begun to take and recommend vitamin supplements. In the January 1993 issue of *Medical Tribune*, editor Bill Ingram said:

"Vitamins in general and vitamin E in particular have a disease fighting role and a place in the generalists practice. That is the sum and substance of the scores of responses received from generalists urged by this newspaper to make their views known. Here are several of their comments:

"Recommended daily allowances (RDAs) for vitamins are a joke . . . Retaining these archaic yardsticks, based on the prevention of deficiency diseases . . . is senseless. Most people now take vitamins

C, E and beta-carotene because of mounting evidence of their efficacy in preventing everything from colds and cataracts to coronaries
and cancer. The amounts required are many times greater than the
RDAs which don't even exist for the beta-carotene."

Paul J. Rosch, M.D., Yonkers, New York.

"I'm a board certified cardiologist. In response to the article concerning the use of vitamins, I place all of my patients on antioxidant
vitamins, C-500—1000 mg. twice daily, and also vitamin E as well as
multivitamins."

David Southern, M.D., Valley College, New York.

"I prescribe vitamins and other nutrients for my patients well in
excess of the RDA and I take substantial amounts myself. Again, far
in excess of the RDA.

"I believe the RDAs have almost no meaning except in the case of
the theoretically healthy individual who does not eat properly."

Norman Borgman, M.D., Miramar, Florida.

"I agree with many of the other observers that vitamin supplements do help, particularly antioxidants. We're exposed to a lot of
pollution in our environment (and antioxidants) also help to neutralize pollutants . . . When it comes to evaluating the vitamins, I don't
want to wait around until scientists decide these things. There's
enough evidence to warrant taking vitamins now.

I don't want to wait around until scientists decide these things.

"Years in the future when the authorities finally decide it is ad-
vantageous I'll be years ahead."

Harvey Rose, M.D., Carmichael, California.

"I'm a little disturbed about the experts saying that you shouldn't
take this and you shouldn't take that. I've been taking multiple dose,
mega dose vitamins for the last 20 years. I went through cancer of

the prostate without any trouble and I attribute that to the fact that I was taking tremendous doses of vitamin C.

"I take approximately 5000 mg. of vitamin C daily, 800 IU of vitamin E and so on right down the line.

"Mega doses of the vitamins have served me well and have certainly not caused me any harm."

Retired doctor.

More About Antioxidants and Other Vitamin Supplements

On March 3, 1994, on the "Today Show," co-host Katie Couric pointed out that the value of vitamin supplements has been debated for years. But she also said that recent studies in the scientific literature show that diets which are rich in the antioxidant vitamins, such as C, E and beta carotene, may play a part in preventing certain illnesses, including cancer and heart disease. Yet, she told viewers that these nutrients could be found in many fruits and vegetables, and some seafoods. She also said:

> "They're available as over-the-counter vitamin supplements. But the question of who should take these supplements and how much they should take confuses many Americans."

She then introduced Daniel Perry, Director of the Alliance for Aging Research and Dr. Jeffrey Blumberg of the Antioxidant Research Laboratory of Tufts University. During the interview, Couric asked Perry why his organization feels the need to come up with specific recommendations for nutritional supplements.

Americans want to take responsibility for their own health.

In responding, Perry said that Americans want to take responsibility for their own health and to do all that they can to experience successful aging. And to accomplish these goals they need information.

When Couric asked him how old a person should be to start taking increased amounts of supplements, Perry said:

"Really it's for adults. Healthy aging really starts much earlier than retirement age. People should begin as soon as they are adults to maximize their diet, exercise and follow good health habits in order to achieve a quality of life in old age."

Couric then directed her comments and questions to Dr. Blumberg and asked him what an antioxidant vitamin is and what it does in the body?

In his reply, Blumberg pointed out that antioxidants are a wide class of compounds and that vitamin C, E and beta carotene are among the most important and effective members of the class.

In his continuing comments, Blumberg explained that while oxygen is important to life, that oxygen has a dark side leading to the production of a compound called free radicals which can be hazardous to virtually every cell in the body. And he said:

"These free radicals can injure these cells, leading to disease, and antioxidants protect it against free radicals and thus reduce our risk for these important diseases like cancer and heart disease."

During a back and forth discussion, Couric presented a graph to show the supplements Blumberg and Perry were recommending. They included:

Vitamin C	250 to 1000 mg. a day
Vitamin E	100 to 400 IU daily
Beta carotene	17,000 to 50,000 units daily

The discussion then turned to ways of increasing vitamin intake by diet alone. Blumberg stated it would take 15 oranges a day to provide 1000 mg. of vitamin C. He also noted you'd have to eat 24 cups of almonds to get the recommended amount of vitamin E and

5 cups of carrots and 6 cups of butternut squash to get enough beta carotene. So he said, "It becomes practical then to consider antioxidant supplements as a way to get that much of these vitamins."

However, in his continuing discussion, Blumberg said:

> "Nutrient supplements are not nutrient substitutes. There are really two messages here for good health. You do have to eat a healthy, well-balanced diet. There are lots of things other than vitamins in the diet. But to get these optimal amounts, you really do need to consider the use of supplements."

> ### *You do have to eat a healthy, well-balanced diet.*

In his concluding comments, Perry pointed out that the ranges he and Blumberg are recommending are safe and are supported by a growing body of scientific evidence. And in his concluding remarks, he said:

> "We're the first national organization to make this kind of specific recommendation of a daily intake. We expect that others will come forward. The issue is now before Congress in terms of health claims labeling. So there's a growing body of desire on the part of the American people for this information and we think the times will change."

Nutritional Supplements and Cataracts

Based on information I've received from various sources, including professional and lay journals, cataracts may be prevented by the consumption of additional amounts of vitamin C and other antioxidants. In his easy-to-read and understand book, *Free Radicals in Disease Prevention*,[5] David J. Lin cited studies which provide support for antioxidant supplementation in preventing cataracts. Here is an excerpt from one of these studies.

"One hundred seventy-five cataract patients were individually matched with 175 cataract-free subjects in a study at the University of Western Ontario . . . Investigators analyzed the results and discovered that the cataract-free group consumed more vitamin E and vitamin C than did the cataract group . . ."[6]

Another investigation[7] carried out at the USDA Human Nutrition Research Center on Aging suggested a relationship between antioxidants and cataracts. In this study, investigators found that cataract patients were particularly low in beta carotene, vitamin C and vitamin E.

Nutritional Supplements and Heart Disease

Elsewhere in this book, I referred to the pioneer work of Nathan Pritikin. This California businessman helped countless people reverse disabling coronary heart disease without surgery. His program featured a low-fat, high-complex-carbohydrate diet and exercise.

Pritikin's observations were, to a large extent, ignored or rejected in the 1970s. Yet, in the 1980s, they gained gradual recognition from many physicians, including heart specialists. One such physician, Joe D. Goldstrich, served for a number of years as chief cardiologist and medical director of the Pritikin Longevity Center in California.

In 1981, Goldstrich published a book, *The Best Chance Diet*, in which he reiterated the Pritikin approach. Because he found that a lot of people couldn't (or wouldn't) stick to the diet, he kept searching for better answers. In 1994 he published another book entitled, *The Cardiologist's Painless Prescription for a Healthy Heart and a Longer Life*. In the preface of this book, he said:

"It's been a long journey, and now, for the first time, I see a very bright light at the end of the tunnel. Coronary heart disease is both preventable and reversible. It is easier to prevent than it is to reverse, but both are definitely possible. I base these conclusions on the fact that THE MOST IMPORTANT BREAKTHROUGHS IN CARDIOVAS-

CULAR DISEASE IN THIS CENTURY HAVE OCCURRED IN THE PAST THREE YEARS."

In his continuing discussion, Goldstrich pointed out that diet is extremely important and he said that if he had coronary heart disease he would become a vegetarian overnight. Yet, he said:

"Most people can't or won't make all the sacrifices that are necessary to maximize diet therapy. If you're willing to make a few changes in your diet and add nutritional supplements to your regimen, you can make a big difference . . . *The central theme of this book is that coronary heart disease can be prevented and its progression stopped through the use of antioxidant supplements* [emphasis added]."[8]

> *Coronary heart disease can be prevented . . . through the use of antioxidant supplements.*

More On the Vitamin Controversy

According to an article reported in the April 14, 1994, edition of *The New England Journal of Medicine,* a study funded by the NIH's National Cancer Institute (NCI) showed that vitamin E and beta carotene produced "no reduction in the incidence of lung cancer among male smokers after 5 to 8 years of dietary supplementation."

Participants in the study consisted of 29,133 male smokers, 50 to 69 years of age from southwestern Finland. But here, too, there is another side of the coin, as noted by John L. Stegmaier, editor of the newsletter of the Well Mind Association of Greater Washington, Inc. Here are excerpts from his comments.

"Almost immediately, the report provoked skeptical and critical reactions from a variety of sources, including *Newsweek* writer, Geoffrey Cowley, who said that the findings don't prove that supplements are worthless or dangerous. The lesson is simply that pills are no substitute for common sense."[9]

Stegmaier also cited the comments of Drs. Hal Hiebert, Joan Priestley and Bernard Rimland of the International Scientific Advisory Council. These professionals described the study as badly flawed. Here are some of the deficiences which were cited.

- It used ⅛ to 1/40 the dose of vitamin E that had been shown by more than 20 previous studies to lower the risk of lung cancer in smokers.
- It used 1/10 the dosage of beta carotene recommended for the treatment of lung cancer in long term smokers.
- It used as subjects people living in Finland, despite the fact that both the *British Medical Journal* and the *American Journal of Clinical Nutrition* consider it one of the least desirable countries in the world for cancer/nutrition studies. The Finns have one of the world's highest rates of per capita alcohol consumption by smokers, and alcohol interferes with the utilization of Vitamin E and beta carotene; and the soil in Finland contains extremely low levels of selenium. This trace mineral in combination with other nutrients plays a role in preventing cancer.

To Supplement or Not to Supplement

This was the title of a three-quarter page discussion in the March 25, 1994, issue of *USA Today*. In this report, Nanci Hellmich interviewed eight different "experts." These included Surgeon General Dr. Joycelyn Elders and John Foreyt, director of the nutrition research clinic, Baylor College of Medicine, who said, "I don't take vitamins. I don't see any need for them. I get the vitamins I need from what I eat."

Others interviewed include Dr. Blumberg; Jane Fonda; Dr. Kenneth Cooper, founder of the Cooper Aerobic Center in Dallas; Dr. Robert Heaney, Calcium researcher at Creighton University; Dr. James H. Moller from the American Heart Association; and, Sonja

L. Conner. All of them take and recommend antioxidant nutritional supplements.

Dr. Cooper commented:

"I take vitamin E because research suggests it may keep LDL cholesterol from oxidizing, depositing on artery walls. Vitamin C enhances the beneficial effects of vitamin E. And there are no long term side effects of taking these vitamins at these doses . . . In my new book, *The Antioxidant Revolution,* I mainly concentrate on the three antioxidants that we have studied extensively—that is vitamin C, E and beta carotene."

My Comments

I agree 100% with the authorities who emphasize that taking a bunch of vitamin pills and continuing to eat diets loaded with junk foods, sugar and fats, will not enable a person to enjoy good health. Yet, I continue to take and recommend vitamin and mineral supplements for other members of my family and for my patients. Those I recommend for my adult patients with yeast-connected health problems contain:

Vitamin A	5,000–10,000 IU	Calcium	500 mgs.
Beta-carotene	15,000 IU	Magnesium	500 mgs.
Vitamin B_1	25–100 mgs/daily	Inositol	100 mgs.
Vitamin B_{21}	25–50 mgs/daily	Citrus bioflavonoids	100 mgs.
Niacinamide	100–150 mgs/daily	PABA	50 mgs.
Pantothenic acid	100–500 mgs/daily	Zinc	15–30 mgs.
Vitamin B_6	25–100 mgs/daily	Copper	1–2 mgs.
Folic acid	200–800 mcg.	Manganese	20 mgs.
Vitamin B_{12}	100 mcg.	Selenium	100–200 mcg.
Biotin	300 mcg.	Chromium	200 mcg.
Choline (Bitartrate)	100 mgs.	Molybdenum	100 mcgs.
Vitamin C	1000–10,000 mgs.	Vanadium	25 mcgs.
Vitamin D	100–400 IU	Boron	1 mg.
Vitamin E	400–600 IU		

When supplements are prescribed by a knowledgeable professional, the amounts may vary considerably from those I've outlined, and his or her experience, expertise and clinical judgment will override my recommendations. Although the use of vitamin/mineral supplements continues to be "controversial," interest and support for their use appear to be increasing.

REFERENCES

1. Ulene, A. and Ulene, V., *The Vitamin Strategy*, Ulysses Press, Berkeley, CA, 1994.
2. *Executive Health*, P.O. Box 8880, Chapel Hill, NC 27515.
3. Cranton, E. and Passwater, R., *Trace Elements, Hair Analysis*, Keats Publishing Company, New Canaan, CT, 1984.
4. Good, R., as cited in Crook, W.G., *The Yeast Connection*, Third Edition, Professional Books, Jackson, TN and Vintage Books, New York, 1986; p 371.
5. Lin, D.J., *Free Radicals and Disease Prevention*, Keats Publishing, New Canaan, CT, 1993.
6. Robertson, J.M., et al, "A possible role for vitamins C and E in cataract prevention," *Amer. J. of Clin. Nutr.*, 1991; 53:346s–351s.
7. Jacques, P.F., et al, "Epidemiologic evidence of a role for the antioxidant vitamins and carotenoids in cataract prevention," *Am. J. of Clin. Nutr.*, 1991; 53:352s–355s.
8. Goldstrich, J.D., *The Cardiologist's Painless Prescription for a Healthy Heart and a Longer Life*, 9-Heart-9 Publishing, 8215 Westchester Dr., Suite 307, Dallas, TX 75225, 1994.
9. Stegmaier, J., The Well Mind Association of Greater Washington, Inc., 11141 Georgia Ave., #326, Wheaton, MD 20902.

29

Chemicals in Your Home and Your Workplace

If your health problems are yeast connected, you'll have a better chance of overcoming them if you get rid of the chemical pollutants in your home—and workplace. The first part of this task you can do something about. Although the second part is more difficult, the job is getting easier.

Increasing Recognition of the Importance of Indoor Air Pollution

During the past decade, in spite of skeptics, the importance of indoor chemical pollutants has been recognized by a growing number of professionals and nonprofessionals. I've found evidence of such recognition in a commentary by Andrew Skolnick, published in the *Journal of the American Medical Association* entitled, "Even the Air in the Home Is Not Entirely Free of Potential Pollutants." Here are excerpts.

> "A 10-year study by the U. S. Environmental Protection Agency (EPA), Washington, DC, shows that, for some pollutants, the air outside may be safer to breathe than the air in the home.
> "Speaking at the American Lung Association's Second Annual Science Writers Forum in Annapolis, Maryland, Lance A. Wallace, Ph.D., an evironmental scientist at the EPA, said that most exposure

number of known or suspected carcinogens appears to come primarily from personal activities rather than from industrial sources.

"The risks Americans may face from some of the pollutants dumped and leaked into the environment by industry may be less than the risk from activities in the home, such as smoking, showering, using room deodorizers and storing and wearing dry-cleaned clothes. Wallace says, quoting the comic strip 'Pogo':

'We have met the enemy and he is us.'"[1]

We have met the enemy and he is us.

Further recognition of the importance of chemicals in making people sick came in a comprehensive 17-page report in the *Chemical & Engineering News* by Bette Hileman. In her article published in the July 22, 1991, issue of *C & EN*, Hileman touched on the people who were so severely affected by chemical sensitivities that they had to live like hermits. She commented:

"... Most people allegedly suffering from multiple chemical sensitivity (MCS) have a far less debilitating form of the disease. The majority manage to keep their jobs and maintain a fairly normal home life ...

"... They usually try to avoid the chemical exposures they believe make them feel sick, such as rooms that have been newly carpeted or recently sprayed with pesticides ...

"... They may not be able to tolerate the smell of new clothing in a department store or the odors in the aisles of cleaning products in the supermarket and so they avoid those places.

"Advocates for MCS patients believe there may be millions of people in the U.S. suffering with frequent headaches or other symptoms who are not aware their problems are caused by their surroundings."[2]

In an article, "Do Buildings Make You Sick?" Michael J. Hodgson, M.D., MPH, discussed the insidious threat posed by indoor air pollutants. Such pollutants, which are found in apartment complexes, office buildings, hotels and houses, can present serious risks to our health. And he said:

"Since the mid-1960s, secretaries, executives, computer operators, maintenance workers and others have complained of symptoms and diseases that have been traced back to the workplace . . . Every year people miss up to 500,000 work days because of these illnesses."[3]

In a 1991 book, *Chemical Exposures—Low Levels and High Stakes,* Nicholas A. Ashford, Ph.D., J.D., and Claudia S. Miller, M.D., M.S., discussed the role chemical pollutants play in causing a wide variety of symptoms. In their book, they identified four major groups of people who had hypersensitivity to low levels of chemicals. Included were occupants of tight buildings.

In preparing their landmark work, Ashford and Miller interviewed key figures in the field and reviewed the relevant literature of the last 40 years. In a review of this book in the October 2, 1991, issue of the *Journal of the American Medical Association,* James E. Cone, M.D., MPH, commented:

"Clinicians and policy makers would do well to read and heed the advice of this book, for many of us are faced with the problem of how to best evaluate patients affected by this disorder, currently without adequate guidance about the best means of diagnosis, treatment and, most important, prevention."[4]

In a recent article in *Woman's Day,* "Are You Allergic to the Modern World?"[5] Sue Browder gave a clear picture of the problem experienced by many people who complained of fatigue, achy muscles, headaches, mental fogginess and other symptoms which are caused by chemical sensitivities. And she cited the observations of a number of physicians and scientists, including Lance Wallace who told her about the new carpet which was installed in EPA headquarters which made more than 100 people sick.

> **Seventy percent of patients seeking treatment for MCS are women.**

She also cited the observations of Dr. Leo Galland, who said that about 70% of patients seeking treatment for MCS are women. She also said that some doctors think this high proportion of women is because their bodies contain a higher proportion of fat than men's, and toxins tend to collect in fat.

Theron Randolph, M.D.

This brilliant pioneer physician was graduated from the University of Michigan Medical School over 60 years ago. Following his graduation, he received many years of specialty training in internal medicine, allergy and immunology. Even before he became aware of chemical sensitivities, Randolph found that he could help many chronically ill patients by changing their diets.

> **Randolph was "fired" from the faculty of Northwestern University Medical School.**

Because his approach was in sharp contrast to that of his academic peers, he was "fired" from his position on the faculty of Northwestern University Medical School. Yet, the world famous otolaryngologist, George E. Shambaugh, Jr., praised him.

In an editorial entitled, "Ahead of His Time,"[6] Shambaugh compared Randolph's brilliant and original contributions to those of the nineteenth century obstetrician/gynecologist, Ignaz Semmelweiss. Like Randolph, this Austrian physician was "kicked off" the staff of a Vienna hospital because he advised young doctors to wash their hands before carrying out pelvic examinations of women in labor.

In the introduction to a book co-authored with Randolph, Ralph W. Moss, Ph.D., said:

"In 1951 Randolph made what was probably his greatest discovery, and one which was to get him into even greater professional difficulties than his previous findings. After studying a number of his patients . . . he came to the conclusion that man's increasing pollution of the environment with chemicals was a major source of chronic illness . . .

"Randolph had discovered [that] . . . seemingly harmless chemicals in use in our homes, offices and work places every day in 'non-toxic' doses were responsible for a variety of mental, emotional and physical problems, from headache to depression to multiple muscle and joint pains and aches."[7]

The Importance of Randolph's Observations Is Recognized by Others

Gradually—oh so gradually—Randolph's observations spread to a small group of other physicians and in 1965, along with a few of his colleagues, a Clinical Ecology Study Club was formed to study and discuss the problems of people who were made ill by chemicals in the environment.

Within a few years, this small club became the nucleus of a new organization, the Society for Clinical Ecology, which subsequently adopted the name, The American Academy of Environmental Medicine.* And today, in the mid-1990s, the importance of Randolph's observations is receiving increasing recognition.

> ### The advance of knowledge hasn't been easy.

The advance of knowledge hasn't been easy. And if you complain of symptoms following exposure to perfume, gas stoves and to-

---

*For information about this organization write to AAEM, 4510 W. 89th St., Prairie Village, KS 66207.

bacco smoke, you're apt to be labeled as a "hypochondriac" or "psychoneurotic." I'm happy to report that the situation is changing, and changing rapidly. Here are the observations of several of Randolph's followers.

William Rea, M.D., Dallas, Texas

After graduating from medical school, Bill Rea prepared for a career as a cardiac surgeon. Then, an event happened that changed his personal and professional life. His home was sprayed with insecticides, which made him and other members of his family sick.

After recovering from his acute symptoms, Rea noted that he was sensitive to many different environmental chemicals—chemicals that did not bother other people. I recall clearly the first time I met him at a medical conference. He brought along aluminum foil to put on the seat of his chair. Here's why. Chemicals emanating from the plastic seats would trigger his symptoms.

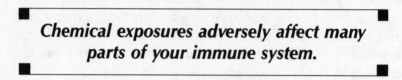

Chemical exposures adversely affect many parts of your immune system.

Studies by Dr. Rea and others show that chemical exposures adversely affect many parts of your immune system. The more chemicals you're exposed to, the greater are your chances of developing health problems. If chemical exposures bother you, Dr. Rea's barrel concept will help you understand what's happening. In explaining his concept to me, he said:

> "Chemicals you're exposed to resemble pipes draining into a rain barrel. The barrel represents a resistance. If you continue to be exposed to chemicals, the barrel overflows and you develop symptoms.
>
> "Infections of various types, including viral and yeast infections, may also precipitate a 'leak' in your barrel, even when the barrel isn't full."

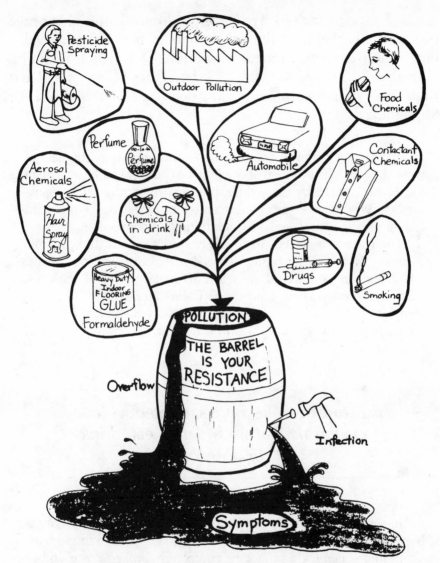

Adapted from William Rea M.D. Used with permission.

Doris Rapp, M.D., Buffalo, New York

During the last two decades this pediatric allergist and immunologist with impeccable academic credentials has helped thousands of patients with food and chemical sensitivities in her practice. She's also helped millions of others by her books, her videotapes* and her appearances on national television, including "Donahue," "Sally Jessy Raphael," the "Today Show" and "Larry King Live." In her recent bestselling book, *Is This Your Child?* Dr. Rapp said:

> "The impact of the global total disregard for our environment affects all of us. The problem of world wide chemical pollution can no longer be ignored by the public, physicians, educators or legislators. . . . We can no longer remain oblivious of the increasing pollution of our air, water, soil, food, clothing and homes. . . .
>
> "There are over 300,000 toxic and hazardous waste dumps in our country. Every day 50 billion gallons of liquid hazardous wastes are deposited in disposal sites. Unfortunately, 85% of these are said to be located above aquifers or water-storage areas. . . . Every year 100 billion gallons of liquid hazardous wastes are absorbed into our ground water. . . . *Safe water must become everyone's concern.* . . .

Fat stores can become saturated with . . . chemicals that we breathe, eat, drink or absorb.

> "In time, our fat stores can become saturated with the smorgasbord of chemicals that we breathe, eat, drink or absorb through our skin. Some chemicals cannot be completely broken down and removed by means of our expired air, perspiration, saliva, urine, and bowel movements. We must wonder how long our bodies, as well as those of our children, can handle our progressively increasing chemical overload."[8]

---

*Dr. Rapp's videos are available from the Practical Allergy Research Foundation (PARF) in Buffalo. For information call 1–800-787-8780.

Sherry Rogers, M.D., Syracuse, New York

In her lectures, scientific articles and books, Dr. Rogers describes her own environmentally-induced illnesses. And she said that once she found answers she made it her business to become an expert in the field and help advance the knowledge of those who want full health.

In her books and in her audio- and video-tapes, Rogers comprehensively reviews the many indoor and outdoor pollutants that play an important part in making people sick. These include formaldehyde, toluene, xylene, trichlorethylene, hydrocarbons and other outgassing chemicals.

She also has reviewed many reports from the medical literature. In a summary of several of these articles, she pointed out that:

1. Chemicals like benzene, toluene, phenol, xylene and formaldehyde tend to be in most homes and offices to varying degrees.
2. Because these are all fat-soluble chemicals, they easily pass through cell membranes into the bloodstream when they're inhaled.
3. Once these chemicals enter the body, they pass easily into the brain, which she says is "the most lipid organ of the body." The most common brain symptoms include depression, inability to think straight, exhaustion, dizziness and headache.

If you're "sick all over," and aren't finding answers—especially if you're bothered by chemical fumes or odors and would like to learn more, get copies of her books and video-tapes from Prestige Publishers, Box 3161, 3502 Brewerton Rd., Syracuse, NY 13220. 1–800-846-6687.

Why More People Are Developing Multiple Chemical Sensitivities

During the last ten years I've learned a lot from Alan Scott Levin, M.D., Adjunct Associate Professor of Immunology and Dermatology, University of California (SF) School of Medicine. I've heard him talk at a number of conferences, and my grandson, Trey Harness, and I stayed in his home during a recent trip to California. In discussing the increasing incidence of multiple chemical sensitivity syndrome with me, Dr. Levin said:

"We are the first generation in the history of the world that has been exposed over a lifetime to synthetic and toxic chemicals in our food, air, water and products we use. Before 1940 everyone lived on organic foods; pesticides weren't invented yet.

"There were no toxic waste dumps, preservatives in foods, antibiotics, malathion spray, chlorinated water, tight buildings, aerosol sprays, synthetic carpeting, formaldehyde products, or major cosmetics and perfume industries.

We are a more vulnerable population, not as biologically strong.

"The AIDS epidemic, sexual permissiveness, the birth control pill, widespread legal and illegal drug use, sedentary living, and convenience foods have changed the way we live. We are a more vulnerable population, not as biologically strong."

I've also received information and help from another California physician, Carol Jessop, M.D. I first met this board-certified internist and assistant clinical professor of medicine at the University of California in San Francisco in April 1989, on the occasion of her presentation at a CFS conference. Following the conference, we began to correspond and in November 1990 I heard her speak again at a CFS/CFIDS conference in Charlotte, North Carolina.

Because of our friendship and her interest in yeast-related health problems and chemical sensitivities, I asked her to write the foreword to my 1992 book, *Chronic Fatigue Syndrome and the Yeast Connection*. Here are excerpts.

"Since 1950 we've seen the development and overuse of antibiotics; the use of hormones and birth control pills; the development of immunosuppressive drugs; the introduction of various chemicals and toxins into our environment; and significant changes which have occurred within our diets, leaving us foods tainted with pesticides, depleted in nutritional value and loaded with sugars and dyes.

"Can we really continue to believe these changes have not affected the well being of some, and eventually perhaps all of us?"[9]

What You Can Do to Lessen Your Exposure to Indoor Air Pollutants and Lead a Less Toxic Life

While physicians and other professionals are arguing about indoor air pollution and chemical sensitivity, you can take these steps in your home to lessen your exposures.

1. *Don't smoke and don't let other people smoke in your home.* People in homes where others are smoking experience twice as many respiratory infections and other health problems as individuals in smoke-free homes. Moreover, such infections set up a vicious cycle of other health problems. Also, as you've probably heard, people exposed to second-hand smoke have recently been found to have higher levels of cancer-causing chemicals in their urine.

2. *Don't spray insecticides in your home.* Also, store insecticides, paint thinners and other toxic chemicals in the outside shed or garage. Don't keep them under the kitchen sink or in the basement where fumes can leak into the house.

3. *Buy all natural fibers.* Wool, cotton and silk. If you buy permanent press clothing, or sheets, wash them before using.

4. *Air dry-cleaned clothes* and bedspreads and drapes outside before bringing them into your house.

5. *Avoid—in every way possible—odorous toxic or potentially toxic substances in your home.* These include paints, formaldehyde, gas cooking stove, and many chemically produced perfumes and colognes.

6. *Do 30 to 40 minutes of aerobic exercise a week* followed, if possible, by a sauna. If you feel your body is loaded with toxic

chemicals, you may need the help of a professional who can carefully guide this "sweating out" therapy.

7. *Get an air purifier* to remove dust, molds and some chemicals.
8. *Drink lots of bottled water (in glass)* to help your body excrete chemicals.
9. *Have your home tested.* According to a spring 1994 article from the Gannett News Service, chemical risks in your home are often hard to track down. In discussing the problem, the article stated:

"In cases where chronic symptoms, such as headache, nausea, fatigue, weaknesses and visual problems persist, experts advise having the home tested."

And they cited the comments of Dr. Robert Simon, president of Toxicology International, a firm which screens homes for 40 pesticides and other chemicals, ranging from outlawed chlordane and DDT to chlordane's replacement, Dursban. The cost of this screening: $150.

Chlordane was cited as being a particular problem because it contains 103 chemicals. Although it did a great job killing termites, it still got into the air and into the carpets, which can steadily release it over time.

If you suspect that your home is contaminated from pesticides and other chemicals, you can call the Indoor Air Quality Information Clearing House, (1-800-438-4318) for advice on getting help. The EPA also runs a pesticide hotline (1-800-858-7378) and a lead hotline (1-800-LEAD-FYI).

Other sources of information include:

American Academy of Environmental Medicine, 4510 W. 89th Street, Prairie Village, KS 66207; the National Center for Environmental Health Strategies, 1100 Rural Ave., Voorhees, NJ 08043; the Practical Allergy Research Foundation, 1–800-787-8780.

You can also get a free booklet, *The Inside Story: A Guide to Indoor Air Quality,* by sending a postcard to Consumer Products Safety Commission, Washington, DC 20207.

An Important New Book

In gathering information for *The Yeast Connection and the Woman*, I sought information from many sources. Included were knowledgeable and interested physicians and books—superb books—which I've cited and quoted in various chapters.

> ## If you're bothered by tobacco smoke, perfume and other odors, this book is for you.

As I was finishing the "last lap" of my manuscript, I spent two hours reading Lynn Lawson's magnificent new book, *Staying Well in a Toxic World.*[10] *It is authoritative, carefully documented and as readable as a paperback novel!* In a prepublication review of the book, I said, "If you're bothered by tobacco smoke, perfume and other odors, this book is for you. It is carefully researched and clearly written by a woman who's been there. I highly recommend it."

Here are a few of the chapter titles.

- Warning: Your job may be hazardous to your health
- Warning: Your home may be hazardous to your health
- In and Under the Rug
- Which Pesticides Are Safe? Fighting the deadly dandelion
- Shooting Arrows at the Storm: What is wrong with modern medicine?

In the chapter "Warning: Your home may be hazardous to your health," Lawson tells the story of a family who became sick when they moved into a new house. And she summarizes the things that people need to do to build a safe home. She then talks about the furnishings in the house and at the end of the chapter she gives nine headings of things to do. She also recommends a number of books.

In the chapter "In and Under the Rug," she touches on toxic carpets and Senate Bill #657 (The Indoor Air Quality Act of 1989). She points out that a number of the people who came to testify were made ill by the carpets in the room.

Additional Sources of Information

Here are a few of the dozens and dozens of books recommended by Lynn Lawson:

Your Home, Your Health and Well-Being by David Rousseau, William J. Rea, M.D., and Jean Enwright, Berkeley, CA, Ten Speed Press, 1989.

The Non-Toxic Home and Office: Protecting Yourself and Your Family from Everyday Toxic and Health Hazards by Debra Lynn Dadd, Los Angeles, Jeremy P. Tarcher, 1992.

Success in the Clean Bedroom: A Path to Optimal Health by Natalie Golos and William J. Rea, M.D., Rochester, NY, Pinnacle Publishers, 1992.

Clean and Green: The Complete Guide to Non-Toxic and Environmentally Safe Housekeeping by Annie Berthold-Bond, Woodstock, NY, Ceres Press, 1990.

Toxic Carpet III by Glen Beebe, Toxic Carpet Information Exchange, P.O. Box 39344, Cincinnati, OH 45239.

Chemical Exposure and Human Health: A reference to 314 chemicals, with a guide to symptoms and a directory of organizations by Cynthia Wilson, Jefferson, NC, McFarland & Company, 1993.

The Allergy Self-Help Book by Sharon Faelten and the editors of *Prevention Magazine,* Emmaus, PA, Rodale Press, 1983.

Chemical Sensitivity: A Guide to Coping with Hypersensitivity Syndrome, Sick Building Syndrome and Other Environmental Illnesses by Bonnye L. Matthews, Jefferson, NC, McFarland & Company, 1992.

The Healthy Home: Attic to Basement Guide to Toxin-Free Living by Linda Mason-Hunter, Emmaus, PA, Rodale Press, 1989.

Pest Control You Can Live With: Safe and Effective Ways to Get Rid of Common Household Pests by Debra Graff, Earth Stewardship Press, P.O. Box 1316, Sterling, VA 22170.

A Chemical Free Lawn by Warren Schultz, Emmaus, PA, Rodale Press, 1989.

Raising Children Toxic-Free: How to Keep Your Child Safe from Lead, Asbestos, Pesticides and Other Environmental Hazards by Phillip Landrigan, M.D., and Herbert Needleman, M.D., 1994.

Non-Toxic, Natural and Earthwise by Debra Lynn Dadd, Jeremy P. Tarcher, Inc., Los Angeles, CA, 1990.

The Cure Is in the Kitchen by Sherry Rogers, M.D., Prestige Publishers, Box 3161, Syracuse, NY 13220.

Chemical Exposures—Low Levels and High Stakes by Nicholas A. Ashford, Ph.D., and Claudia A. Miller, M.D., Van Nostrand, Reinhold, New York, 1991.

She also listed many other sources of help for people with chemical sensitivities, including the following:

The Human Ecologist: This superb 36-page journal is published quarterly by HEAL (Human Ecology Action League), P.O. Box 49126, Atlanta, GA 30359–1126. Copies are free to members. Yearly membership dues, $20; Canada/Mexico, $25.

Informed Consent: The Magazine of Health, Prevention and Environmental News: This up-to-the-minute 66-page glossy magazine is published bi-monthly by the International Institute of Research for Chemical Hypersensitivity, P.O. Box 1984, Williston, ND 58802–1984. 701–774-7760. $18/year.

National Coalition Against the Misuse of Pesticides (NCAMP), 701 E Street, S.E., Suite 200, Washington, DC 20003; 202–543-5450; publishes *Pesticides and You.*

National Center for Environmental Health Strategies (NCEHS), 1100 Rural Avenue, Voorhees, NJ 08043; 609–429-5358; publishes newsletter, *The Delicate Balance,* Mary Lamielle, Editor.

Environmental Health Network (EHN), P.O. Box 1155, Larkspur, CA 94977; 415–331-9804; publishes newsletter, *The News Reactor,* Susan Molloy, Editor.

Environmental Health Association of Dallas, P.O. Box 388, Forestburg, TX 76239; publishes newsletter, *Twentieth Century Living*, Peggy Dunlap, Editor.

A Final Comment

Rush to your bookstore and buy a copy of *Staying Well in a Toxic World*. If they don't have it in stock, ask them to order it, or call or write her publisher, The Noble Press, Inc., 213 W. Institute Place, Suite 508, Chicago, IL 60610. 1–800–486-7737.

REFERENCES

1. Skolnick, A., "Even Air in the Home Is Not Entirely Free of Potential Pollutants: Medical News and Perspectives," *JAMA*, December 8, 1989; 262:3102–03, 3107.
2. Hileman, B., "Multiple Chemical Sensitivity," *Chemical & Engineering News*, July 22, 1991; pp 26–27. Copyright 1991, American Chemical Society.
3. Hodgson, M.J., "Do Buildings Make You Sick?" *Executive Good Health Report*, P.O. Box 8880, Chapel Hill, NC 27515.
4. Cone, J.E., Book Review, *JAMA*, October 2, 1991; 266:13: 1858–59.
5. Browder, S., "Are You Allergic to the Modern World?" *Woman's Day*, April 1, 1992.
6. Shambaugh, G.E., "Ahead of His Time," *Archives of Otolaryngology*, February 1964; 79:118–119.
7. Randolph, T.G. and Moss, R.W., *An Alternative Approach to Allergies*, Harper & Row, New York, 1989; p 50.
8. Rapp, D., *Is This Your Child?*, William Morrow, New York, 1991; pp. 262–264.
9. Jessop, C., in the Foreword to Crook, W.G., *Chronic Fatigue Syndrome and the Yeast Connection*, Professional Books, Jackson, TN, 1992.
10. Lawson, L., *Staying Well in a Toxic World*, The Noble Press, Chicago, IL, 1993.

30

◆

Lifestyle Changes

◆

Are you bothered by fatigue, headache, depression, muscle aches and/or a whole "laundry list" of other complaints? If your answer is "yes," it would be great if you could take a shot or a pill that would make these symptoms vanish. I don't need to tell you there are no such "magic" shots or pills.

You can begin to overcome some of your symptoms when you change your diet and get rid of chemical pollutants in your home. There are also many other things you'll need to do. You'll need to take charge of your health and say to yourself, *If it's going to be, it's up to me.*

I'm not saying that pills, shots and medical advice aren't needed. Far from it. In a recent conversation, George Miller, M.D., a Pennsylvania gynecologist, said:

> "When a woman comes in to me who feels 'sick all over,' I usually spend about an hour taking a history. Then, of course, I carry out a physical examination and do appropriate laboratory tests. Then, after I review these findings, put them together and come to a conclusion, I sit down with the patient and I say:
>
> " 'Chances are good—even excellent—that you can regain your health and get your life back on track; and I will help you. *I'd like to tell you about the 70/30 rule which I go by. This means that 70% of what needs to be done will be your responsibility and the remaining 30% will be mine.'* "

In several of my previous books and booklets I casually mentioned "lifestyle changes." They included exercise, stopping smoking and spending less time in front of the TV set and more time outdoors.

Yet, I only skimmed the surface. So I decided to dig deeper and obtain more information and pass it along. I'll begin by citing comments by Dean Ornish, M.D., the young California physician who has been and is revolutionizing the management of heart disease.

Comments by Dean Ornish, M.D.

In a chapter from his recent book entitled, *Dean Ornish's Program for Reversing Heart Disease,* Dr. Ornish discussed the need people have for contact with others—and for group support. He also pointed out that egocentric people are especially apt to experience health problems. So are people who are cynical or hostile. Such individuals are apt to feel isolated. And, he said:

> "Anything that promotes a sense of isolation leads to chronic stress and often illnesses like heart disease. Conversely, anything that leads to real intimacy and feelings of connection can be healing in the real sense of the word: to bring together, to make whole."

He presented all sorts of fascinating data from the scientific literature—data which dealt with both human beings and animals. Here are examples.

- Rabbits who were individually petted, held, talked to and played with on a regular basis by a technician developed less heart disease than genetically similar rabbits.
- A *New England Journal of Medicine* article which reported that 2320 male survivors of heart attacks who were "socially isolated" had more than four times the risk of death from heart disease than men with low levels of stress and isolation.
- A Stanford University study of women with metastatic breast cancer which showed that women who attended weekly group support meetings had *twice* the survival rate of a control group.
- An Ohio State University College of Medicine study which

showed that patients who scored above average in loneliness had significantly poor immune functioning.

In summarizing his thoughts and recommendations, Ornish said, "Isolation can lead to illness, where intimacy can lead to healing. Isolation comes in several forms:

- Isolation from our feelings, our inner self and inner peace
- Isolation from others
- Isolation from a higher force . . .

"The chronic stress in Twentieth-Century America is not only from the increased pace of modern life, but also from the isolation, loneliness and lack of love and support that so many people experience.

"Stress comes not only from what we do, but also how we *react* to what we do. How we react, in turn, is a function of how we perceive ourselves. When we perceive ourselves as only isolated and alone, then we're likely to feel chronically stressed . . . Anything that helps us transcend and transform this perceived isolation can be healing. The rest of this book shows how."[1]

In his book Ornish provides many fascinating details, including yoga techniques, improving communication skills, meditation and visualization.

Relaxation and Meditation

In a special health issue of *USA Weekend* (January 2, 1994), the feature article was entitled, "Stress Busters, Real Stress, Real People, Real Advice—You asked for help juggling family, money, school and work. Inside, experts offer stress busting strategies that you can start today."*

One of the articles in this health issue entitled "Count Down to Relaxation," featured 42-year-old Anna L. S. Battle of Trenton,

---

*Copyright, 1994, *USA Today*. Reprinted with permission.

New Jersey, a head nurse at Ewing Residential Treatment Center for troubled youths. According to the article:

"Anna Battle has had it up to *here*. She is continually under stress from her work with tough youngsters. She worries that budget cuts will soon have her doing more work for less pay. What's more, cold winter weather keeps her from fishing, her favorite stress buster. She's a prime candidate for relaxation therapy says Herbert Benson, who literally wrote the book on the subject [*The Relaxation Response*]."

In discussing Battle's problem, Herbert Benson, M.D., pointed out that she was reacting in a natural physiological way to her stress. He called it the "fight or flight" response.

And such a response increases a person's heart rate, blood pressure, metabolism and blood flow to the muscles. It also temporarily shuts down some body functions and depresses the immune system.

In a further discussion of Battle's problem, Benson pointed out that because she cannot eliminate her problems without eliminating her job, she must learn to deal with the symptoms. And he said:

"That's where the relaxation response comes in. . . . It's therapeutic, preventative and cost-effective at the same time."

Yet, Benson warned readers that there's no substitute for a doctor's care, and he said:

"First make sure there's nothing [wrong] that isn't better treated with our modern marvelous medicine. It would be tragic and totally inappropriate to start with this."

He also pointed out that more and more physicians and prestigious medical institutions (including Harvard Medical School) are now interested in mind/body medicine.

How Do You Meditate?

A number of my patients have tried it and some say it's easy to do, while others say, "It didn't help me." If you'd like to try it, here are some of Dr. Benson's suggestions as summarized in *USA Weekend*.

1. **Pick a mental focusing device.** A word or phrase, religious or secular. Most of Benson's patients choose something religious: "Hail Mary, full of grace"; "Allah be praised"; "*Sh'ma Yisroel*." The specific words are unimportant.
2. **Assume a comfortable position or activity.** You may sit quietly or listen to music; others might prefer to exercise.
3. **Close your eyes,** to help you focus.
4. **Relax muscles,** to counter physical tightness.
5. **Breathe slowly and naturally, and repeat your focus word or phrase,** replacing the fight-or-flight response with a calm-down attitude.
6. **Assume a passive attitude.** This may be the hardest step, because we're keyed to "doing something." Don't be discouraged if outside thoughts intrude. Just say, "Oh well," and return to your discipline. Why get stressed over stress-busting?
7. **Continue for 10–20 minutes.** Make the time—think how much time you waste worrying.
8. **Practice once or twice a day.**

More Interest and Support of the Relaxation Response

According to Leslie Miller in a cover story in the July 28, 1994, Life Section of *USA Today*, meditation is now becoming mainstream.*

In her article, Miller pointed out that people have been meditating in this country for a long time. Yet, she said:

> "Although Americans now flock to classes and retreats, few outside religious communities were meditating here before Maharishi Mahesh Yogi introduced transcendental meditation to the U.S. in 1959."

---

*Copyright, 1994, *USA Today*. Reprinted with permission.

Miller also cited the observations of a number of professionals, including Benson and Jon Kabat-Zinn, founder of the Stress Reduction Clinic, University of Massachusetts Medical Center.

She also said that 30 clinics now use stress reduction, and that a Kansas corporation has offered meditation to stressed out executives. And in quoting Kabat-Zinn, she said:

> ### *Meditation is a way to cultivate sanity and well-being and wisdom.*

"Americans now know there's no magic answer to all life's problems . . . Meditation is a way to cultivate sanity and well-being and wisdom in one's life that you can't get from watching television or taking a pill."

Comments by Elson M. Haas, M.D.

In his 1140-page, comprehensive, easy-to-read and understand book, this San Rafael, California, physician touches many important bases. And in a section entitled "Personal and Planetary Survival," he lists "88 Survival Suggestions," including 15 lifestyle changes. Here are a few of them.

- **Create** a good exercise program. This includes regular exercise, stretching and at least 30 minutes of vigorous activity several times a week.
- **Avoid** excessive sun exposure. With the depletion of the ozone layer and the effect of ultraviolet light, the risks outweigh the benefits.
- **Practice** some sort of stress reduction daily. Meditate, lie down without sleeping, or just sit with eyes closed, breathe deeply, relax for at least 15 to 20 minutes.
- **Reduce** or avoid alcohol use. Alcohol depresses the senses and reduces immune resistance. In addition, chemicals are used in processing most alcohol products.

- **Avoid** habitual drug use, such as consumption of caffeine in coffee, tea or colas, and regular sugar use.
- **Drink** more clean water and less soda, coffee, juice and alcoholic beverages.
- **Wear** more natural-fiber clothes (cotton, rayon and silk), especially if you're sensitive to synthetic materials.
- **Buy** and use organic foods, those that are grown without chemicals, fertilizers and pesticides.
- **Minimize** soft drink use. Substitute water or a combination of fruit juice and carbonated mineral water.
- **Take** antioxidant nutrients.
- **Eat** more cruciferous vegetables and rotate foods to avoid allergic/sensitivity reactions.
- **Obtain** natural lighting or full spectrum lights at work.
- **Take** regular breaks from a computer—walk and stretch, drink water and get fresh air.
- **Learn** some healing arts, such as massage, herbal therapy and nutrition for yourself and others.
- **Plant** a garden and grow your own food.
- **Learn** *to meditate. You can become your own stress counselor and can be more attuned to your inner nature.*[2]

My Comments

During the past couple of years, I've received many more reports about the importance of lifestyle changes of all sorts. Then a few weeks before I completed my last revision and editing of my manuscript, I received a letter from a California lawyer, Rosemary (not her name), which says it all. Here are excerpts.

"About two years ago I wrote to you desperate and depressed about my health and financial situation. Thanks to an insightful health food store clerk, I picked up a copy of your book. I'm writing to thank you. I went to a kind and caring doctor a full day's drive from my home. He listened and didn't dismiss my aches and pains as 'hysteria' or 'depression.'"

In her letter Rosemary told me how she had taken the various antifungal drugs, yet she made little progress and was forced onto disability. She said, "I could only aspire to do the morning dishes and walk the quarter mile to the post office with my toddler." And she said, "No firm would hire me." Then she said:

"In April this year I accepted my new lifestyle limitations. I weaned myself off the Diflucan and Prozac. I slowed down even as I sped up. I now have a real full-time practice . . . I'm now a single mother, but I have a live-in housekeeper/nanny, so I don't work the 'double shift.'

I walk one to one-and-a-half miles twice a day, rain, shine or snow.

"I walk one to one-and-a-half miles twice a day, rain, shine or snow. (I live by a ski resort.) I still fall asleep sometimes when stressed. (My husband just filed for a divorce a week ago.) I also wanted to share another book which has helped me and two of my CFIDS clients.

"I'm a spiritual person, but private in my beliefs. I'm not a 'New Ager' by any stretch. However, the book, *The Celestine Prophecy,* by James Redfield gave me a concept . . . of immense proportions: Since we, humans, are all made up of the same stuff as the rest of the world, instead of getting our energy just from food or from other people, we can get it from everything around us.

"I may not have put the concept as eloquently as I could, but please understand the ramifications. For someone whose daily existence pleads for energy, I was like a person dying from thirst while swimming in an ocean of fresh water.

"I now meditate outside, in nature, every morning, re-charging my batteries. I monitor my food and my relationships. Like a drained rechargeable battery, I must recharge more often. But in two months it takes less and less effort. Dr. Crook, thank you. Your book literally saved my life since I was on the verge of suicide when I found it. If there's ever *anything* I can do, call on me, please."

REFERENCES

1. Ornish, D., *Dean Ornish's Book for Reversing Heart Disease*, Ballantine Books, 1990; pp 85–103.
2. Haas, E.M., *Staying Healthy with Nutrition*, Celestial Arts, Berkeley, CA, 1992; pp 487–497.

31

Exercise

Whether your health problems are yeast connected, or whether they aren't, you'll need to exercise if you want to enjoy good health. All three of my daughters walk almost every day. Nancy said, "If I don't get my exercise, I can tell it. I do not feel good."

Exercise Helps You Overcome Depression and Fatigue

According to Charles W. Smith, M.D.,* it is especially important for patients with depression and chronic fatigue to exercise. And he especially recommended aerobic exercises which require the use of oxygen to produce energy. And, he said:

> "Exercises that are regarded as predominantly aerobic are those that are performed at a moderate effort level and use continuous movement of large muscle groups. Anaerobic exercise involves bursts of speed or intense effort that create energy needs that temporarily outstrip the body's ability to deliver oxygen to the muscle."

Aerobic exercises he recommended include walking, running, aerobic dance, swimming, cross-country skiing, bicycling and rowing.

And, in his continuing discussion, he urged physicians to recognize the importance of choosing activities that suit the patient so that the exercise program is more likely to be continued. And he

---

*Professor of Family and Community Medicine and Executive Associate Dean for Clinical Affairs, University of Arkansas for Medical Sciences, Little Rock, Arkansas.

said, "If the importance of enjoyment of exercise is forgotten, it will soon be discontinued."[1]

In commenting on the immediate benefits of exercise, gynecologist Joe S. McIlhaney, Jr., said:

> "There are several direct rewards for anyone who starts a regular program of exercise.
> "FEELING BETTER. When patients complain to me of feeling tired and not having much energy, I assure them if they will begin exercising, within two weeks they will feel like different people."[2]

He points out that exercise also helps people increase their mental alertness and control their weight, and that studies have shown that people who exercise develop fewer illnesses and are less apt to have accidents.

Exercise Helps Strengthen Your Bones

In his 1994 book, *Preventing and Reversing Osteoporosis,* Alan Gaby, M.D., Baltimore, said:

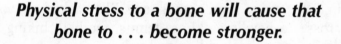

> ***Physical stress to a bone will cause that bone to . . . become stronger.***

> "It has long been known that bones develop in a way that resist the forces acted upon them. This means that repeated application of a physical stress to a bone will actually cause that bone to remodel and become stronger."

Gaby cited an international study of hip fractures in women from different countries which showed that physical activity, or lack of it, played a key role in determining whether a fracture would occur.

He also cited another study of 46 menopausal women. "Those who were physically fit had greater bone mineral content in the femur and the spine than women of the same age who were less fit."In his continuing discussion of various forms of exercise, he pointed out that although all forms of exercise promote better health, that weight bearing exercises, including walking, running, jumping on a trampoline, or playing tennis or basketball, are the best ways to strengthen your bones. He concluded:

> "What is most important is that you engage in some form of regular exercise, perhaps 30 minutes at a time, 3 or 4 times a week. To promote optimal health, exercise should be started early in life and continued on into your later years. When my sedentary patients begin an exercise program, they almost always begin to feel better in many ways within a month or two."[3]

In a chapter, "Women in Motion," in the new *Our Bodies, Ourselves* by the Boston Women's Health Collective, Janet Jones said:

> "A lot more of us women are out in the world moving around and *it feels good*. We're swimming, walking, dancing, jogging, power lifting, fencing and hiking."[4]

Jones also listed 36 other physical activities that women are engaged in. They range from team sports like basketball, volleyball and lacrosse to bowling, skiing, tennis, football, biking, karate, scuba diving, horseback riding and golf.

She pointed out that a century ago middle class women didn't exercise because it was considered "unladylike." Times have changed. Women today know exercise helps their muscles, hearts and bones.

Exercise Helps Prevent Cancer

On a September 1994 program on the "Today Show," Kate Couric interviewed Leslie Burnstein who said that women who participated in one to three hours of exercise a week over their reproductive lifetime had a 20% reduction in breast cancer. And those who participated in more activity each week showed a 60% reduction in breast cancer.

> **Those who participated in more activity each week showed a 60% reduction in breast cancer.**

In responding to the question from Couric about how exercise helps, Burnstein said it affects hormones that are important in determining a woman's breast cancer risk. Modifying these hormones that are produced over the reproductive lifetime of women lowers their risk. In her continuing discussion, Burnstein said her studies found that exercising during adolescent years was especially important. It also provided significant protective effects for women who began exercising later in their lives.

Exercise Helps Prevent Heart Disease

An article in the April 1994 *Mayo Clinic Healthletter* cited an August 1993 report in the *Journal of American College of Cardiology* which described some of the beneficial effects of exercise. Adults who exercised vigorously five or six times a week for a year partially reversed the buildup of cholesterol and fatty acids in their arterial walls.

I was glad to see this report about the possibility of reversing blocked arteries without surgery. This subject has interested me for many different reasons. As I have mentioned elsewhere in this book, I was a member of Nathan Pritikin's Advisory Board for almost 10 years.

During visits to Pritikin's Longevity Research Institute, I talked to a number of people who had been disabled by chronic disease, including chest pain, diabetes and arthritis, who had regained their health and their life on a program which featured walking and dietary changes.

The second reason for my interest in the subject is what I call the "epidemic" of by-pass surgery in hospitals around the country. I'm not saying that some of these operations aren't necessary. Yet, I'm concerned about them for many reasons. Here's one of them.

Six of my friends died during (or shortly after) by-pass surgery and another friend developed Alzheimer's almost overnight following surgery.

Of course, exercise alone won't keep you from developing heart disease, but when you combine it with diet and lifestyle changes, your risk of developing heart disease will be greatly lessened.

Exercise Helps Your Reproductive Organs

In a further discussion of exercise in *The New Our Bodies, Ourselves*, Janet Jones pointed out that until recently women were taught that exercise could damage their "internal organs." But today, exercise helps women, including those with PMS and during and after pregnancy.

> *But today, exercise helps women, including those with PMS and during and after pregnancy.*

She did, however, insert a word of caution for those who run over 30 miles a week, or train heavily. She pointed out that overly vigorous exercise may result in infrequent or absence of menses. And she advised women who experience menstrual irregularities to cut back on your workouts to see if you will resume your cycles.

Susan M. Lark, M.D., in her book, *PMS—Self-Help Book*, in discussing exercise, said:

"When I was a teenager exercise was never mentioned as a possible treatment for PMS. I was only told about aspirin, hot water bottles and bed, none of which was effective. When my menstrual cramps would occur, I would go to bed and simply brave out the pain, hoping it wouldn't last too long. I wish I had known about the benefits of a well conditioned body."

In her continuing discussion, she said she had learned about personal benefits of exercise as well as the help it had given many of her patients. The benefits she cited included lessening of fluid retention, prevention of back pain, improved posture, relief of anxiety and irritability and other psychological effects. And she said:

"Walking at a fast pace and fresh air can be particularly beneficial. Try to walk in the early morning sunlight to increase your levels of natural vitamin D. Swimming is excellent for all around toning and for cardiovascular health. Other enjoyable sports include bicycling, tennis and moderate jogging."[5]

So there you have it. If you want to look good, feel good and overcome health problems of any sort, you'll need to exercise regularly.

REFERENCES

1. Smith, C.W., Jr., "Exercise: Practical Treatment for the Patient with Depression and Chronic Fatigue," *Primary Care*, 1991; 18:2:271–281.
2. McIlhaney, J.S., Jr. with Nethery, S., *1250 Health-Care Questions Women Ask*, Baker Book House Company, Grand Rapids, MI, and Focus on the Family Publishing, Colorado Springs, CO, 1992; p 816.
3. Gaby, A., *Preventing and Reversing Osteoporosis*, Prima Publishing, P.O. Box 1260 BK, Rocklin, CA 95677, pp 219–224.
4. Jones, J., in the Boston Women's Health Collective, *The New Our Bodies, Ourselves*, Touchstone, Simon and Schuster, New York, 1992; pp 65–78.
5. Lark, S.M., *PMS—Self-Help Book*, Celestial Arts, P.O. Box 7327, Berkeley, CA, 1984.

32

<hr>

The Mind/Body Connection

<hr>

During my years in medical school at the University of Virginia, I spent most of my time learning about the body. My courses included anatomy, bacteriology, biochemistry, pathology, medicine, surgery, obstetrics, pediatrics and a smattering of psychiatry.

I was especially fascinated as I studied and treated patients with disorders ranging from high blood pressure, heart and kidney disease to meningitis, diabetes, and epilepsy. But "mental" problems that I learned a little about from lectures and visits to a psychiatric ward were only of passing interest to me.

After leaving Virginia, I served a rotating internship at the Pennsylvania Hospital in Philadelphia. I delivered babies, sewed up lacerations in the emergency room, assisted at surgical operations, treated people with heart failure, kidney stones, diabetes and other disorders and worked in the lab.

Army Experiences Which Made Me Aware of the Mind/Body Connection

After a few months of general practice, I entered the army medical corps in August 1943. During one of my assignments, I served for seven months on the psychiatric staff of an army hospital in Oklahoma. I worked with and under Dr. Kurt Adler, a son of the famous Viennese psychiatrist. While there, I learned for the first time that emotional stress could cause physical symptoms.

One soldier I remember well (I'll call him Tom) was transferred from a hospital in France. His complaint was numbness and paralysis which developed following a blow to his right shoulder during a bombing raid. Although on examination Tom showed no objective evidence of an injury, he seemed unable to move his arm.

> ### When Tom touched a lighted cigarette to the back of his hand, he said, "I can't feel it. It doesn't burn."

Moreover, he experienced no sensation of pain when he was given a shot. Tom also took a lighted cigarette and touched it to the back of his hand and said, "I can't feel it. It doesn't burn." Yet, his paralysis and absence of sensations of pain in his hand did not follow a neurological pattern. My chief, Dr. Adler, called it "glove" anesthesia. And he said:

> "Dr. Crook, problems of this sort often develop in people who have experienced a severe fright or other emotional trauma which causes them to develop anxiety. When this anxiety is 'converted' into physical symptoms, we call it 'conversion hysteria.' And we may be able to confirm my tentative diagnosis by giving Tom an intravenous injection of a sedative/tranquilizer."

To my amazement, during and following this injection, Tom was able to use his arm and sensation in his hand returned. Yet, the paralysis and numbness were replaced by severe anxiety.

A short time later, I was sent to Texas where I was assigned to the staff of the 178th General Hospital. Our unit left the States in October 1944 and after about 6 weeks in a staging area in England, we moved on to Rheims, France. There we "took over" the care of American soldiers who had been sent to this 2000-bed general hospital. I was assigned to an infectious disease ward consisting mainly of patients with pneumonia. And because the battle front was over a hundred miles away, I went to bed each night feeling safe and sound.

Then, along with all the other doctors on the hospital staff, I was awakened about 2:00 A.M. I think it was on the morning of December 20th. Colonel Monte Belot, the head of our hospital, made the following solemn announcement:

"Elements of the German army are breaking through American lines in Belgium and heading toward the Meuse River. We need physicians from our hospital staff who will volunteer to go to the front."

I was one of only four officers on the hospital staff under the age of 30. So I slowly raised my hand. So did three other young officers. We were told that we would be taken to operations headquarters at 10:00 A.M. where we would learn what we would do and where we would go.

During the months following my indoctrination into the army, I received training of various sorts designed to convert a civilian doctor into a soldier. Included were drills and marches and crawling through an obstacle course under the cover of live ammunition.

> **I could feel a tingling in my neck, shoulders and arms, and a burning in my stomach.**

Yet, when I heard Dr. Belot's announcement I was frightened—really frightened. I was unprepared psychologically to fulfill this new assignment. My heart rate which was usually 60/minute jumped to 120. My mouth became dry and I could feel a tingling in my neck, shoulders and arms, and a burning in my stomach.

My fellow officers who were also given this new assignment seemed almost as scared as I was. Happily, during the next few hours, as we talked and shared our feelings, my anxiety lessened and I felt better. Yet, my symptoms didn't really go away until my colleagues and I met with another colonel at operations headquarters who told us what we would be doing.

Along with two medical corpsmen from our hospital, I was assigned to temporary duty with an engineering battalion. Its mission: Blow up the bridge across the Meuse River in case the German advance got to the river.

About 6:00 P.M., under the cover of darkness, we headed north from Rheims and on into Belgium. We arrived about midnight in a town five or six miles from the Meuse River. I have to admit that I was still scared, but my severe physical symptoms had gone away and I slept like a log the rest of the night.

The next morning we learned that the German advance had been turned back by American ground and air forces. And after a few days in a charming little Belgian town, I was able to return to my duties at the hospital.

As I reflect on what happened, I'm sure it was the uncertainty—the "not knowing"—along with my fear—that caused my physical symptoms. *My work with Tom in Oklahoma, and my brief personal experience in World War II, made me a more understanding and empathetic physician in dealing with my patients over the years. It also provided me with information about the "mind/body connection"—a subject I'm hearing more about today.*

My Experiences During Medical Training and in Practice

After being discharged from the army and several months in general practice, I went to Vanderbilt where I served a pediatric internship and residency. After leaving Vanderbilt, I served as Chief Resident at the Sydenham Hospital in Baltimore, an infectious disease facility affiliated with Johns Hopkins.

There I saw and treated children and adults with many diseases, including diphtheria, polio and meningitis. During my last month in Baltimore, I worked in the children's cardiac clinic at Hopkins.

In these hospital experiences I received little exposure to the role psychological factors could contribute to illness.

I then returned to Tennessee and hung out my shingle to practice general pediatrics. Because there were no other full-time pediatricians in my community, my office was loaded with patients right from the word "go." I made many house calls and saw a few patients in the hospital. I soon obtained an associate, and then other associates, and we all stayed busy seeing well children and those who appeared to be affected by "physical" diseases.

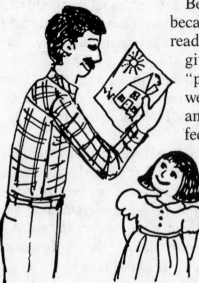

Because of my army experiences and because of seminars I took and articles I read, I was aware of the importance of giving children and their parents "psychological vitamins." Included were reassurance, praise, smiles, hugs and other expressions of approval, affection and encouragement.

As the years went by, I developed a strong interest in allergies and sensitivities of various sorts, including those which were caused by adverse reactions to foods. Symptoms in these children included fatigue, headache, irritability, short attention span, muscle aches and hyperactivity—symptoms which parents and most professionals blamed on psychological causes.

> **I found that I could relieve symptoms which were supposedly "emotionally induced" using elimination diets.**

When I found that I could relieve these supposedly "emotionally induced" symptoms using elimination diets, I said to myself, "The importance of psychological factors is often overrated."

I continued to feel that way on through the 1960s and 1970s. During these years, because of my interest in allergies and in environmental illness, I began to see more and more adult patients—especially women with complex medical problems, including food and chemical sensitivities.

Although I helped many of these patients using a comprehensive program which featured nutrition, control of environmental pollutants and avoidance of foods that caused sensitivity reactions, there were some patients I failed to help. At least I didn't help them as much as I would have liked.

Then came what to me was a real "breakthrough." In 1979, I learned about the observations of C. Orian Truss, the Alabama physician who first described the relationship of yeast to many chronic health problems. And in the early and mid-1980s, I saw and helped several hundred patients—most of whom were women—using a restricted diet and antiyeast medications.

I Learn More About the Mind/Body Connection

Although I was aware that psychological factors could contribute to the health problems in some of these patients, I didn't really pay much attention to them until about 10 years ago.

At that time, during a trip to California, I had dinner with the late Doctor Phyllis Saifer, a leader in studying patients with food and environmental sensitivities and yeast-related health problems. During and after dinner, Phyllis talked about many things, including the role psychological factors played in many of her patients. And, she said, in effect:

> "Although food and chemical sensitivities and candida play an important role in making people sick, *I've found in my own practice that many people with these problems—especially women—give a history of having been physically or sexually abused. And such abuse weakens the immune system and makes them more apt to develop other health problems.*"

About the same time I read and re-read Norman Cousins' article published in the *New England Journal of Medicine*[1] and his books, *Anatomy of An Illness*[2] and *The Healing Heart*.[3] I also listened to several of his tapes. In the mid-1980s I visited Mr. Cousins in his UCLA office on two occasions. He told me jokes and many stories.

One that really impressed me had to do with a football game. Here's a summary.

An announcement came over the loud speaker stating that a cola beverage in the drink machines had been contaminated with a poison. Immediately, people all over the stadium developed severe abdominal cramping. Many vomited and had diarrhea. Some were so severely affected that they were carried out on stretchers and taken to the hospital.

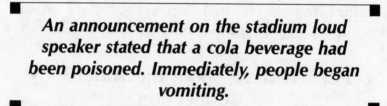

> ***An announcement on the stadium loud speaker stated that a cola beverage had been poisoned. Immediately, people began vomiting.***

Then, about 40 minutes later, another announcement came over the loudspeaker stating that the beverage was perfectly safe and that the previous announcement had been in error. All of the vomiting and other signs of illness immediately stopped.

During our conversations, Mr. Cousins also told me about his work with groups of people with arthritis, cancer and other chronic disabling and painful illnesses. And he said:

"I always tell them jokes and after about the third joke I have them laughing so hard they have to hold their sides. Then when my session with them is completed, I ask, 'How many of you are still hurting as much as you were when you walked into this room?' and no hands are raised."

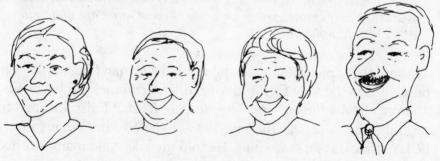

In the third edition of *The Yeast Connection,* I cited the comments of my friend, the late Charles May, M.D., who said, "Billy, many of your patients get better because they have faith in you and what you're doing rather than because of the diet you put them on."[4]

I disagreed with Dr. May at the time (1976), mainly because he was skeptical of my observations about the relationship of food sensitivities to fatigue, headache, muscle aches and other symptoms. I also disagreed with numerous professionals in the mid-1980s who said, "The chronic fatigue syndrome is caused by depression." I felt that these critics were ignoring the role of viral infections, food and chemical sensitivities and other organic causes of CFS, including the yeast connection.

Yet, because of the observations of Mr. Cousins and others, including Michael Weiner* and Bernard Siegel,[6] I did not completely ignore the role of psychological factors in people with CFS. And in my 1992 book, *Chronic Fatigue Syndrome and the Yeast Connection,*[7] I included a four-page chapter discussing the importance of psychological support. And more and more in recent years, in talking to my patients and to people who write and call me, I say:

"You need caring, empathetic people to encourage you, work with you and help you, including family members and professionals. Support groups consisting of people who are experiencing similar problems can also help.

"You need to be noticed, praised and encouraged. You need smiles, touching, holding, patting and petting. Physical contact stimulates the release of endorphins, a chemical which lessens anxiety and pain."

You did a great job!

---

*In his book, *Maximum Immunity,*[5] Weiner described a study carried out on cadets at West Point to see how psychological factors influence their susceptibility to infectious mononucleosis. Their findings: Those who developed this illness were found to have experienced greater academic pressure than the resistant group of cadets.

My Further Education in Mind/Body Medicine

In the fall of 1992, Jessica Rochester, Ph.D., a good friend and a member of the advisory board of the International Health Foundation called me and said in effect:

> "Billy, I really do like your new CFS book. Congratulations on a job well done. Yet, there's a lot of fascinating new information about the mind/body connection. I hope you'll look at it as you gather information for your next book. I think you'll be especially interested in books by Dr. Larry Dossey."

Then, in March 1993, at a meeting of the American Holistic Medical Association in Kansas City, I heard many fascinating discussions of the mind/body connection, including presentations by Drs. Dossey, Deepak Chopra and James Gordon.

When I came home from the meeting, I began reading anything and everything I could get my hands on that had to do with the relationship of psychological stimuli to physical and organic symptoms. One book that I found especially fascinating was *Meaning and Medicine* by Dr. Dossey.[8] In this book he tells fascinating and often dramatic stories which show how thought and emotions *do* influence the body—and can make the difference between life and death. Here are a couple of them.

A man who was highly allergic to penicillin was given a placebo pill which he thought was penicillin. Within a few moments he died of shock.

Pollen sensitive people began to sneeze when they looked at a picture of a hay field.

Mind/Body Medicine Comes into the Mainstream

Along with many other Americans, I saw a number of TV programs on mind/body medicine hosted by Bill Moyers. I subsequently got a copy of his book, *Healing and the Mind*. Here are excerpts from the book jacket which will give you an idea what this book is all about.

"Ancient medical science told us our minds and bodies are one. So did philosophers of old. Now modern science and new research are helping us to understand these connections. In *Healing and the Mind*, Bill Moyers talks with physicians, scientists, therapists and patients—people who are taking a new look at the meaning of sickness and health. In a series of fascinating and provocative interviews, he discusses their search for answers to perplexing questions: How do emotions translate into chemicals in our bodies? How do thoughts and feelings influence health? How can we collaborate with our bodies to encourage healing?"

The people Moyers interviewed included a number of renowned American professionals from major medical centers. One chapter of the book told of a visit Moyers made to China with Dr. David Eisenberg, an instructor in medicine at Harvard Medical School. Subjects observed and investigated there ranged from acupuncture to an indepth look at "chi." In commenting on Chinese medicine, Moyers said:

> *Herbal medicine, massage, exercise, meditation are part of this complex medical system.*

"I suspect that acupuncture is what we think of first when we conjure up a picture of Chinese medicine. But herbal medicine, massage, exercise, meditation and an appreciation for 'balance' in lifestyle are also part of this complex medical system, which I have come to explore precisely because it refuses to make distinctions between mind and body."[9]

A short time later, while I was Christmas shopping and browsing through a bookstore, I picked up a copy of a big, beautiful book entitled *Mind/Body Medicine—How to Use Your Mind for Better Health*. I took it home and read most of it.

In the preface, the authors pointed out that some popular magazine articles, ads and brochures which come in our third-class

mail, hailing medical miracles and touting breakthrough products, are fraudulent and exaggerate what medical science is finding to be the actual relationship between the mind and physical
health. And they said there is "much to be wary of." Yet, they also
said:

> "But if some entrepreneurs and journalists have overinterpreted
> the meaning of mind/body medicine, *others have not taken this
> growing field seriously enough* . . . [emphasis added] Mind/body
> medicine does not offer miracle cures any more than nutrition and
> exercise do. And yet, like those other 'lifestyle' approaches, it has
> much of real value to offer the ill and the well alike."

In their continuing discussion, these authors pointed out that
more and more medical centers, including prestigious ones, are
offering mind/body interventions to their patients. In the concluding comments of their preface, they said:

> "Another crucial part of being an active patient discussed in the
> book's final chapter is to find the best way to communicate with
> your physician to make yourself your doctor's close ally in your own
> medical care. Ultimately, one of the most appropriate roles for mind/
> body medicine is to add a humane dimension to conventional medi-
> cal treatment."

Included in this book were chapters by many different profes-
sionals from major American medical centers, including Stanford,
Cornell, the University of Michigan, Vanderbilt, Harvard, Johns
Hopkins and many others. I especially liked a chapter by Kenneth
R. Pelletier, Ph.D., of the Stanford University School of Medicine
who, in talking about prevention and treatment, said:

**Meditation, visualization, hypnosis,
biofeedback and relaxation techniques may
help prevent and treat a variety of illnesses.**

"Meditation, visualization, hypnosis, biofeedback and numerous relaxation techniques already show promise in helping prevent and treat a variety of illnesses . . . Other studies have suggested that humor, positive emotions and hypnotic suggestion may alternatively affect the immune response."[10]

A short time before I finished the manuscript of this book, I picked up a copy of a 753-page, 1994 book entitled, *Women's Bodies, Women's Wisdom.*[11] In this book, Dr. Christiane Northrup, a former president of the American Holistic Medical Association, provides women and those who care for them with a tremendous amount of information.

Included is a discussion of how she and her colleagues at their Holistic Health Center use their dramatic discoveries in mind/body medicine to show women how to heal by listening to their own bodies' wisdom.

In a chapter entitled, "Steps for Healing," the author lists 12 steps. Here are a few of them.

- Respect and release your emotions; learn to listen to your body
- gather information
- forgive
- acknowledge a higher power or inner wisdom

In discussing this latter step, Northrup said that our bodies are permeated and nourished by spiritual energy and guidance. She also said that having faith and trust in this reality is an important part of creating health. When a woman has faith in something greater than her intellect or her present circumstances, she gets in touch with her inner source of power.

Comments of Professionals

During early 1994 as I gathered material for this book, I interviewed a number of professionals who were helping people with candida-related health problems using a comprehensive treatment program. Here are comments of several professionals who emphasize the importance of psychological factors.

Jessica Rochester, Ph.D., Montreal, Quebec, Canada: "There's a wonderful emerging paradigm in medicine with evidence of this in two areas. The first is increased awareness of the importance of nutrition, lifestyle, exercise and relaxation in relationship to health. The second is the considerable data available demonstrating the connection between the consciousness (the mind or soul or spirit) and the physical part of us, the body.

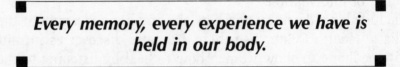

Every memory, every experience we have is held in our body.

"I try to help people develop their inner strengths so that they can look at the patterns that brought them to where they are in their lives now. Also where they would like to go from here ... Everything is held in the cells of our body which are made out of what we eat, drink and breathe. But beyond that, every memory, every experience we have is held in our body."

Bethany Hayes, M.D., Yarmouth, Maine: "When I see a woman who's been troubled by chronic yeast infections, I'm always interested in finding out when it started and what was going on in her life. I find it's common that it started right after an abusive relationship, rape or incest.

"So I'm very much aware of how women's experiences in life affect their immune system and how important their immune system is in treating chronic disorders—including yeast-related problems."

Jessie Lynn Hanley, M.D., Malibu, California: "Our immune system is an extension of ourselves. When a person's self-image is weakened, the immune system is adversely affected. I've found that abused people are especially apt to have weakened immunity.

"Many other patients may also need emotional help—I'm referring to those who experience trouble coping with the sometimes drastic, but vital, diet changes which temporarily add to their self-image fragility.

"In helping each of these patients, psychological support is extremely important. I *always* do some counseling and I refer some of my patients elsewhere for additional help."

Elson Haas, M.D., San Rafael, California: "The four cornerstones of preventive medicine are nutrition, exercise, managing stress and attitude. I believe that attitude is the most important of these. When people have a good attitude toward life, they want to get better. They tend to exercise. They want to do things in a loving, positive way for themselves. To me that is crucial to preventing illness and supporting long-term health."

Marcelle Pick, R.N.C., NP, Yarmouth, Maine: "Over the years if people are not looking at what's going on with them emotionally, they'll continue to be plagued with yeast problems. I can do everything with diet and supplements, and it doesn't change things if their self-esteem is really poor or they are not willing to look at what is going on in their lives that is definitely contributing to this chronic problem."

O. Jack Woodard, M.D., Albany, Georgia: "Although I help many of my patients using nystatin and diet, I tell my patients that anything I prescribe for them will work better if they're using the mind/body connection to enhance healing.

"There are three approaches. The first is to gain knowledge. And powerful, well-researched material is now available in print and on tape. I especially like Wayne Dyer's book, *Real Magic.*

"Second is meditation. This enables a person to access a dimension of reality that triggers the self-healing mechanisms of the body. Third, people need to discover their purpose in life. Nothing turns on the healing power of the body like fulfilling one's purpose every day."

Prayer—An Effective Therapeutic Intervention

During the past decade I've received thousands of letters. Some came from people seeking information and help, while others told me how they overcame their health problems.

In one such letter (the longest one I included in *The Yeast Connection*), Karen described the multiple health problems she had experienced over a period of many years.

Her symptoms included cystitis, recurrent vaginal yeast infections, joint pains, swelling, visual disturbances, abdominal bloating, constipation, fatigue, inability to concentrate, numbness, tingling, excessive intestinal gas and heart palpitations.

I kept a headache that never left.

"I kept a headache that never left. Sometimes it was mild, other times it was severe. *I felt so horrible I would pray, Lord Jesus how can I keep living this way?* ... Then in October 1981, through a sort of unique coincidence (it was definitely an answer to my prayers), I first learned about yeast-related illness. Soon afterward I was put on a comprehensive treatment program to help me control candida, improve my immune system and regain my health."[12]

Since that time I've received many other letters from people who have said, "Without any question prayer played a key role in enabling me to regain my health."

Observations by Larry Dossey, M.D.

This physician, who is co-chairman of the recently established Panel on Mind/Body Interventions, Office of Alternative Medicine, National Institutes of Health, Bethesda, Maryland, has discussed the effectiveness of prayer in several of his books, including *Healing Words: The Power of Prayer in the Practice of Medicine*.[13] And in a recent article, "The Role of Prayer in Health and Healing," published in the March 1994 issue of *Health Confidential*, Dr. Dossey said:

"Probably since the earliest days of human kind, people have prayed for those who are sick. The world of Western science—with its national analytical orientation—has tended to avoid the issue of prayer and its relationship to healing, even dismissing it as mere superstition.

"Yet, numerous scientific studies support the connection between prayer and healing—as I was astonished to discover several years ago."

In his article, Dr. Dossey told of his initial skepticism about the possible effects of prayer; yet, after reviewing dozens of scientific studies which showed that prayer could have an important influence in healing, he incorporated prayer into his medical practice.

He pointed out that people can pray for themselves, or they can pray for others. And he cited three studies where people who didn't know they were being prayed for showed significant improvement, as compared to people who weren't prayed for. And he pointed out that this was a "double-blind" study. The doctors and other hospital personnel didn't know which patients were being prayed for; neither did the patients.

In answering the question *"Why does prayer work?"* Dossey said:

"So far research has only identified that prayer works—not why it works. Yet, this is hardly a new situation in medicine. When penicillin was discovered, no one had any idea why it cured infection. There are countless examples in medical history of treatments that were used because data proved them effective—whether the mechanism could be explained or not."

In discussing how to pray, he pointed out that there is no one right way to pray. And that prayer can be "directed" or "nondirected." And he said:

"Studies suggest that while both types are effective, nondirected prayer yields more dramatic results . . .

"If you have the impulse to connect with a power beyond human understanding, don't worry too much about how to do it. Just honor the impulse."[14]

My Comments

In Chapter 8 of this book, I briefly summarized the steps you'll need to take to regain your health. These steps included changing your diet and controlling chemical exposures; making lifestyle changes; taking nutritional supplements and anticandida medication; and, tracking down hidden food sensitivities.

I also said you'll need love, praise, touch, hugs, laughter and other psychological nutrients to strengthen your immune system and to work with a kind and caring, knowledgeable physician.

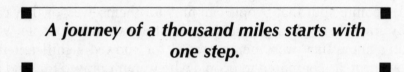

A journey of a thousand miles starts with one step.

Accomplishing all of these things won't be easy, but you can get started today. Remember the old Chinese proverb of Confucius who said, "A journey of a thousand miles starts with one step."

Read again parts of Chapter 6, including the comments of Dr. Truss and the stories of my patients Sarah, Janet and Karen. They'll give you hope, courage and confidence. Also read the story of Linda, who through "networking" found a warm, kind, caring physician. With the help and collaboration of nurse colleagues, Linda and her family were able to find needed help.

Read also Joyce Frederick's almost unbelievable story (the longest one in this book) in Chapter 21, Terry Oldham's story in Chapter 13 and Anita's story in Chapter 16.

There *are* kind and caring physicians and other health professionals "out there." And their numbers are gradually increasing. So keep networking and searching. Look also for support groups in your community. In most cities you'll find them listed in the newspaper. If you don't find a candida support group, you may find allied groups, including CFS, FMS, MCS and other groups.

You'll also find magazines and books in your health food store which are loaded with information that can help you. See also suggestions in Chapter 49, Alternative Medicine and in Part Nine, Other Sources of Information (page 706).

REFERENCES

1. Cousins, N., "Anatomy of an Illness (As perceived by the patient)," *N. Engl. J. Med.*, 1976; 295:1458–63.
2. Cousins, N., *Anatomy of an Illness*, Bantam Books, New York, 1981.
3. Cousins, N., *The Healing Heart*, Avon Books, New York, 1983.
4. Crook, W.G., *The Yeast Connection*, Third Edition, Professional Books, Jackson, TN and Vintage Books, New York, 1986; pp 251–252.
5. Weiner, M.A., *Maximum Immunity*, Houghton Mifflin, New York, 1986; pp 45–50.
6. Siegel, B.S., *Love, Medicine and Miracles*, Harper & Rowe, New York, 1986. And Siegel, B.S., *Peace, Love and Healing*, Harper & Rowe, New York, 1989.
7. Crook, W.G., *Chronic Fatigue Syndrome and the Yeast Connection*, Professional Books, Jackson, TN, 1992; pp 236–239.
8. Dossey, L., *Meaning and Medicine*, Bantam Books, New York, 1991.
9. Moyers, B., *Healing and the Mind*, Doubleday, New York, 1993.
10. Goleman, D. and Gurin, J., *Mind/Body Medicine—How to Use Your Mind for Better Health*, Copyright 1993 by Consumers Union of U.S., Inc., Yonkers, NY 10703–1057. Excerpted by permission from Consumer Reports Books, January 1993.
11. Northrup, C., *Women's Bodies, Women's Wisdom*, Bantam Books, New York, 1994; pp 485–543.
12. Crook, W.G., *The Yeast Connection*, Third Edition, Professional Books, Jackson, TN and Vintage Books, New York, 1986; pp 224–227.
13. Dossey, L., *Healing Words: The Power of Prayer in the Practice of Medicine*, Harper, San Francisco, 1993.
14. Dossey, L., in *Health Confidential*, Board Room Reports, 55 Railroad Ave., Greenwich, CT 06830, March 1994, pp 5–6.

33

Nonprescription Antiyeast Medications

Ideally, your own family physician, internist, gynecologist, dermatologist, or other specialist, will help you and work with you. And, even if your physician is skeptical of "the yeast connection," perhaps he or she will prescribe nystatin or one of the azole drugs, Diflucan, Sporanox or Nizoral.

These antiyeast medications literally punch holes in candida cell membranes. They knock them out and keep them from multiplying and raising large families. Moreover, the azole drugs may also keep the little round yeast cells from putting out branches (mycelia) which can burrow beneath your mucous membranes.

But suppose you do not have a knowledgeable medical doctor (M.D.) or osteopathic physician (D.O.), what then? You may be able to find help from other licensed health professionals, including N.D.s, D.C.s, R.N.s and R.D.s. Fortunately, there are also nonprescription substances and products which help limit or retard the growth of candida in the digestive tract.

> **There are nonprescription substances which help limit the growth of candida in the digestive tract.**

In gathering new material on the management of yeast-related disorders for this book, I sought information and help from many sources. Included were books on natural and alternative medicine and physicians and other professionals who are treating candida-related health problems using nonprescription medications. Here's some of the information I found.

Books on Alternative, Herbal and Natural Medicines

In their comprehensive book, *Encyclopedia of Natural Medicine,* Michael Murray, N.D., and Joseph Pizzarno, N.D., in discussing candidiasis, described a number of nutritional and herbal compounds including:

caprylic acid	lactobacillus supplementation
garlic	Pau d'Arco (La Pacho or taheebo)
German chamomile	ginger, thyme and rosemary
berberis	

In discussing caprylic acid, they said, "Caprylic acid, a naturally occurring fatty acid, has been reported to be an effective antifungal compound in the treatment of candidiasis. Since caprylic acid is readily absorbed in the intestines, it is necessary to take time-released or enteric-coated caprylic acid formulas to allow for gradual release throughout the entire intestinal tract."

In discussing garlic, they said, "Garlic is especially active against *C. albicans,* being more potent than nystatin, gentian violet and six other reputed antifungal agents."

In discussing berberis, they said, "It is an effective antimicrobial agent against a wide range of organisms, including *Candida albicans.* Its action on *Candida albicans,* as well as on disease causing bacteria, prevents the overgrowth of yeast that commonly follows antibiotic use. It appears to be effective in normalizing the content of the gut by acting against both disease-causing bacteria and the yeast. Its activity against the yeast is quite potent."

In discussing ginger, rosemary and other common spices, they said, "They contain some of the most powerful candida killing substances available."[1]

In their remarkable, comprehensive and informative 1068-page book, *Alternative Medicine—The Definitive Guide*, the authors discussed many herbal anticandida agents. These included golden seal, Oregon grape and barberry, as well as cinnamon, rosemary, tea tree oil, fennel and licorice. And they cited the observations of a number of professionals, including James Braly, M.D., of Ft. Lauderdale, Florida, and Leon Chaitow, N.D., D.O., of London, England. Here are excerpts.

"Dr. Braly's first line of attack on candidiasis is caprylic acid, only after which, if there's no improvement, will he use drugs. Since caprylic acid is readily absorbed into the system, it should be taken in enteric or sustained relief forms.

"Dr. Braly also likes golden seal root extract, standardized to 5% or more of its active ingredient, hydrastine, 250 mg., twice daily. In a recent study, golden seal seemed to work better in killing off candida than other common anticandida therapies . . .

Both bifido bacteria and acidophilus should be supplemented during candidiasis treatment.

"According to Dr. Chaitow, both bifido bacteria and acidophilus should be supplemented during candidiasis treatment to help repopulate the bowel and for antifungal therapy."

The book also discussed other herbal remedies, including garlic and Pau d'Arco, yet, they said:

"Many products claiming to contain Pau d'Arco have only trace amounts, or even none of the herb . . . When purchasing products with Pau d'Arco, be sure they contain Lapachol, an organic compound known for its antibiotic action."[2]

In his book, *The Scientific Validation of Herbal Medicine*, Daniel B. Mowrey, Ph.D., also talked about golden seal root and its major constituent hydrastine. And he said that these products "have been repeatedly proven through global research first to reduce inflammation of mucous membranes (vaginal and uterine)—and to destroy harmful bacteria and other germs."

According to Mowrey, this herb was remarkably successful in treating patients during cholera epidemics in Calcutta, India, in the 1960s. And he said, "During those sieges berberine proved more effective, with fewer side effects than antibiotics."

In treating vaginal yeast infections, he recommended two capsules four times a day, supplemented with capsules of garlic. Supplemental potassium was also suggested, along with this herb. He said that the mode of action of this herb and other herbs was to "soothe inflamed and infected mucous membranes and inhibit discharges."

In the introduction of this book, Mowrey cautioned readers:

"The information contained in this book is intended for educational purposes only. It does not provide the knowledge to diagnose, prescribe or treat any disease . . . Many persons on their first encounter with the information presented in this book are tempted to throw out their medications and start using nothing but herbs . . . Please do not do that.

> **In my opinion people should ease into the use of herbs.**

"In my opinion people should ease into the use of herbs, and ease out the use of traditional medicines only where possible, especially if their health problems are severe. A sudden switch of health regimen can be hazardous. I use the word 'treat' to describe the relationship between an herb and its users. The word is not a synonym for 'cure.' It implies only that the herb is used by certain people in an 'attempt to cure.' There's a big difference between treat and cure: while cure involves a successful treatment, treat does not imply success; it only suggests the attempt."[3]

In his 1993 book, *Healing Through Nutrition,*[4] Melvyn Werbach, M.D., discussed other herbal remedies, including echinacea. He pointed out that this herb was used widely in this country by native Americans and early settlers. He said that even though echinacea does not kill germs, it stimulates the body to fight the infection.

I found more information about herbs in a beautifully illustrated book published in England entitled, *The Complete Medicinal Herbal.* According to the author of the book, Penelope Ody:

"A traditional healing herb of native Americans that has entered the European herbal repertoire, golden seal, was used by the Cherokee for indigestion, local inflammations, and to improve the appetite. The herb was introduced into Europe in 1760—and was listed in the United States Pharmacopoeia until 1926."[5]

Another herbal remedy, tea tree oil, was said to be effective when used in the vagina in treating yeast infections.

Antiyeast Medications
Garlic

Garlic has been widely used for medicinal purposes for centuries; for example, Virgil and Hippocrates mention it as a remedy for pneumonia and snake bite. In looking through the Index Medicos, I found numerous articles from American and foreign literature describing the inhibitory action of garlic on candida organisms.

To learn more about the effect of garlic on *Candida albicans,* in the mid-1980s I consulted Moses Adetumbi, Ph.D., who at that time worked in the Department of Biology at Loma Linda University, Loma Linda, California. Dr. Adetumbi sent me two reprints and several abstracts on the effectiveness of garlic as an antifungal, antimicrobial and pharmacological agent.

Then in the early 1990s, a number of the participants at the First World Congress on the Significance of Garlic and Garlic Constituents, presented scientific reports which documented the effectiveness of garlic as a useful anticandida agent.

Chopping, steaming and food processing does marvelous things to garlic.

In a news report of this conference, Joy Ashchenbach, in an article in the April 20, 1991, *Rocky Mountain News* quoted Herbert Pierson, Head of the National Cancer Institute, "Designer Foods Program," who said, "Chopping, steaming and food processing does marvelous things to garlic."

Ashchenbach also quoted Eric Block of the State University at New York, an authority on garlic's chemistry, who said:

> "Undisturbed, the garlic bulb has limited medicinally active compounds. Cutting triggers the formation of a cascade of compounds that are quite reactive and participate in a complex sequence of chemical reactions. Ultimately an amazing collection of chemical compounds is produced."

In another report on this conference (*New York Times*, September 4, 1990), columnist Jane Brody said:

> "Garlic does not have to be consumed raw to be effective; in fact, raw garlic is more likely than cooked or processed forms to cause adverse reactions. Furthermore the characteristic odor of garlic or its freshness are not critical to its health benefits; aged, deodorized forms seem to work as well or better than pure unadulterated fresh garlic."

In summarizing reports at the conference, Brody listed a number of the therapeutic effects of garlic, including suppressing cholesterol synthesis, lowering the levels of triglycerides and combating *Candida albicans*. In the concluding paragraph of her article, she said:

"While scientists continue to sort out the benefits and risks of garlic, and its constituents . . . researchers suggested that those who can tolerate garlic would be wise to eat it at least every other day in cooked form. An alternative for those wishing to avoid garlic breath is regular use of aged garlic extract, a deodorized supplement sold in health food stores under the trade name Kyolic."

Further comments on the 1990 World Congress on Garlic were made by Osamu Imada, Ph.D., visiting scientist, University of Texas, who said:

"More than 50 scientists from 15 countries presented their recent research findings on garlic at the Congress. The beneficial effects of aged garlic extract have become the center of the presentations at the congress. Fourteen of the 46 presentations were related to the efficacy of aged garlic extract."

More recently, researchers from Loma Linda University, Loma Linda, California, reported the effectiveness of aged garlic extract against *Candida albicans* infections in mice. After candida exposure, one group was treated with aged garlic extract, while the other group was given a garlic-free control. The treatment with aged garlic extract hastened the clearance of candida cells from the blood and reduced their growth in the kidney.

In addition, germ-killing activity of macrophages ("big" white cells which eat up germs) was observed in the mice treated with aged garlic extract. According to Dr. Lau, this study suggested that the control of *Candida albicans* may be mediated through the enhancement of phagocytic (germ eating) function by garlic extract.

As you probably know, many different garlic products, including odor free garlic, are available from health food stores. Which garlic preparation is best? The arguments and claims of many resemble those of the various automobile makers. Yet, I've been especially impressed by copies of presentations that I've read which document the efficacy of aged garlic extract (Kyolic).

Caprylic Acid

This substance, a short chain saturated fatty acid, was studied some 40 years ago by Dr. Irene Neuhauser, the University of Illinois, and found to have antifungal activity.[6] Because caprylic acid is a food substitute, it's available without a prescription. Moreover, it's now being marketed by a number of different companies under various brand names.

> **Because caprylic acid is a food substitute, it's available without a prescription.**

During the past decade, a number of health professionals have found that caprylic acid products are effective in controlling candida in the intestinal tract. Moreover, some of the professionals I've talked to say, "It's just as good as nystatin."

To learn more about the use of this antiyeast agent, I interviewed Laura Shelton, N.D., of Bellingham, Washington. Here are excerpts from my interview:

"My favorite anticandida remedy is Mycopryl, a caprylic acid product which comes from coconut oil and is bound to calcium and magnesium. In my experience it works much better than any of the other caprylic acid products.

"I use the '680' size capsule and I work people up very slowly, depending on how bad their symptoms are. This helps avoid the 'die-off' reaction. I start on one capsule the first day, two a day for three days and then work them up slowly to two to four capsules, three times a day. I continue that dose for two to four weeks.

"Then most people can stop the medication and stay on a no-yeast, no-sugar diet, along with other anticandida herbal remedies, including garlic, Pau d'Arco (taheebo tea) or the citrus seed extract."

Citrus Seed Extract

I first heard of the efficacy of this herbal remedy in controlling candida from Drs. Leo Galland and Charles Resseger, who said:

"These extracts are as effective as nystatin and caprylic acid and other nonabsorbed antifungal agents in treating patients with candida-related complex. In addition, they're also effective in treating patients with giardiasis and some other intestinal parasites."

Other physicians I've talked to have found citrus seed extract to be helpful, especially as a follow-up to the prescription antifungal medications. Yet, they've cautioned that the liquid preparations must be well diluted so as to avoid gastric irritation. During a recent conversation, Dr. Galland said:

"ParaMycrocidin liquid is bitter and compliance was a problem. It's now available in capsule and the usual dose is 100 mg. twice a day after meals. Side effects include occasional gastric irritation . . . Also, at times, flushing. If the patient flushes on the grapefruit seed extract, the dose should be reduced."

Dr. Galland also uses a preparation which combines grapefruit seed extract with berberine and another preparation which combines grapefruit seed extract, berberine and the herb artemisia—especially for patients who may also have parasites.

I found further information about Citricidal in a booklet sent to me from Bio-Chem Research, Lakeport, California. Here are some of the advantages they listed for this product.

"Citricidal is an extremely potent and effective alternative to the toxic and environmentally harmful chemicals used in a diverse spectrum of consumer, commercial and agro-industrial products . . . Citricidal is currently used in international markets as a sanitizing and disinfection agent, as a fungicide, antibacterial, antiparasitic, antiviral and preservative in food and cosmetics. Citricidal should be handled with care in full strength. Avoid contact with the eyes and avoid breathing vapors at full strength. Any direct contact with the skin should be thoroughly rinsed with cool water."

The hundred-page brochure describes tests on various microorganisms, including *Candida albicans*. Moreover, they included a scientific report by Dr. Gruia Ionescu. Here are excerpts.

"Serial dilutions of a citrus seed extract (ParaMycrocidin) were highly effective at concentrations ranging from 0.5 to 2 p.c. against a large number of Gram positive, Gram negative and yeast strains in vitro . . . By using ParaMycrocidin capsules in a dosage of 150 mg., three times a day, we noticed a significant activity against several pathogenic intestinal strains in our patients. The extract was mostly effective against *Candida,* Geotrichum sp. and hemolytic *E. coli.*"[7]

Tanalbit *

This internal intestinal antiseptic consists of natural tannins, combined with zinc. It has been found to be effective in the management of yeast overgrowth in the intestine, acute and chronic diarrhea, colitis, constipation and spastic colon.

Here are the comments of James Brodsky, M.D., Chevy Chase, Maryland.

"I've found that Tanalbit has helped a number of my patients, who aren't responding to nystatin as well as I think they should or those who cannot tolerate nystatin. The usual dose is three capsules, three times a day. I've experienced few if any side effects . . . especially when it is taken with meals."

In discussing Tanalbit, Murray R. Susser, M.D., Santa Monica, California, said:

"I've been using Tanalbit on candidiasis for about eight years. I've, of course, used many other treatments, including nystatin, caprylic acid and Diflucan. I find that Tanalbit is a very consistent product. It gives good therapeutic results with little side effects.

"I find it especially useful when I'm treating parasites with powerful drugs like metronidazole (Flagyl) and Iodoquinal. These parasitics often cause yeast overgrowth, as well as their own peculiar side effects.

"I find that I can minimize the yeast overgrowth without increas-

---

*Tanalbit can be purchased without a prescription from some health food stores and pharmacies, or can be ordered from Scientific Consulting Services, 466 Whitney St., San Leandro, CA 94577.

ing side effects by including Tanalbit. I've not done it as data collection, but I've observed this phenomenon hundreds of times."

Mathake

This herbal product, which is widely distributed in the tropics, was introduced in the U.S. in the mid-1980s by Michael Weiner, Ph.D. During a 1993 interview, Dr. Richard Noble of Hillsboro, Oregon, said:

> "Mathake is a very affordable, easy to use medicine. It doesn't taste terrible. It's portable, it doesn't require refrigeration. All that it takes is boiling water and a tea bag of the mathake herb.
>
> "Mathake has to all intents and purposes replaced nystatin in my practice. Moreover, the cost is 1/3 to 1/2 the cost of nystatin. Used for a 6 to 12 weeks period, combined with the yeast, mold and sugar-free diet, probiotics and nutritional support, mathake will help many patients with mild gastrointestinal yeast overgrowth and resulting health problems.
>
> "For individuals with chronic vaginitis, sinusitis and other persistent or long-standing candida-related health problems, Diflucan, a systemic medicine is a far better choice."

Probiotics

Probiotics are a group of friendly bacteria that help us stay well. They include *Lactobacillus acidophilus* and bifidobacteria. These bacteria, which are found in yogurt, were first identified about 100 years ago. And in 1908, Metchkinoff, a Bulgarian, recommended a daily consumption of yogurt because he felt it promoted good health and long life.

> **These bacteria . . . were first identified about 100 years ago.**

During the years since that time, preparations of these friendly bacteria have been used by both physicians and nonphysicians to treat complaints ranging from constipation and diarrhea to skin problems.

When I was an intern and resident at Vanderbilt, over 40 years ago, we treated some of our babies with resistant diarrhea with human breast milk (which contained lots of lactobacilli). Then, in the '60s and '70s, along with my pediatric peers, I often prescribed a powdered lactobacillus preparation to control diarrhea, which developed following broad spectrum antibiotic drugs.

At the first conference on the relationship of superficial yeast infections to chronic illness (Dallas 1982), the role of lactobacilli in competing with candida was discussed and a knowledgeable participant during an informal luncheon address commented:

> "Giving preparations of live lactobacilli may help your patients with candida overgrowth in the digestive tract, especially if you give them every day."

During the '80s and early '90s, many professionals I've talked to tell me that they use preparations of various probiotics to help control candida in their digestive tract. Although they are not potent agents for "knocking out yeast," most people I talk to find that they help.

In introducing their discussion of probiotics, the authors of the book, *Alternative Medicine,* said:

> "Inside each of us live vast numbers of bacteria without which we could not remain in good health . . . There are several thousand billion in each person . . . Most of them living in the digestive tract. If they were all placed together the total weight of these 'friendly' bacteria would come to nearly four pounds . . .

> **These bacteria . . . perform many important functions in the body.**

> "These bacteria . . . perform many important functions in the body . . . However, not all of the friendly bacteria perform the same

functions, some being far more useful and plentiful than others. Certain bacteria help to maintain good health, while others have a definite value in helping us regain health once it has been upset.

"These dual protective and therapeutic roles help explain why the word 'probiotics' was coined, since it means 'for life.'

"They manufacture some of the B vitamins . . . They manufacture the milk digesting enzyme *lactase*, which helps digest calcium rich dairy products. They actually produce antibacterial substances which kill or deactivate hostile disease-causing bacteria. Some bacteria, such as bifidobacteria, and acidophilus have been shown to have anticarcinogenic features.

"They improve the efficiency of the digestive tract."[8]

In her book, *Food—Your Miracle Medicine,*[9] Jean Carper cited the research studies of Dr. Eileen Hilton, who found that yogurt eaters have a three-fold lower incidence of vaginitis than the non-yogurt eaters. Yet, she pointed out that yogurt, to be effective, must contain *live,* active acidophilus bacterial cultures.* She also suggested that you can make your own yogurt using acidophilus cultures sold in many health food stores.

In the 1992 edition of, *The New Our Bodies, Ourselves—A Book By and For Women,*[10] the authors said that as an alternative to antibiotics for vaginitis, many women are turning to natural and herbal remedies. They pointed out that such remedies restore the normal vaginal flora and promote healing.

During the past decade, much of the information I have learned about nutrition has come from Jeff Bland's monthly audio-tapes, *Preventive Medicine Update.* I've also "picked Jeff's brain" on several occasions.

In discussing probiotics with him a couple of years ago, I asked him if he used plain *Lactobacillus acidophilus* or a combination product. In responding, he said:

---

*In a presentation at the October 1994 Annual Conference of the American Academy of Environmental Medicine, Beatrice Trum Hunter said that the vigor of yogurt cultures diminishes with age. So when you purchase yogurt check the expiration date on the carton.

"I think we all recognize that *the most important criteria for activity of probiotic substances is that there must be an adequate number of live organisms,* they must be reasonably resistant to oxgall (bile) and they must be able to adhere to the gastrointestinal epithelium. If any one of these three criteria is not met, then the activity of the product is limited."[11]

You can find many probiotic products in your health food store; and, I recommend them as a nutritional supplement for my patients, especially those who are taking broad-spectrum antibiotic drugs.

Brand names include Vital-plex, Vital-dophilus, Kyo-dophilus, Primeplex, Kala, BifidoBiotics, Geneflora, Maxidophilus, Acidophilus DDS1, Flora Balance, GI Flora, Primadophilus, *Saccharomyces boulardii** and Superdophilus. The usual dose is ¼ to ½ teaspoon of powder or one to two capsules, one to four times a day.

You can usually obtain these and other products from your health food store, the National CFIDS Buyer's Club 1-800-366-6056 and from the pharmacies listed in Chapter 34.

Comments About Nonprescription Medications by Health Professionals

James Brodsky, M.D., Chevy Chase, Maryland: In discussing nonprescription antifungals, especially citrus seed extract, he said, "Although I use them, I don't generally start most patients on citrus seed extract unless they have evidence of parasites.

"Yet, I have other patients who have no parasites who don't do very well on nystatin alone. In such patients, I may try them on citrus seed or grapefruit seed extract. Although I don't use a lot of it, I use more than I did a couple of years ago."

Marcelle Pick, R.N.C., NP, Yarmouth, Maine: "I tend not to use nystatin. I use mostly grapefruit seed extract. I also use Biocidin, which is a gentian violet preparation. It works extremely well for

---

*See More About Probiotics in Part Nine.

things like yeast, and other pathogens in combination with yeast. I also use caprylic acid products and Artemisia Forte in dealing with parasites."

Joan Priestley, M.D., Anchorage, Alaska: "In treating my yeast patients I still use the old standbys. My first line is garlic and acidophilus and getting the sugar and alcohol out of the diet. Also nutritional supplements.

"Then I like Pau d'Arco (taheebo tea) in all its forms. I also tell people to chew whole fennel as seeds because there's something in them that's very good against yeast. I also like caprylic acid products and I put my patients on borage oil as opposed to evening primrose oil because it's cheaper. I also use fish oils and zinc.

"It takes about six months to get them back to normal health and graduated from the program. For the 25% who don't seem to be improving, I pull Diflucan out as my ace in the hole."

Elson Haas, M.D., San Rafael, California: In discussing nonprescription antifungals, this California physician said, "The one I use most commonly now is ParaMycrocidin, the grapefruit seed extract. The usual dose is 100 mg. capsules, twice a day after meals. Yet, I continue to use nystatin more than any other antifungal medication."

Ken Gerdes, M.D., Denver, Colorado: This Colorado physician generally relies on nystatin and Diflucan for antifungal therapy, yet he said, "I'm becoming more impressed with citrus seed extract and I trust the liquid more than the capsules. I had one patient buy some of the over-the-counter citrus seed extract and got no benefit from it. Then she tried a different preparation, Paracan 144, and it helped her. I'm not sure if it's just a difference in the manufacturer or a difference in dose. But I'm not sure that they're all the same."

Ronald Hoffman, M.D., New York, New York: During a recent conversation with me, Dr. Hoffman told me that he had been working recently with a traditional Chinese herbalist and acupuncturist. In discussing it, he said, "He was an obstetrician and gynecologist on the faculty of the University of Shanghai who has come over to the United States. With each patient we see, regardless of what they come for, he does the pulse reading and the traditional Chinese diagnosis which includes looking at the tongue. As he's working with me we've come to realize that we're talking about the same thing, using a little different terminology when we talk about candida.

"His favorite herbal formula is called Jenchena, a popular formula in Chinese medicine. It's a commonly used bitter herb, which happens to have antifungal properties."

Paul Jaconello, M.D., Toronto, Ontario, Canada: Like many other physicians, Dr. Jaconello uses diet, Sporanox and other antifungal medications during the early weeks of therapy. After the patient improves, he also uses nonprescription medications, including citrus seed extract and garlic.

Jacqueline Krohn, M.D., Los Alamos, New Mexico: In discussing the treatment of patients with the candida-related complex in her book, *The Whole Way to Allergy Relief and Prevention,** Dr. Krohn said, "*Lactobacillus acidophilus* preparations will supplement 'good' bacteria so that colonies can be re-implanted on the intestinal tract mucosal lining as the candida is killed."[12]

Dr. Krohn also recommends fatty acid preparations that have fungicidal properties, including Caprystatin. It comes in enterically coated tablets that release the caprylic acid slowly—total dose varies from person to person. She suggests that her patients begin with one tablet a day and work up to six to nine tablets; and, that they take them on an empty stomach and do not use them if pregnant. She feels that this product is a potent and effective preparation.

She then discusses Kaprycidin-A, which releases the caprylic acid in the stomach and upper intestine. She suggests taking Kaprycidin-A and Caprystatin together.

She also recommends ParaMycrocidin (grapefruit seed extract),

---

*Dr. Krohn's book is superb in every way. Of the dozens of books I reviewed, it ranks at the top of the list. It is a comprehensive, up-to-date, self-care guide for any person with yeast-related health problems, food allergies and chemical sensitivities.

She also provides her readers with a detailed discussion of other antifungal agents, including grapefruit seed extract, mathake, taheebo tea, garlic, Orithrush (a buffered form of sorbic acid which can be used as a mouthwash or vaginal douche), golden seal and tea tree oil for use in douches.

available from Allergy Research, Inc., in two strengths, 75 mg. and 125 mg. Other products which she uses and recommends include Mycocidin, an organic fatty acid (undecylenic acid) derived from castor bean. (Must be prescribed by a physician.) Suggested dose, one pearl daily, gradually increases up to nine to twelve pearls daily.

Allen Spreen, M.D., Jacksonville, Florida: "I use taheebo tea all the time. Also garlic. I think they help. I also use FOS and acidophilus together. Although some patients note an increasing amount of gas out of both ends of the GI tract, I like FOS.

"According to the scientific literature, acidophilus thrives on FOS. By contrast the other organisms in the gut, including candida, are not able to break it down. My patients love to take it and I do seem to be getting good results with it.

"I would like to comment briefly on the natural zinc, tannin compound, *Tanalbit,* which I used instead of caprylic acid and nystatin. It's cheaper and nonprescription. Die-off symptoms are common which implies efficacy to me. Moreover, poor responders are switched to Diflucan unless yeast vaginitis is a chief complaint, in which case I start with Diflucan.

"Another observation: killing the vaginal 'bad guys' does not seem to prevent recurrences. So I recommend reintroducing the vaginal 'good guys.' Years ago in Europe this was done with inserted applications of yogurt—wetting a tampon (or inserter) and covering with acidophilus powder seems to help. If vaginal itching is paramount, introducing garlic oil the same way can be very therapeutic—at least that's what my patients report."

Walter Ward, M.D., Winston-Salem, North Carolina: In discussing nonprescription antifungal agents, Dr. Ward especially recommends the Mycopryl brand of caprylic acid. He said, "In our patients who take Diflucan, if they're doing well, after two, four or six weeks, we switch them over to Mycopryl. We use the Mycopryl 400, one capsule, three times a day the first week; two capsules, three times a day the second week and three capsules, three times a day the third week.

"Then, as they improve, we put them on a maintenance dose of one capsule, three times a day. Then, as they improve further and become asymptomatic, we reduce the dose."

Gus Prosch, Jr., M.D., Birmingham, Alabama: "About four years ago I began using Tanalbit. It's still my number one choice. I always start every patient out on Tanalbit and I'm getting about 90% effectiveness.

"I'm convinced it is superior to other antifungal agents in the treatment of candida infections. My usual dose is two capsules, three times a day for four months, along with a special diet, probiotics and nutritional supplements. I then start gradually cutting back the dose."

Gerald Deutsch, D.C., Tempe, Arizona: "After trying many different products, we found that Tanalbit seemed to be as effective as nystatin . . . I found that by avoiding all yeast-containing products, fruits, or anything that ferments or has been fermented, and grains of all types provides for a more rapid control of the candidiasis . . .

"Based on symptomatology and chronicity, we utilize Tanalbit at one to three caps with meals. There's a natural improvement as the weeks go by. With the very strict dietary controls and the use of Tanalbit, results are usually demonstrable in 10–15 weeks. There is a very large percentage of total recovery using this protocol. I would certainly recommend it to all who need to avail themselves of this type program. I utilize Tanalbit for four months, one per meal after the candidiasis has cleared. This helps to maintain the integrity of the digestive tract."

REFERENCES

1. Murray, N. and Pizzarno, J., *Encyclopedia of Natural Medicine*, Prima Publishing, Rocklin, CA, 1991; p 86.
2. The Burton Goldberg Group, *Alternative Medicine—The Definitive Guide*, Future Medicine Publishing, Pyallup, WA, 1993; pp 591–592.
3. Mowrey, D.B., *The Scientific Validation of Herbal Medicine*, Cormorant Books, 1986; pp 272–273.
4. Werbach, M., *Healing Through Nutrition*, HarperCollins, New York, 1993; pp 327–330.
5. Ody, P., *The Complete Medicinal Herbal*, Dorling Kindersley, New York, 1993; p 67.
6. Neuhauser, I., *Arch. Int. Med*, 1954; Vol. 93.

7. Ionescu, G. et al, "Oral Citrus Seed Extract in Atopic Eczema: In vitro and in vivo studies on intestinal microflora," *J. of Orthomol. Med.*, 1990; Vol. 5 No. 3.
8. The Burton Goldberg Group, *Alternative Medicine—The Definitive Guide*, Future Medicine Publishing, Pyallup, WA, 1993.
9. Carper, J., *Food: Your Miracle Medicine*, HarperCollins, New York, 1993; p 450.
10. Boston Women's Health Collective, *The New Our Bodies, Ourselves—A Book By and For Women*, Touchstone, Simon & Schuster, New York, 1992; p 605.
11. Bland, J., quoted in Crook, W.G., *Chronic Fatigue Syndrome and the Yeast Connection*, Professional Books, Jackson, TN, 1992; p 262.
12. Krohn, J., Taylor, F.A and Larson, E.M., *The Whole Way to Allergy Relief and Prevention*, Hartley and Marks, Point Roberts, Washington, 1991; pp 197–208.

34

◆

Prescription Antiyeast Medications

◆

The Fascinating Story of Nystatin

If your health problems are yeast connected, especially if you've been helped by nystatin, you'll be interested in knowing how it was discovered and where it got its name.

You'll be especially interested if you're a woman. Here's why. Two brilliant pioneer female scientists collaborated in discovering this remarkable antifungal substance. The story of nystatin is told in a 1981 book, *The Fungus Fighters*, by Richard S. Baldwin.

In the foreword on this book, Gilbert Dalldorf recalls the story of the "wonder drug," *penicillin*. He said:

> "Medical history was changed by what appeared to be at first a chance discovery: a mold growing on a culture plate kept common bacteria from growing."

Soon afterward (in 1943), bacteriologist Selman Waksman, after years of searching, found a second antibiotic in the soil. Its name . . . streptomycin. In his continuing comments, Dalldorf had this to say:

> "Sparks from the Fleming and Waksman discoveries started a blaze in the Albany laboratory of the New York State Department of

Health. There, mold researcher Elizabeth Lee Hazen, began to look for an agent that might be useful in controlling fungus diseases."[1]

Working with organic chemist Rachel Brown during the years 1948–50, Hazen found many antifungal substances in the soil; however, most of them proved toxic not only to yeasts, but to laboratory animals.

Then, while vacationing with friends on a farm in Warrenton, Virginia, Elizabeth Hazen dug a soil sample and took it back to her laboratory. In this soil she found a mold which "knocked out" other yeasts and molds (including *Candida albicans*). Moreover, tests showed that this substance did not harm the animals.

Soon afterward, E.R. Squibb & Sons met with Hazen and Brown and arranged to take this new fungus fighting substance, study it, patent it and produce it.

Early in 1951, Hazen and Brown signed an agreement with Squibb to develop the new drug. They named it nystatin (pronounced ny-state-in) in honor of the New York State Department of Health. In their agreement with Squibb, their royalties were put in a special Brown-Hazen scientific and educational fund. Neither of these women asked for or received any personal financial gain from their discovery.

During the next decade, nystatin was produced in 18,000 gallon vats and marketed in many forms, including vaginal suppositories, foot powders, oral tablets and ointments. It was made available to physicians and patients (on prescription) all over the world. A patent, obtained in 1957, continued in force until 1974.

During these years royalties totaling 6.7 million dollars were paid to the Brown-Hazen fund and used to fund research on fungous diseases throughout the world.

Elizabeth Hazen died at the age of 89 in 1975; Rachel Brown died in 1980 at the age of 81. They were gratified by the help nystatin afforded women with vaginitis and people of both sexes with yeast-related digestive disturbances. Neither lived long enough to learn that their discovery would help millions of people with candida-related health disorders.

A Special Word to the Physician About Nystatin Powder

If you're prescribing nystatin powder* for many of your patients, ask your pharmacists to order it in bulk. They can obtain it from the following sources.

Lederle Laboratories, 300 Precision Dr., Horsham, PA 19044. 1-800-LEDERLE. It can be obtained in quantities of 150 million units, 1 billion units and 2 billion units.

Paddock Laboratories, 3101 Louisiana Ave. No., P.O. Box 27286, Minneapolis, MN 55427. (612) 546-4676. Fax (612) 546-4842. It can be obtained in quantities of 50 million units, 150 million units, 500 million units, 1 billion units, 2 billion units, 5 billion units.

If you're prescribing nystatin powder for your patients only occasionally and your pharmacist does not wish to stock it, your patients can fill their prescriptions from the following pharmacies:

Wellness Health & Pharmaceuticals
2800 S. 18th St.
Birmingham, AL 35209
(800)227-2627

Bio Tech Pharmacal**
P.O. Box 1992
Fayetteville, AR 72702
(501)443-9148 (ask for Dale Benedict)
(800)345-1199

N.E.E.D.S.
527 Charles Ave., 12A
Syracuse, NY 13209
(800)634-1380

College Pharmacy
833 N. Tejon St.
Colorado Springs, CO 80903
(800)888-9358.

Freeda Pharmaceuticals
36 E. 41st Street
New York, NY 10017
(212)685-4980
(800)777-3737

Medical Tower Pharmacy
1717 11th Ave. South
Birmingham, AL 35205
(205)933-7381

Willner Chemist
330 Lexington Ave.
New York, NY 10016
(212)685-0441
(800)633-1106

The Apothecary
5415 Cedar Lane
Bethesda, MD 20814
(800)869-9159
(301)530-0800

---

*Elmer Cranton, M.D., comments: "I've found that Squibb Mycostatin and some imported nystatins are quite bitter. Lederle nystatin (Nilstat) tastes better. I prefer it."
**Does not fill single prescriptions. Supplies nystatin powder to other pharmacies.

One-eighth tsp. of powder = 500,000 units = 1 tablet. The approximate cost for 500,000 units of nystatin in powder form ranges from 15¢ to 30¢ (in 1995).

Do Not Use Nystatin Topical Powder

For many years nystatin powder has been available in combination with talc and other ingredients. And many physicians have prescribed it for their patients with jock itch, diaper rashes and athlete's foot. Yet, in spite of instructions on the package which say "For topical use only," on a number of occasions during the past decade, people have taken their nystatin powder prescription to a pharmacy and have been given the topical nystatin.

Although a pharmacist friend of mine told me that taking the topical powder orally would not be hazardous, it's obviously better to obtain "the real thing."

Why You Should Not Use Nystatin Suspension

Nystatin suspension (Nilstat, Lederle and Mycostatin, Squibb) has been available for many years. Moreover, these products are often prescribed by pediatricians for infants with oral thrush. Although they sometimes seem to be effective, I do not recommend them. Here's why. They're loaded with sugar and research studies carried out by a number of investigators show that sugar greatly increases the growth of *Candida albicans*.

Nystatin Enemas

Several years ago, during a visit to New Zealand, I spent the day with Dr. Bruce Duncan who, for over a decade, has been interested in yeast-related health problems, food and chemical sensitivities and more especially in the role multiple, hidden or latent viruses play in making people sick.

During my visit with Bruce and his professional colleague, Joan R. Smith, as you might guess, we talked about yeast-related health problems. And Dr. Duncan said in effect:

"I've found nystatin to be a highly effective medication for patients with yeast-related problems. Our studies show that oral nystatin is broken down by gut organisms and may not reach the colon. So my practice is to combine oral nystatin with nystatin enemas."

> ## *So my practice is to combine oral nystatin with nystatin enemas.*

I hadn't given the matter of nystatin enemas much thought until early 1994 when I received a copy of a fascinating book by Duncan and Smith entitled, *The Hidden Viruses Within You.* Although a major part of the book was devoted to the management of viral infections, nystatin enemas were covered in a comprehensive manner. Here are excerpts.

"Oral nystatin and amphotericin B are broken down by gut organisms. No evidence of nystatin was found in the colon contents of a patient who had taken 36 tablets by mouth . . . No nystatin reaches the sigmoid colon, just above the rectum, where most of the candida live* . . . It is better to anticipate the effect of oral nystatin and begin enemas between the fourth to the sixth week. Half of the oral dose is continued and the other half is given as an enema.

"Patients react to the suggestion of nystatin enemas in a variety of ways, from 'tell me why and how,' embarrassment and a few feel disgusted at the thought. Explaining why, how to use the enema and continuing encouragement have nearly all people using enemas and delighted with the increased recovery . . .

"Enemas are very cost effective. There is no need to double or triple the dose you are taking by mouth. Keep to the eighth of a teaspoonful of powder, four times a day until considerable relief occurs or your physician advises you to abandon the therapy. Patients who

---

*Elmer Cranton, M.D., comments: "This may not be entirely true. Perianal itching and rash from yeast is relieved by oral nystatin and oral amphotericin B. Improvement in these symptoms would not occur if these medications were inactivated. Another possible explanation: constipation and slow bowel transit time which allow time for bacterial inactivation."

have carried out enema therapy in a useful manner are unanimous that it is more effective than nystatin by mouth as a long term treatment."[2]

The Effectiveness of Nystatin As a Therapeutic Agent

Many physicians interested in candida-related health problems use nystatin in treating their patients. In a number of conversations with me during the past 15 years, candida pioneer, Dr. C. Orian Truss, has emphasized the effectiveness and safety of this antifungal medication. And in the conclusion of his most recent scientific report, he said:

> "Chronic superficial yeast infections may lead to generalized symptoms. A six week therapeutic trial of nystatin and diet is adequate to establish or reject the diagnosis of this, the 'superficial candidiasis syndrome.'
>
> "This simple, safe and relatively inexpensive six weeks therapeutic trial will identify yeasts as the cause of this complex of symptoms, and stop the very large expense entailed in the repeated investigation of these symptoms."[3]

Dr. Truss tells me he prefers oral and vaginal nystatin because he has found it effective and so safe. He bases this opinion not only on his own experience, but on reports in the medical literature during the past several decades.

According to the 1992 *Physicians' Desk Reference (PDR)*:

> "Nystatin is virtually nontoxic and nonsensitizing and is well tolerated by all age groups, including debilitated infants, even on prolonged administration. Large oral doses have occasionally produced diarrhea, gastrointestinal distress, nausea and vomiting."

Nystatin is virtually nontoxic and nonsensitizing and is well tolerated by all age groups.

In looking at this volume (which lists thousands of prescription drugs), I read about the many adverse reactions which could accompany the use of most of these drugs. Although I did not make a page-by-page search of the *PDR*, nystatin was easily the safest of all prescription medications. Here's additional information from the *PDR* about nystatin.

"Nystatin is an antifungal antibiotic which is both fungistatic and fungicidal, *in vitro* against a wide variety of yeasts and yeast-like fungi. It is a polyene antibiotic of undetermined structural formula, that is obtained from *Streptomyces noursei* . . . It is the first well-tolerated antifungal antibiotic of dependable efficacy for the treatment of cutaneous, oral and intestinal infections caused by *Candida albicans* and other candida species.

"Nystatin probably acts by binding to sterols in the cell membrane of the fungus with a resultant change in membrane permeability, allowing leakage of intracellular components. It exhibits no appreciable activity against bacteria, or trichomonads.

"Following oral administration, nystatin is sparingly absorbed with no detectable blood levels when given in the recommended doses. Most of the orally administered nystatin is passed unchanged in the stool . . .

"*Candida albicans* demonstrates no significant resistance to nystatin in vitro on repeated subculture in increasing levels of nystatin . . .

"No adverse effects or complications have been attributed to nystatin in infants born to women treated with nystatin."[4]

To obtain further information about the experiences of physicians with nystatin, I interviewed a number of candida clinicians in 1993 and 1994. Here are excerpts.

James Brodsky, M.D., Chevy Chase, Maryland: "Nystatin is my number one antifungal medication and I've used it for over 10 years. My present practice is to start the nystatin and the diet simultaneously. The average duration of full therapy is four to six months with a tapering period of six months to two years. Yet, it is not unusual for me to see patients who after two to four years are still taking one or two nystatin capsules a day. They feel more comfortable when they take it. Then some use it intermittently on an as needed basis.

"I've had patients who've been off nystatin for years, then they come back because their symptoms have returned. Moreover, I'm seeing patients now that I treated back in the early '80s who did well for seven or eight years, and now they've come back to be re-treated. Maybe they're not as bad, and most of them aren't, but they're starting to see a return of symptoms and they want to go back on the program.

"If a patient isn't doing really well after two months, I look at the possibility of sensitivity to foods, especially wheat and corn. Then, if they're still not doing well I add Diflucan, Sporanox or Nizoral. Moreover, *I've combined the nystatin with these drugs and have not found a problem with the combination* [emphasis added].

"Of course, if they receive no benefit at all from the nystatin, I'll drop the nystatin and use the systemic antifungal alone, or with a nutritional antifungal such as caprylic acid or one of the citrus seed extract preparations. If their response to nystatin is partial, as I've already noted, I'll continue the nystatin and add the systemic antifungal."

Aubrey Worrell, M.D., Pine Bluff, Arkansas: "I like to start with nystatin tablets since patients seldom, if ever, have a die-off reaction. Here's a possible explanation. The tablets make it down into the lower part of the intestinal tract, maybe even to the colon before they start wiping out the candida. By contrast, the powder may start working in the mouth, esophagus and stomach very quickly, so that's what gives the bigger die-off reaction.

"Once my patients have been on the tablets for several weeks, I then switch them over to nystatin powder if they're not doing well. Although I sometimes use Nizoral and Diflucan, I reserve these medications for the people who do not respond to the nystatin."

George Kroker, M.D., LaCrosse, Wisconsin: *"I began using nystatin in the late '70s, and I find that it is still an excellent drug— perhaps the only antifungal medication they need* [emphasis added]. During the past several years, however, I've been impressed with the value and effectiveness of the azole drugs.

"So in some of my patients—especially those with severe symptoms—I begin them on Diflucan, then in two or three weeks after they improve, I'll go to a maintenance dose of nystatin, two to four million units a day and stay with that. This often works very well."

George Miller, M.D., Lewisburg, Pennsylvania: "When my poly-symptomatic patients come in I, of course, take a good history. I tell my patients I'm going to do something very unusual—'I'm going to listen to you.' (Many times, it seems to me the patients go to the doctors and they start writing out lab slips before hearing the patient's story.)

"If their problems seem to be yeast-related—as they often are—I put them on the diet for the first week, then I add Diflucan the second week. Then I put them over on the nystatin.

"After they've been on the nystatin for 30 days, I re-evaluate them and decide whether they need allergy testing for inhalants, foods or chemicals."

The Systemic "Azole" Anticandida Drugs—Nizoral, Diflucan, Sporanox

These highly effective anticandida medications are synthetic compounds which are classified as imidazoles (Nizoral) or triazoles (Diflucan and Sporanox), according to whether they contain two or three nitrogen atoms, respectively, in the five-membered azole ring. Their antifungal effects are targeted primarily at ergosterol, the main sterol in the fungal cell membrane.

According to a recent review article in the *New England Journal of Medicine*, discussing these drugs:

> "The depletion of ergosterol alters membrane fluidity, thereby reducing the activity of membrane-associated enzymes and leading to an increased permeability and inhibition of cell growth and replication. Other antifungal effects of azoles include . . . the inhibition of the morphogenetic transformation of yeast to the mycelial form."[5]

Nizoral (ketoconazole)

This potent anticandida medication, available only on prescription, was introduced into the U.S. in 1981. Using this medication in my practice in the 1980s, I was able to help over 150 of my patients; moreover, many of these patients had not improved on nystatin.

As is the case with any medication, Nizoral may occasionally cause adverse side effects. These include elevated liver enzymes, and in rare instances, hepatitis. Yet, in reviewing the experiences of dozens of physicians during the past decade, I've received no reports of dangerous side effects of this medication, except when it was prescribed in large doses.

In the third edition of *The Yeast Connection*, I quoted Allan Lieberman, M.D., N. Charleston, South Carolina, who commented:

> *"I use Nizoral as my drug of choice in treating every patient in whom I suspect a candida-related health disorder.* I've treated hundreds of patients in this manner and have never experienced a severe reaction. Nizoral acts promptly . . . and sometimes a patient feels better after the first dose, and often the response is dramatic.

I treat the average patient with Nizoral for seven days. On the fifth day I add nystatin while continuing the Nizoral.

"I treat the average patient with Nizoral for 7 days; occasionally in a patient with severe problems I continue the medication for 10 days. On the fifth day I add nystatin while continuing the Nizoral.

"A significant advantage of Nizoral is that it provides a prompt therapeutic trial which helps me determine if my patient's health problems are related to *Candida albicans*. In addition, it causes fewer 'die-off' type reactions. *It is an extremely useful drug."*[6]

Diflucan, one of the cousins of Nizoral, became available on prescription in the U.S. in 1990, and most (but not all) physicians now prefer it to Nizoral. Then still another related azole drug, Sporanox, was licensed for general use in 1993. To find out more about Dr. Lieberman's current observations, I called him in January 1994. Here are excerpts from our conversation.

"Many of my patients respond dramatically to any of the antifungal medications, no matter what the diagnosis is. And I continue to put patients in whom I suspect a yeast-related problem on a 14-day course of an antifungal. Although I think all three of these systemic antifungal medications are useful, Nizoral and Diflucan are not always interchangeable, nor equally effective in all patients.

"To my surprise, I've seen patients who did not respond to Diflucan, but who responded to Nizoral. I haven't seen it often, but I've seen it often enough to realize that if I'm treating a patient with Diflucan and she isn't doing well, I do not stop there if I suspect the problem is yeast-related. Instead I go back to Nizoral.

"I've also found Sporanox to be a useful drug and is probably equivalent to Nizoral. Yet, I've seen more reactions with Sporanox and I feel they might be coming from the colored capsule."

And in an April 1994 letter to me, Dr. Lieberman commented:

"In the course of 15 or more years of using antifungal therapy, *I have found yeast and fungi to be the single most contributory cause in several clinical conditions*. These include ulcerative colitis, psoriasis, depression and the attention deficit/hyperactivity disorder. Therapeutic trials resulted in complete resolution in some of these cases. As you cannot tell who will respond, a therapeutic trial seems indicated where history is suggestive."

I also cited the comments of Francis Waickman, M.D., an Akron, Ohio, physician who enthusiastically recommended Nizoral. He said that he gave all of his patients with yeast-related problems 200 mg. once a day for two weeks and that 90% of them showed significant improvement. He then switched them over to nystatin.[7]

To get an update on his experiences in using antifungal medication, I called him in October 1994. Here are excerpts from our conversation.

> *In my experience, and that of my physician associates, Nizoral continues to be an excellent drug.*

"In my experience, and that of my physician associates, Nizoral continues to be an excellent drug. We have run into no liver problem with Nizoral except in one patient whose pharmacist husband gave her six times the usual dose!

"We feel we get better response to Nizoral and Sporanox than we do to Diflucan. We've had our best results using Nizoral or Sporanox for about two weeks, then we change over to nystatin. And after about six or eight weeks on nystatin, we'll add the probiotic Vitalplex. After three months we try to get the patient off the nystatin and just continue with the Vitalplex and most patients do quite well.

"However, we do run into some patients who go downhill after we stop the Nizoral or Sporanox and go to the nystatin. But when we again give them the absorbed antifungals, they do well. So we have a small number of patients—I'm not sure how many—that we cannot get off the absorbable antifungals without having symptoms."

Possible Adverse Effects of Nizoral

Although Nizoral is generally well tolerated, in one person out of about 10,000 who take it, hepatitis or other serious adverse reactions may occur. Accordingly, blood tests to monitor liver function should be carried out at monthly intervals—more often if the patient is given doses larger than 200 mg. (one tablet) daily.

Here are further comments which appeared in the *New England Journal of Medicine* about the possible toxicities of Nizoral and other azole drugs.

"The main difference in potential toxicity between ketoconazole (Nizoral) and the newer triazoles relates to the effects of this class of drugs on steroidogenesis.

"When given in daily doses exceeding 400 mg., ketoconazole may reversibly inhibit the synthesis of testosterone (and therefore estradiol) and cortisol, resulting in a variety of endocrine disturbances, including gynecomastia (enlarged breasts in the male), oligospermia (deficient sperm production), loss of libido, impotence, menstrual irregularities, and very rarely, adrenal insufficiency.

"By contrast, fluconazole and itraconazole, when given in recommended doses do not inhibit steroidogenesis."[8]

Endocrine Dysfunction Related to Nizoral

A 45-year-old professional (I'll call her Laura) gave a 3½ year history of recurrent urinary and vaginal infections and *vulvodynia* (burning vulva). In her efforts to obtain help, she saw many physicians in her own city, including gynecologists, urologists, allergists, dermatologists and psychiatrists. She also consulted specialists at a world famous clinic in the upper midwest.

In September 1989, after research of her own at a university library, she discovered an article by Dr. Marilynne McKay[9] describing the response of women with vulvodynia to anticandida therapy. A few months later she saw her physician who prescribed Nizoral, 200 mg. daily.

While taking Nizoral, Laura's vaginal and vulvar symptoms were controlled. Yet, she developed other problems. Her psychiatrist called me and we discussed various aspects of Laura's problems. He also asked her to write me and provide me with further information about her history.

And in a January 16, 1993, letter to me she said: "As my psychiatrist probably told you, I'm currently experiencing difficulties with orgasm . . . The pleasurable sensation accompanying an orgasm began to slowly diminish four years ago when the vulvodynia and bladder symptoms were most severe."

In her continuing discussion in her letter to me, she said that she had continued to use Nizoral on a fairly regular basis for over two years. And she said, "Any time that I stopped using Nizoral, or cut the dosage, my symptoms seemed to reappear after approximately ten days. Yet, I have been very concerned about the long term use of Nizoral. I would appreciate any input you may have regarding my current situation."

Because of the known tendency of Nizoral to cause endocrine disturbances in some patients, after reviewing Laura's history, I called her physician and suggested the substitution of Diflucan for the Nizoral.

In a letter to me in May, 1993, Laura reported that less than a week after changing from Nizoral to Diflucan her sexual dysfunction ceased to be a problem. She continued to take Diflucan for many weeks and the burning vulva, fatigue and other symptoms improved to such a degree that she tapered off the Diflucan and changed over to nystatin.

And in her November 1, 1993, letter to me, Laura said:

> "I'm doing *GREAT*. And I feel that the primary source of my yeast problem is in my intestinal tract and nystatin keeps it under control. I really appreciate your efforts in educating the public about yeast-related problems. I wish more physicians took it seriously."

Nizoral is a useful drug; yet, like all medications, it may cause adverse side effects. Based on Laura's story and the reports I've had from other sources, the endocrine disturbances caused by Nizoral are reversible and disappear or subside when the medication is stopped.

Diflucan—A Highly Effective Anticandida Medication

I'd heard little or nothing about this medication until the September 1988 Candida Update Conference in Memphis, sponsored by the International Health Foundation. At that conference, two British physicians, Stephen Davies and Jean Monro, commented:

> "A new antifungal agent is being widely used in the United Kingdom. Its name: Diflucan. It's a great drug and we've found it has played a key role in helping many of our patients with candida-related health problems."

On a trip to Europe in September 1989, I visited Dr. Davies, a researcher who, along with two colleagues, published findings of their investigations of the candida/human interaction. Included were studies of the relationship of candida to alcohol production in the intestinal tract.[10] During our visit, Davies said, *"Diflucan is an exciting first class medication."*

He also made copies of a 25-page Pfizer booklet which provided more information. One of the reports which impressed me stated that *a single Diflucan tablet was more effective than a whole week of suppositories in helping women with vaginal yeast infections.*

In the spring of 1990, Diflucan was licensed for use in the United States. However, the initial recommendations by the manufacturer focused entirely on treating patients with AIDS, cancer and other illnesses. These disorders cause such severe disturbances in the immune system that candida "jumps aboard." Many research papers published in the last several years show that Diflucan is superior to (and safer than) intravenous amphotericin B in treating these immunosuppressed patients.

Even though Diflucan was released primarily for use in treating patients with severe immunosuppression, word of its effectiveness in treating patients with the candida related complex and chronic fatigue syndrome spread to physicians and patients throughout North America. In a November 2, 1993, Third Quarter Report, William C. Steere, Jr., CEO of Pfizer stated:

> "In early August Pfizer received an 'approval' letter from the U.S. Food and Drug Administration for use of our antifungal agent Diflucan in the treatment of vaginal yeast infections caused by Candida (vaginal candidiasis) . . . In U.S. clinical trials, which included more than 800 women with vaginal candidiasis, a single 150 mg. oral Diflucan tablet proved to be well tolerated and as effective as seven days of intravaginal therapy . . .

The oral dosage form eliminates the inconvenience associated with intravaginal agents.

> "In the 57 countries where Diflucan is already available for vaginal candidiasis, more than 9 million women have received single dose treatment. The oral dosage form eliminates the inconvenience associated with intravaginal agents. In addition, since one tablet provides the full course of therapy, patient compliance with Diflucan is virtually ensured."

During the past three years, more and more physicians have prescribed Diflucan and have confirmed its effectiveness. Here are some of the reports I've received.

Sidney M. Baker, M.D., Weston, Connecticut: "I started using Diflucan before it was on the market in the U.S. and by now I have prescribed it for over a thousand patients. I have not seen a single significant toxic effect—even in children. I have seen only a handful of GI disturbances—some of them persisting for a while after the patient comes off of it. I have seen dry mouth and a few people have claimed they were getting dizzy or light headed who had to stop.

"But this is merely a handful and it's amazing considering that one is bound to see a certain amount of die-off with any antifungal drug . . . When a person continues to take Diflucan and the side effect goes away and when the side effect mimics symptoms of their illness, that's pretty good evidence for die-off. I'm really impressed by this medication—yet I do think it's very dose-sensitive. Some people may need to take doses as large as 400 mg. a day to obtain maximum benefit.

"When I first started using Diflucan, I did so cautiously and used 50 mg. once a day. Now I give patients 200 mg. a day for 21 consecutive days. If this program doesn't provide them with significant help, I figure a yeast problem isn't apt to be their main difficulty."

Charles S. Resseger, D.O, Norwalk, Ohio: "I've now treated over 6000 patients with Diflucan with doses of 100 to 600 mg. a day up to 18 months. I've never seen an adverse reaction other than an occasional mild one after four months in therapy."

Philip K. Nelson, M.D., Sarasota, Florida: "I've had the opportunity of working with CFIDS patients over the past two years and seeing their response to both diet and antifungals has been impressive.

"That is not to say that all CFIDS patients will benefit from this approach, but certainly many do and with this illness we accept improvement from many sources.

"Many people have trouble sticking to your diet completely, but even avoidance of simple sugars has been a great help. I have been using a program of Diflucan, two tablets initially followed by one tablet every other day for a total of three weeks (12 tablets total). I then go directly to Nilstat TID for two weeks out of each month indefinitely. This has apparently succeeded in clearing the gut. This same regimen has helped many of my patients with recurrent vaginal candidiasis. I think most experts agree that vaginal candidiasis has a bowel reservoir."

Serafino Corsello, M.D., New York, New York: "I was ignorant about the yeast/human interaction until January 1981. At that time I heard Orian Truss talk and I said to myself, 'Baloney.' Then, as fate would have it, about five days later a patient came in with all the symptoms that Dr. Truss talked about. I called Dr. Truss and his observations truly changed my life."

In her continuing discussion, Dr. Corsello talked about the comprehensive program she uses in treating her patients, including dietary changes which result in cleansing of the intestinal tract. She also gives magnesium, antioxidants, Omega 3 and Omega 9 fatty acids, lactobacillus and other nutritional supplements. Then she said:

"After about a month I go to Diflucan 100 mg. a day for seven to ten days then 100 mg. twice a day for a month. I've found that along with a comprehensive treatment program, Diflucan plays an important role in helping many people regain their health."

Ken Gerdes, M.D., Denver, Colorado: "I'm using more and more Diflucan. I feel like it's a very positive, capable kind of drug that does a good job against yeast. And sometimes it's the only drug that will help. I've seen several patients (probably three or four) where I've followed Sid Baker's lead of going up to 400 mg. a day. And they seem to gain additional benefits in that gap between 200 and 400 mg.

"In an occasional patient I start with 400 mg. or 200 mg. a day and then taper the dose on down. Usually people who get full benefit from these larger doses want to stay on it. I'm happy to report that I've seen little or no liver function problems with Diflucan."

Walter Ward, M.D., Winston-Salem, North Carolina: "I see 12 to 16 new patients a week. Half of them are yeast-related. I'm using an awful lot of Diflucan. Yet, for my chronic patients with skin problems I'm still staying with Nizoral because it seems to penetrate the skin a lot better.

"A word about Diflucan side effects. I've seen them only rarely, yet I've had a couple of patients who popped up with strange mental problems. One was a very religious lady who started cussing like a sailor and started doing strip-teases—very inappropriate."

Richard Noble, M.D., Hillsboro, Oregon: "In managing my patients with candida-related problems, during the first month I change their diet, recommend nutritional supplements and make suggestions for lifestyle changes.

"When they come back for a recheck, I generally prescribe 200 mg. the first day, then 100–200 mg. a day for three weeks. At that time I re-evaluate the patient's response and during the second three weeks I may vary the dose, depending on the woman's symptoms and the time of her cycle. In some women, I continue to give it daily and others I give it twice a week.

"Usually by the end of six weeks patients have shown enough improvement that Diflucan may no longer be necessary and I follow it with herbal remedies, including Mathake herbal tea and citrus seed extract.

"One of the problems with Diflucan, however, is what I feel to be the excessive cost."

Gary Oberg, M.D., Crystal Lake, Illinois: "During the first week I put patients on a diet eliminating all simple sugars and fruits. Then I begin antifungals. The great majority I treat with Diflucan, 100 mg. a day. If the dose is helping, I generally leave them on this medication for several months or so.

I've now given it to several hundred patients with only minimal side effects.

"I've now given it to several hundred patients with only minimal side effects—a few GI upsets and a few who had alterations in their menstrual cycle.

"Yet, I find it important to treat other predisposing factors. If I just treat the yeast problem and don't do anything else, I find it hard to get patients off the medication without relapsing.

"I've found little use for the nonprescription antifungal agents. All the over-the-counter antifungal agents don't seem to hold a candle to the glorious reports I receive from patients who have taken Diflucan."

Aubrey Worrell, M.D., Pine Bluff, Arkansas: "Diflucan is a little more effective than Nizoral, and safer. I generally give Diflucan 200 mg. a day for up to two weeks. Then I'm apt to shift over to nystatin. I haven't seen any adverse side effects in patients who have taken it."

Leo Galland, M.D., New York, New York: "I usually have my patients follow a diet for a week before starting antifungals. And in my adult patients with candida-related problems, I generally give Diflucan 200 mg. daily for three to six weeks. Then if the patient improves, I try to see if they can be maintained on a nonabsorbed antifungal, either nystatin or citrus seed extract, an agent which I've found very helpful and equally as effective as nystatin."

George F. Kroker, M.D., La Crosse, Wisconsin: "I generally start patients on Diflucan two tablets on the first day and then one tablet daily for two weeks in many of my patients. At the end of two weeks, I often switch them over to a maintenance dose of nystatin.

"I have not had any significant side effects involving liver toxicity or hepatitis. And I had one patient who had elevated liver enzymes on Nizoral who could take Diflucan without problems."

Compassionate (free) supplies of Diflucan are available. The person requesting this medication must have a clinical and/or laboratory confirmation of infection by *Candida albicans;* the patient must be uninsured, that is, not covered by private insurance, Medicaid, Medicare, the state AIDS Drug Assistance Program or any other third-party payer; the patient's annual income must be less than $25,000 if single with no dependents, $40,000 if married or with dependents.

Diflucan tablets must be prescribed; the IV dosage form is not available through this program. The drug must be taken in an outpatient setting. Inpatient use in an acute or chronic care setting is not recovered. To obtain further information, call Roerig Division, Pfizer, Inc., 1-800-869-9979.

Sporanox—Another Highly Effective Anticandida Medication

This systemic azole drug is a cousin of Nizoral and an even closer cousin of Diflucan in that both are "triazoles." As is the case with Diflucan, Sporanox (itraconazole) was extensively studied prior to its release in the U.S.A. in the spring of 1993. Here are excerpts from a 1989 article.

"Itraconazole was shown to be extremely effective in a wide range of superficial and more serious 'deep' fungal infections when administered once or twice daily. Generally, greater than 80% of patients with superficial dermatophyte or yeast infections are cured by itraconazole. . . Preliminary findings also indicate that itraconazole may hold promise for the prophylaxis of opportunistic fungal infections . . . in women with chronic recurrent vaginal candidiasis.

"Following oral administration of itraconazole peak plasma concentrations are reached within 1½ to 4 hours . . . Itraconazole is widely distributed in the body, achieving concentrations in some tissues up to ten times higher than corresponding plasma concentrations. Itraconazole can be detected in stratum corneum up to four weeks after discontinuing therapy, which probably reflects the drug's affinity for sebum and keratinocytes.

"The elimination half-life and healthy volunteers is about 20 hours after a single load dose of 100 mg. and approximately 30 hours after two to four weeks treatment with itraconazole, 100 mg. daily.

"Overall, itraconazole, 100 mg. once daily, has proven to be optimal dosage in dermatophytoses producing a greater than 80% cure or marked improvement (against a number of skin fungal infections).

"Adverse effects—itraconazole is well tolerated by most patients, the most common side effects relating to gastrointestinal disturbance . . . It appears to be devoid of effects on the pituitary-testicular-adrenal axis. Rarely transient increases in liver enzymes have occurred.

"Recommended dose in most situations is 100 mg. once daily at mealtime. For vaginal candidiasis recommended dose is 200 mg., once daily for three days."[11]

In another report, "Discovering Antimycotic Drugs: Today and Tomorrow," the authors commented:

"The new triazole, itraconazole, appears to be an even more effective agent with a broader spectrum of action than ketoconazole.

"During the past five years itraconazole has been distributed throughout 48 countries. Cure rate greater than 80% in candidiasis.

"Of the 15,000 patients who have been treated with itraconazole, only 7% experienced side effects, gastrointestinal complaints and headaches were the most frequently reported of these.

"In the study of patients with acute vaginal candidiasis, several treatment regimens have been tested. Length of treatment is varied from one to five days in total dose from 200 to 800 mg. The mycologic results clearly demonstrate that a minimum total dose of 400 mg. should be given to obtain acceptable results. Excellent results in a large number of patients have been obtained with a dosage of 200 mg. once daily for three consecutive days.

"In a group of patients with chronic vaginal candidiasis, 30 patients were treated with 200 mg. of itraconazole for three days, followed by one single dose of 200 mg. every first day of their menses for six consecutive cycles. This regimen resulted in a cure.

"Usually these patients will have experienced at least two episodes of candidiasis during this period. However, this prophylactic, itraconazole regimen kept 80% of the patients free of candida infection and symptoms of candidiasis.

"Once the prophylaxis was discontinued, relapses or reinfections reappeared in some patients, two to three months later.

"Of 1,276 patients, 6.2% reported side effects—nausea was the most frequent complaint. No consistent abnormalities in results of blood biochemical tests have been observed."[12]

Because I had not used Sporanox in my own practice in treating patients with candida-related health problems, I interviewed a number of practicing physicians in late 1993 and early 1994. Here are the observations of some of these physicians.

James Brodsky, M.D., Chevy Chase, Maryland: "I continue to have good results with Sporanox, yet I must say I don't see a tremendous difference between Diflucan, Sporanox, or Nizoral for that matter. I think there are some people who will respond well to one and not to the other and that there are other patients in which it will be vice versa. Yet, I've been pleased with all three of the drugs in this family.

"I still reserve these drugs for patients who do not respond well to nystatin. I don't think they should be first line drugs. Since they're systemic, there's a potential toxicity, although it's small. So I generally always start patients on nystatin."

Carol Jessop, M.D., El Cerrito, California: "I've used all the azole drugs and I've found them extremely helpful. Yet, there are some people who tolerate Diflucan better than Sporanox and vice versa. I can't explain why.

"Generally my choice of drugs has to do with the patient's insurance. As you may know, the insurance company may tell you which drug you can order.

"I had some patients on Diflucan originally, they sign up for insurance and it covers only Sporanox, and they tell me it's not the same for them. So they have to decide to pay out of pocket for it, or get compassionate care from Pfizer. Yet, I've also had good luck with Sporanox and I can think of two or three patients who felt quite strongly that Sporanox was not as helpful to them as Diflucan, yet I've seen it the other way around also."

Ronald Hoffman, M.D., New York, New York: "My impression is that Sporanox is a drug of choice in skin problems. It seems to get into the skin tissues more effectively than Diflucan."

Elmer Cranton, M.D., Yelm, Washington: "I've been using this drug in the same dose I used to use Diflucan. I use a 200 mg. loading dose on the first day and then 100 mg. a day. I have not found it necessary to use 200 mg. a day of Sporanox. Two Sporanox a day would be considerably more expensive than one Diflucan a day, whereas using one Sporanox a day is a little bit less expensive than one Diflucan a day—100 mg. dose that is.

"In regard to side effects, including nausea and headache, I can only say that for the last 18 months I've been using Sporanox exclusively and not Diflucan, and I have not seen any side effects. The patients tolerate it well. I still see the kill-off effect, but to no greater extent."

Paul Jaconello, M.D., Toronto, Canada: "I've been using Sporanox for two to three years. I've found it reasonably successful. Patients don't seem to get the die-off they get on Diflucan. My usual dose is one tablet a day for four weeks."

George Kroker, M.D., LaCrosse, Wisconsin: "Sporanox seems to have an excellent tissue penetration and a longer half-life than other azole drugs. It's especially good in people with fungus infections of the nails."

Al Robbins, D.O., Boca Raton, Florida: "Sporanox is a wonderful, safe medication that has been quite beneficial to people with yeast-related health problems, especially those with chemical sensitivity. In some patients it just pulls them completely out of this complex illness that has been devastating them.

"I have my patients take Sporanox out of the capsule and put the beads on their tongue and swallow them with water. Here's my rationale: Some people seem to be sensitive to the ingredients in the capsule. Regarding the dosages, I use four capsules a day for 14 to 30 days.

> *I have also noted that Sporanox helped a number of my patients with musculoskeletal problems.*

"I have also noted that Sporanox helped a number of my patients with musculoskeletal problems. Some of these people had gotten to the point where they could hardly exercise and had gone downhill rapidly. Sporanox has helped them. Of course, Nizoral and Diflucan also helped these patients.

"Although I haven't seen many adverse reactions, Sporanox seems to cause more of them than Diflucan. When the Sporanox works it seems to work better. It also is quite effective in patients with problems involving their skin, nervous system, muscles and joints."

William Shrader, M.D., Santa Fe, New Mexico: "Although Diflucan is my first choice, I've also found that Sporanox is a useful medication. I've given it to at least 150 patients. I usually give 100 to 200 mg. a day and it seems to me that the larger dose works better."

Charles Resseger, D.O., Norwalk, Ohio: "I'm still as enthusiastic about Diflucan as ever. It works beautifully for most people. I also like Sporanox and the combination of the two drugs has enabled me to clear up many patients who didn't clear up on Diflucan alone . . .

"I've treated about 50 people who were 'just on the edge' and I've been able to turn their lives around by using both drugs at the same time. Also, I've found I can use a smaller dose of Diflucan when I add Sporanox 100 mg. a day.

"In my usual patient I begin on systemic antifungal therapy. I start with Diflucan 100 mg. and an absolutely no-sugar diet. In 65% of my patients that will control their yeast problem. For the other 35% I do other things. The first thing I do is to boost their dose of Diflucan up to 200 mg., then I generally add Sporanox 100 mg. a day. Occasionally I have to give even more Diflucan, up to 400 mg. a day.

"However, there are some patients who once required 600 mg. of Diflucan to do well, who now do well with 100 or 200 mg. of Diflucan along with the Sporanox."

Further Comments About the Three Azole Drugs

In their discussion of these drugs, Como and Dismukes pointed out that the peak plasma concentration after a single 200 mg. dose of itraconazole and ketoconazole varied widely among different patients. And they noted that the peak plasma concentrations of itraconazole, but not of ketoconazole, are three to five times higher after 7 to 14 days of treatment (steady state) than after a single dose.

In contrast to itraconazole and ketoconazole, the absorption of oral fluconazole is not altered by the presence of food or gastric acidity. Peak plasma concentrations of fluconazole are proportional to the dose and occur within two to four hours after oral administration. Yet, as is the case with itraconazole, plasma concentrations are approximately 2 to 2½ times higher after 6 to 10 days of treatment than after single doses.

These authors noted that all three of the azole drugs are active against *Candida albicans,* yet they said:

"In vitro susceptibility testing of antifungal drugs against fungal organisms is of questionable value because of the limited correlation of the results of clinical response."

In their continuing discussion, they pointed out that there were variations from laboratory to laboratory. Yet they said that the development of clinically important resistance to azoles, even after prolonged courses of therapy, was rare.

In summarizing their discussion of these drugs, they said:

"The oral azole drugs ketoconazole, fluconazole and itraconazole, represent a major advance in systemic antifungal therapy. Among the three, fluconazole has the most attractive pharmacologic profile ... ketoconazole is less well tolerated than either fluconazole or itraconazole and is associated with more clinically important toxic effects, including hepatitis and inhibition of steroid hormone synthesis. However, ketoconazole is less expensive than fluconazole and itraconazole—an especially important consideration for patients receiving long-term therapy."[13]

Should Nystatin Be Given Along with Sporanox or Diflucan?

Some physicians say such combinations are not necessary. Yet, others hold a different point of view. They feel that the concentration of Diflucan and/or the other azole drugs in the colon may not be high enough to control yeast proliferation. Such physicians feel that the combined administration of the two drugs is not only appropriate, but that it shortens the time antifungal medication is needed.

Elmer Cranton, M.D., Yelm, Washington, a graduate of Harvard Medical School, a founder and past president of the American Holistic Medical Association and Editor Emeritus of the *Journal of Advancement in Medicine,* during a March 1994 conversation with me said, in effect:

"*The combined administration of two drugs is not only appropriate, it shortens the time antifungal medication is needed.* Based on my experience, Diflucan, Sporanox or Nizoral alone must be taken for many months to completely eradicate yeast in the gut.

"Here's why. These drugs are all absorbed in the upper GI tract and taken into the circulation. They go to many parts of the body, including the liver and are excreted in the bile. Yet, the drugs are reabsorbed in the upper part of the small intestine. As a result, therapeutic levels do not reach the colon. Therefore, I strongly urge that nystatin be given in conjunction with the systemic drugs.

"I continue to be surprised that physicians are so reluctant to use two different drugs at the same time which work synergistically and greatly shorten the necessary therapeutic period. *If nystatin and Diflucan are used together (and the same could be said for nystatin and Sporanox, or Nizoral), the body can be rid of yeast much more quickly and efficiently.*

"I personally prefer to use Sporanox and nystatin together for two months. When these drugs are stopped the benefits are lasting and my patients get well. *The majority not only get well, but they stay well. They don't relapse as they often do when only one of these medicines is used at a time.*"

Amphotericin B (Fungizone, Squibb)

In the third edition of *The Yeast Connection*,[14] I included a four-page discussion of this antifungal drug which was first isolated by the Squibb Institute for Medical Research many years ago. I also cited comments from the 1986 edition of the *Physicians' Desk Reference* which stated that this antibiotic is "*substantially more active in vitro against candida strains than nystatin . . . Given orally, it is extremely well tolerated and is virtually nontoxic in prophylactic doses.*"

Like nystatin, it is poorly absorbed from the gut and has a high degree of activity against candida in the intestinal tract. This drug has also been widely used by the intravenous route in the treatment of deep-seated fungal infections.

Comments of Elmer Cranton, M.D.

"As you know, this medication is closely related to nystatin and is the leading oral antifungal medication distributed in Europe. Although for some years I sent my prescriptions to pharmacies in France, it is now available from several pharmacies in the U.S., including Wellness Health & Pharmaceuticals, 2800 S. 18th St., Birmingham, AL 35209, 1-800-227-2627 and College Pharmacy, 833 N. Tejon St., Colorado Springs, CO 80903, 1-800-888-9358.

"Physicians and patients should not confuse the oral form of amphotericin B, which is not absorbed and is nontoxic, with the injectable form which *is* quite toxic. People occasionally read about this drug in the PDR and on noting the side effects of injectable amphotericin B they become alarmed."

Other Comments About Antiyeast Medications

Candida Albicans May Become Resistant to Antifungal Medications

During 1993 several reports were published in the peer-reviewed literature describing the resistance of *Candida albicans* to azole derivative antifungals in patients with AIDS. Here are excerpts from a study by Norwegian researchers.

"The increased importance of yeast and especially *Candida albicans* as a cause of serious infections in hospitalized patients has been documented in several studies. This has resulted in an increased use of systemic antifungal agents . . . One of the new antimycotic agents, fluconazole, was registered for use in Norway early in 1991."

In the abstract of this article, they stated:

"All *Candida albicans* isolates in Norwegian microbiological laboratories in 1991 judged clinically important (except vaginal isolates) were collected. The isolates were tested for susceptibility to fluconazole, with an igar dilution test and a commercially available agar diffusion test. A total of 212 strains (95%) were susceptible to fluconazole."

In discussing the resistant strains which were found in a few patients, they said:

"The twelve fluconazole-resistant isolates originated from eight AIDS patients with oral or esophageal candida infections. Seven of the patients had been given fluconazole for one month or more, often as self-medication. Four had infections that were clinically resistant to fluconazole; one additional patient responded only when the dose was increased."[15]

Another study from Duke University examined yeast strains from the mouths and throats of 87 consecutive patients infected with HIV Type 1 virus. In analyzing the findings of their study, these researchers said:

". . . In vitro testing identified a large group of patients . . . who remained symptomatic while receiving azole therapy. This study supports the ability of an in vitro testing to predict the clinical outcome of mucosal fungal infections. The study also demonstrates that azole resistance of oropharyngeal yeast is a common problem in patients infected with human immunodeficiency virus Type 1; and that this azole resistance has clinical relevance."[16]

My Comments

Although all of these resistant *Candida albicans* strains were taken from patients with AIDS, these findings naturally are a cause for concern. And here are suggested directions to take in treating patients with superficial yeast infections and generalized symptoms.

- If a patient is improving significantly while taking the azole drug, the medication can often be tapered off, or even discontinued, after a few weeks of therapy. The decision, of course, would depend on the judgment of the physician.

- A nonabsorbable antifungal medication could be given along with the azole medication and could be continued after the azole medication is stopped. These medications include nystatin, caprylic acid and/or citrus seed extracts.
- Emphasis on an appropriate diet, especially the limitation of simple carbohydrates so as to discourage yeast proliferation in the intestinal tract.
- The importance of other parts of a comprehensive treatment program should be emphasized, including the avoidance of chemical pollutants, psychological support and nutritional supplements.

For the person who has improved on an antifungal drug (whether it's an azole drug or nystatin), and then gets to a standstill or goes backward, the physician may wish to—

- Change to a different prescription or nonprescription antifungal.
- Have the candida in the stool tested with cultures and sensitivity tests.

Adverse Reactions to Drugs and Other Therapies

Drugs, regardless of how "safe" they appear to be, can cause adverse reactions, either mild or serious. Perhaps the worst reaction I ever experienced in my own practice, came from aspirin—yes, ordinary aspirin.

A 14-year-old boy with a previous history of asthma took two ordinary aspirin tablets for a headache. Within a few minutes he developed a cough and an attack of asthma. The attack was so severe that he was kept in intensive care for 48 hours before he improved.

Another child, an 8-year-old girl (not one of my patients), was troubled by short attention span and hyperactivity. A brain wave test, which was carried out as a part of her medical workup, showed a few abnormal tracings. This finding prompted her physician to prescribe the anticonvulsant drug Dilantin.

After taking this drug for less than a week, she developed a critical illness called the *Stevens-Johnson Syndrome*. The symptoms included an extensive rash and a temperature of 103 to 105, which lasted almost a month. Moreover, she was left with residual damage to her vision. These reactions, and others I've seen in my practice, make me cautious about prescribing any medication unless I feel it is essential for the patient's recovery. Some of my own experiences also make me aware of the possibility of side effects that may develop from medications of various types.

During childhood, I took a tetanus "shot" which at that time was prepared using horse serum. I developed an all-over rash with severe swelling of my face, lips and tongue. Fortunately, my severe symptoms were relieved by injections of epinephrine. Yet, some of my rash remained for over a week.

Some twenty years later, I experienced a similar reaction following a penicillin shot. Then, a few years later I took a drug which caused a depression of my white blood count.

In spite of these reactions, I have prescribed many different medications for my patients over the years. I've also prescribed and recommended nystatin, and the azole drugs, Nizoral, Diflucan and Sporanox for patients with yeast-related health problems.

I especially recommend the azole drugs for patients with severe and long-lasting chronic health problems which appear to be candida- related. And based on the reports I've received from dozens of physicians who are using these drugs, taking them is probably a lot safer than getting in an automobile and driving to a nearby shopping center.

Possible Adverse Reactions to Diflucan

In the spring of 1994, W. A. Shrader, a Santa Fe, New Mexico, physician wrote to Pfizer/Roerig to request information concerning the possible effect of Diflucan on liver function. Here are excerpts from a three-page letter he received from Vincent Mascoli, a registered pharmacist who works with the producers of Diflucan.

"Safety data have been collected for 4,048 subjects who received Diflucan . . . for seven or more days. Diflucan was not associated with any significant pattern of laboratory tests or abnormality indicative of toxicity . . . However, the most frequently reported laboratory abnormalities occurred in tests of liver function. The vast majority were attributable to underlying diseases (malignancy, AIDS), concomitant medications . . . or concurrent illnesses . . . Clinically important abnormalities in at least one liver function test was judged to be possibly related to Diflucan in 2.5% of subjects."

> *Detailed information about possible Diflucan reactions could be found on the package insert.*

In his continuing discussion, Mascoli pointed out that detailed information about possible Diflucan reactions could be found on the package insert which he enclosed. He also pointed out that liver problems related to Diflucan were usually, but not always, reversible on discontinuation of therapy. In his summary paragraph, he stated:

"Clinically significant increases in liver function tests have occurred in some patients receiving Diflucan, although serious hepatic reactions have been rare . . . We have no specific recommendations as to frequency of monitoring liver function tests in patients receiving Diflucan, and suggest that the monitoring schedule be left up to the discretion of the physician . . . Patients who develop abnormal liver function tests during Diflucan therapy should be monitored for the development of more severe hepatic injury."

My Comments

In my opinion, the azole drugs are important, safe medications. I will continue to use them and recommend them. Moreover, as I look through the *Physicians' Desk Reference,* I find that all of the drugs listed can and do cause adverse reactions. Included are drugs prescribed for arthritis, infections, depression, hyperactivity and the attention deficit disorder. Almost all of these frequently prescribed drugs are more apt to cause adverse reactions than the prescription antiyeast medications.

Certainly, taking them where indicated, based on your medical history, is much safer than letting your problems go untreated. Yet, no drug provides a "quick fix" for candida-related health problems. You must be willing to consume an appropriate diet and take other measures to regain your health and get your life back on track.

REFERENCES

1. Baldwin, R.S., *The Fungus Fighters,* Cornell University Press, Ithaca, New York, 1981.
2. Duncan, B. and Smith, J., *The Hidden Viruses Within You,* ViroPrint, Wellington, New Zealand, 1993; pp 73–74.
3. Truss, C.O., Truss, C.V. and Cutler, R.B., "Generalized Symptoms in Women with Chronic Yeast Vaginitis: Treatment with nystatin, diet and immunotherapy vs. nystatin alone," *J. of Advancement in Medicine,* 1992; 5:139–175.
4. Copyright, *Physicians' Desk Reference,* 46th Edition, Medical Economics, Montvale, NJ 07645, 1992; p 605. (Reprinted by permission. All rights reserved.)
5. Como, J.A. and Dismukes, W.E., "Oral Azole Drugs As Systemic Antifungal Therapy," *N. Engl. J. Med.,* 1994; 330:263–272.
6. Lieberman, A., as quoted in Crook, W.G., *The Yeast Connection,* Third Edition, Professional Books, Jackson, TN and Vintage Books, New York, 1986; p 351.
7. Waickman, F., as cited in *The Yeast Connection,* Third Edition, Professional Books, Jackson, TN and Vintage Books, New York, 1986; p 352.

8. Como, J.A. and Dismukes, W.E., "Oral Azole Drugs As Systemic Antifungal Therapy," *N. Engl. J. Med.,* 1994; 330:263–272.

9. McKay, M., "Vulvodynia—A multifactorial clinical problem," *Arch. of Dermatol.,* 1989; 125:256–262.

10. Hunnisett, A., Howard, J. and Davies, S., "Gut fermentation (or the auto-brewery syndrome): a new clinical test with initial observations and discussion of clinical and biochemical implications," *J. of Advan. in Med.,* 1992; 5:139–175.

11. Grant, Susan M. and Clissold, S.P., "Itraconazole: A review of its pharmacodynamic and pharmacokinetic properties and therapeutic use in superficial and systemic mycoses," *Drugs,* 1989; 37:310–344.

12. Jacob, S. and Nall, L., "Discovering Antimycotic Drugs: Today and Tomorrow," *Cutis,* 1990; 45:245–250.

13. Como, J.A. and Dismukes, W.E., "Oral Azole Drugs As Systemic Antifungal Therapy," *N. Engl. J. Med.,* 1994; 330:263–272.

14. Crook, W.G., *The Yeast Connection,* Third Edition, Professional Books, Jackson, TN and Vintage Books, New York, 1986; pp 281–285.

15. Sandven, P., and associates, The Norwegian Yeast Study Group, "Susceptibility of Norwegian *Candida albicans* strains to fluconazole: Emergence of resistance," *Antimicrobial Agents and Chemotherapy,* 1993; 37:2443–48.

16. Camron, M.L., "Correlation of In Vitro Fluconazole Resistance of *Candida* Isolates in Relation to Therapy and Symptoms of Individuals Seropositive for Human Immunodeficiency Virus Type 1," *Antimicrobial Agents and Chemotherapy,* 1993; 37:2449–53.

35

Food Allergies and Sensitivities

Unusual reactions to substances in a person's diet or environment have been recognized for thousands of years. Yet, it wasn't until 1906 that the term "allergy" was coined by the Austrian pediatrician Clemens von Pirquet.[1] He put together two Greek words, *allos*— meaning "other" and *ergon*—meaning "action." To von Pirquet *allergy* meant altered reactivity.

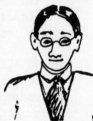

Today, most doctors feel that allergy means "hypersensitivity to a specific substance, which in a similar quantity doesn't bother other people." Incidentally, that's the definition you'll find in Webster's New World Dictionary. However, if you move from one city to another, you may run into different ideas about allergy—how it is defined, how it is diagnosed and how it should be treated.

Some doctors feel the term "allergy" should be limited to those conditions in which an immunological mechanism can be demonstrated using allergy skin tests or more sophisticated laboratory tests. But other conscientious physicians feel that the allergic and hypersensitivity diseases are much broader in scope. For example, the late Frederic Speer, M.D., of the University of Kansas, said:

> "While immunological mechanisms are undoubtedly important in explaining allergic diseases, they don't tell the whole story."[2]

> **Immunological mechanisms are important but don't tell the whole story.**

And Elmer Cranton, M.D., Yelm, Washington, a recent past president of the American College of Advancement in Medicine, said:

> "The assumption is often made that we fully understand the immune system, which is not true. These scientific discoveries are published routinely to add to our knowledge. It is quite possible we still only know a small fraction of the whole story."[3]

Why You Need to Know About Food Allergies/Sensitivities

In gathering material for this book, I sought the help and consultation of many people. Included were colleagues who were knowledgeable and experienced in treating patients with yeast-related health problems and other colleagues who were not. One academic physician in the latter group asked, "Why are you including so much material on food allergies and sensitivities in your book?"

In responding, I cited the observations of a number of clinicians and researchers, including Dr. J.O. Hunter, a Fellow of the Royal College of Physicians, who, in a discussion of food intolerance in the British journal, *The Lancet*, suggested that patients with food intolerances have an abnormal gut flora even though pathogens may not be present. And, he said:

> "If food allergy is not an immunologic disease, but a disorder of bacterial fermentation in the colon, it might be more appropriately named an 'enterometabolic disorder.' This is of more than mere terminological importance: modern microbiology has opened the way to the manipulation of bacterial flora to allow the correction of food intolerances and thus the control of disease."[4]

Another European researcher and clinician, Gruia Ionescu, Ph.D., shares Hunter's views about the relationship of gut flora to food sensitivities. And in an interview with Marjorie Hurt Jones, R.N., editor of *Mastering Food Allergies,* Ionescu stated that he had found candida overgrowth in the gut in approximately half of his allergic patients. He also noted that many people diagnosed with candida infections exhibit intolerances to food.[5]

Still other investigators, including Leo Galland, M.D.[6] and W. Allen Walker, Professor of Pediatrics at Harvard Medical School, have also been studying the gut. Some of Walker's research studies have focused on the role of the mucosal barrier in handling allergens. In a comprehensive review of antigen handling by the gut, he commented:

> "There's increasing experimental clinical evidence that suggests that large antigenically active molecules can penetrate the intestinal surface, not in sufficient quantities to be of nutritional importance, but in quantities that may be of immunologic importance.
>
> "This observation could mean that the intestinal tract represents a potential site for the absorption of bacterial breakdown products such as endotoxins and enterotoxins, proteolytic and hydrolytic enzymes and other ingested food antigens that normally exist in the intestinal lumen."[7]

Neither Hunter nor Walker mentions the possible role that candida overgrowth contributes to normal gut flora. Yet, the observations of Galland, Ionescu and other candida clinicians about the favorable response of individuals with food sensitivities to anti-yeast medications and sugar-free special diets provide support for the yeast connection to food allergies and sensitivities.

Types of Allergies

When you develop an allergy to something you breathe, such as grass, pollen, animal danders or house dust mites, the cause of your symptoms can be suspected from your history and identified through the use of the simple allergy prick test. In carrying out such a test, a physician pricks your skin through a small amount of an allergy extract.

If you are allergic to the test substance in the extract, as for example Bermuda grass, ragweed or cat dander, within a few minutes an itching bump or welt that looks like a mosquito bite will pop up on your skin.

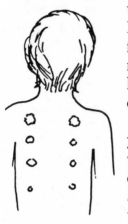

Skin testing will usually produce similar welts if you're allergic to foods such as peanuts, lobster or shrimp. However, if you're obviously sensitive to these foods, you already know it, and skin tests aren't needed. Moreover, skin testing of foods that have caused severe symptoms can be dangerous.

The allergic reactions which take place in your body if you develop sneezing or wheezing when exposed to bermuda grass, ragweed or cat dander are mediated through *immunoglobulin E* (IgE). So are the obvious allergic reactions caused by peanuts or seafoods.

Yet, there are other types of food allergies and sensitivities you need to know about. Such allergies have been called "hidden," "masked," "variable," or "delayed-onset" food allergies. *Allergies or sensitivities of this type are often caused by foods you eat every day.* You'll probably be surprised to learn that you're apt to be sensitive to some of your favorite foods, especially wheat, corn, milk, yeast, chocolate, citrus and coffee.

Moreover, you may be "addicted" to foods that are making you tired or cause headaches, muscle aches or nasal congestion. Like the cigarette or narcotic addict, you may feel temporarily better if you've eaten some of the foods to which you're allergic.

My Experiences in Practice

When I completed my internship and residency training and returned to Tennessee to open my office to practice pediatrics many, many years ago, I knew nothing about hidden food allergies. In fact, I was an *ignoramus* in this area. Two pediatricians in my community, Helen Johnston and the late Barbara Truex, told me that a number of their patients were sensitive to cow's milk and other foods. I didn't believe them. I thought they didn't know what they were talking about.

I continued to be blind to the possibility of food sensitivities in my patients for six or seven years. Then Aileen, the mother of a 12-year-old boy, opened my eyes. Here's what happened: Her son, Tom, was so tired she could hardly get him out of bed for school each morning. Tom also complained of headaches, belly aches and muscle pains, and often was so irritable, Aileen said, "You can hardly stay in the house with him."

Because Tom had experienced problems with milk in infancy and had been drinking a lot of milk for several months before these complaints developed, Aileen took him off milk for a week. At the end of the period, she said, "Tom is like a different child. He bounced out of bed this morning whistling. No headaches, muscle aches or belly aches."

I was astounded because I had learned something that I hadn't known before . . . intolerances, allergies or sensitivities to common foods could provoke systemic and nervous complaints.

A short time later, I came across articles by Albert Rowe[8] and Theron Randolph[9] published in the peer-reviewed medical literature discussing food allergies and sensitivities. They reported that many of their patients improved—often dramatically—when they avoided wheat, corn, milk, egg and other foods.

To learn more about their experiences, I visited Dr. Rowe in California and Dr. Randolph in Chicago. And I was fascinated by what they and their patients told me.

After returning home and thinking about the problems of some of my difficult patients, I said to myself:

"I wonder if a food sensitivity could be responsible for Ed's persistent headaches or Rosemary's fatigue and irritability . . . or

George's lethargy which keeps him from going out and playing with the rest of the gang."

So I began putting a number of my tired, inattentive, irritable patients on a one-week elimination diet. Although I didn't help all of them, I was excited because I began to receive reports from mothers who said:

> "Susie's like a different child. But when she drinks chocolate milk or eats corn chips, wheat or eggs, her symptoms return."

I collected and summarized my findings on 50 of these patients and published them in a major pediatric journal over 30 years ago.[10] *The diagnosis of food sensitivity was made in the following manner: Symptoms and signs were relieved by eliminating suspected foods from the diet for 5 to 12 days and then reproduced by giving the food back to the child, and noting reactions.*
During the past 35 years, I've seen and helped countless patients using carefully designed and properly executed elimination diets. Moreover, I've found that such sensitivities can affect just about any and every part of the body, and they occur commonly in people with yeast-related health problems.

Controversy Over Food Allergies

Many subjects are controversial, including religion, politics, education, abortion and many others. What's more, if you read *USA Today*, you'll see opposing opinions on different issues expressed 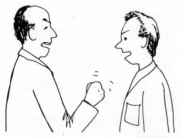 on the editorial page every day. Food allergy is another such controversial subject.

Most of my colleagues in the American Academy of Allergy and Immunology and the American College of Allergy and Immunology, in their discussions of "food allergies," emphasize IgE-mediated adverse food reactions. And they express skepticism over the relationship of food allergies to systemic and nervous system symptoms in children and adults.

Obvious (IgE-mediated) adverse food reactions are important. No doubt about it. And they can and do cause severe and fatal reactions. A heartbreaking example, which continues to occur all too frequently, is the peanut-allergic child who dies of anaphylactic shock within a few minutes or hours after eating a peanut-containing cookie.

In the mid-1970s, I was invited to write an article on food allergy for the *Pediatric Clinics of North America*. Yet, at the time of the invitation, Elliot Ellis, M.D., the editor, told me that Dr. Charles May would be presenting an opposing point of view.

In my article, "Food Allergy—The Great Masquerader," I reviewed the many symptoms I'd seen in my patients with hidden food allergies. They ranged from fatigue, depression, muscle aches and abdominal pain to overactivity, restlessness, inability to concentrate and nasal congestion. And, I said:

> "All it takes to identify this type of food sensitivity is a carefully designed, seven to ten day elimination diet. Carrying out such a diet is amazingly simple—especially if you compare it to complicated medical studies, such as gastrointestinal or genitourinary x-rays, and/or other in-hospital diagnostic procedures . . . *In my experience, hidden food sensitivity is the most common cause of chronic unwellness seen in pediatric office practice.*"[11]

Dr. May, in his article which presented a diametrically opposite point of view, said:

> "Controversy over food allergy leads to unwholesome conflicts in the profession and loss of confidence by the public . . . Our troubles begin when we leap from a suspicion that eating a food causes symptoms to the assumption that these symptoms are due to allergy.
>
> "Until we prove, on scientific, immunologic grounds, that food is responsible for such reactions, rational physicians cannot accept the tension-fatigue syndrome and the other systemic manifestations which are claimed to be due to food allergy.
>
> "Those who claim otherwise fill the literature with clutter . . .

rather than calling food allergy "the great masquerader," we should call it the current crutch for neurotic patients."[12]

In spite of those strong words, the late Dr. May and I remained friends. Yet, we approached the subject of food allergy from points of view just as different as those of coaches of two competing football teams.

In commenting on Dr. May's remarks in an October 1994 letter to me, Dr. Elmer Cranton said:

"Unfortunately, Dr. May's attitude characterizes most physicians today who say, 'Unless we understand how it works, we won't accept the observations.'

"In other words, too often the assumption is made that medical science can now explain all mechanisms of action; therefore, if an observation in practice contradicts currently held scientific theories, it is often rejected."

Support for Food Allergies by Academic Physicians

Because of my strong interest in food sensitivities, I talked about them to almost anyone who would listen. I also reported my observations in professional and lay journals on numerous occasions in the 1970s and 1980s. Yet, as was the case with two of my mentors and heroes, Drs. Albert Rowe and Theron Randolph, few of my medical colleagues seemed to be listening.

Then, through a series of serendipitous events, William C. Deamer, M.D., Chairman of the Department of Pediatrics at the University of California (San Francisco), became a "convert." Here's what happened.

In 1956, I went to northern California to learn more about the observations and experiences of Dr. Rowe. When I told Dr. Amos Christie, my pediatric chief at Vanderbilt, about my planned trip, he encouraged me to stop in and visit his good friend and classmate, Bill Deamer. Dr. Deamer was kind, interested, courteous and cordial, as was his usual custom.

When I told him why I had come to California, he said, "I, of course, know Dr. Rowe and he's a wonderful man. Yet, it seems to me that his patients improve on his diets because of his positive enthusiastic personality."

A couple of years later, Bill Deamer went to Europe on a sabbatical and served as Visiting Professor at a medical school in Switzer-

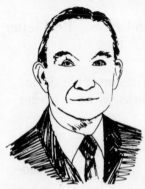

land. As was the custom of his hosts, and others, Bill drank a glass or two of wine each day. After a time, though, he developed a number of symptoms, including headache and fatigue which went away when he stopped drinking the wine.

When Bill returned to California, he stayed away from the wine, but he began drinking unfermented grape juice on a regular basis. Lo and behold, he developed the same symptoms. About the same time, one of his allergy fellows observed a patient whose headache, fatigue, muscle aches, depression and other symptoms were relieved when he stopped consuming corn; and, the symptoms of another patient vanished when he removed milk and dairy products from his diet.

During the 1960s, Dr. Deamer developed an increasing interest in food sensitivities; and, in 1973 he asked me to serve as a Visiting Professor and present my observations to his medical students and staff. Following my presentation in San Francisco, my wife, Betsy, and I visited Bill and his wife, Ellie, at their vacation home in Silverado. And we remained fast friends until his death in the early 1980s.

Observations by William C. Deamer, M.D.

In his award-winning presentation delivered before the Section on Allergy of the American Academy of Pediatrics, Dr. Deamer commented on the deceptive nature of food allergy and the difficulties in diagnosing and treating it.

Deamer noted the unreliability of food skin tests and the value of trial elimination diets in studying patients with fatigue, irritability, headache, abdominal pain, musculoskeletal discomfort, and respiratory symptoms, including asthma and allergic rhinitis. And, he said:

> "There can be no doubt . . . of the role specific foods may play in causing these symptoms nor of the fact that the respiratory tract symptoms may be identical to those caused by accepted antigens.
>
> "It is probable that every pediatrician and physician in general practice sees such cases . . . Despite an extensive bibliography, it may be one of the most under-diagnosed syndromes in practice. Dr. William Crook finds such patients to be numerous in a general pediatric practice. I agree, but it took me a long time to become fully aware of the fact.
>
> "I cannot help but feel that all physicians . . . would do well to become acquainted with the allergic-tension-fatigue syndrome and with the frequency with which foods . . . are responsible for it."[13]

Observations of John W. Gerrard, M.D.

While a member of the faculty of a medical school in the United Kingdom, Dr. Gerrard became interested in patients who showed adverse reactions to wheat and other gluten-containing foods. Although such reactions aren't considered "allergic," his experiences in England prepared him for an interest in other food-related illnesses.

In 1956, he received an appointment as Professor and Chairman of the Department of Pediatrics at the University of Saskatchewan, Saskatoon. And his interest in adverse reactions to wheat continued. Dr. Gerrard, in addition to his academic and administrative duties, also saw a number of children with nasal congestion, bronchitis, bedwetting and other persistent health problems.

He noted that the symptoms in many of these children responded to simple dietary changes, especially the elimination of cow's milk. Moreover, he published his observations on several occasions in the peer reviewed literature in the 1960s.[14,15,16]

At some point, I learned of Dr. Gerrard's observations and we began to correspond. Then, in the late 1960s, I invited him to serve as a guest speaker at the annual meeting of the Tennessee Pediatric

Society and the Tennessee Chapter of the American Academy of Pediatrics.

Because of our shared interest in food sensitivities, during the 1970s John and I roomed together at several medical conferences. And in 1976, I accepted his invitation to serve as a Visiting Professor at the University of Saskatchewan. A year or two later, John and his wife, Betty, visited my wife, Betsy, and me in Tennessee when John served as Visiting Professor for the Jackson, Tennessee, pediatricians.

Dr. Gerrard's interest in food allergies and sensitivities prompted him to publish two books, *Food Allergies—New Perspectives*[17] and *Understanding Allergies*. In these books, Gerrard described patients with nasal congestion, drowsiness, irritability, bed-wetting and other symptoms which were related to common foods. In *Understanding Allergies*, Dr. Gerrard commented on the reaction of his patient, Tim, who had been placed on a restricted diet for two weeks and then given a glass of milk to drink, and in an hour a second glass, he said:

> "Tim promptly became a 'ball of fire.' He went wild and was quite uncontrollable. At first I found it hard to believe that harmless foods could so change a child's personality; but—I'm not fully convinced that in ways we do not yet understand, the allergic child's, and adults too, behavior can be altered and modified . . . as dramatically by foods as it can be altered by drugs."[18]

Behavior can be altered and modified . . . as dramatically by foods as it can be altered by drugs.

Observations by William T. Kniker, M.D.

I first met Ted Kniker* 30 years ago at a small workshop/conference in Texas which was organized by the Borden Company. Par-

*Professor of Pediatrics and Microbiology, Head, Division of Clinical Immunology, Department of Pediatrics, University of Texas Health Science Center, San Antonio.

ticipants included practicing physicians and academicians. Our purpose: discussing sensitivities to cow's milk and designing research studies.

During the years since that time, Ted and I have shared our experiences and ideas in person, by letters and in telephone conversations. In April 1984, I was sitting on the front row when he gave his award-winning Bela Schick lecture at the annual meeting of the American College of Allergists. In this lecture, which was subsequently published in the *Annals of Allergy*, Dr. Kniker said:

> "There are countless—millions—of individuals who have unrecognized adverse reactions to various antigens, foods, chemicals, and environmental or occupational triggers . . . The acquired disease may be limited to body surfaces, or may involve a puzzling array of organ systems causing the patient to visit a number of different specialists who are unsuccessful in recognizing that an allergic or adverse reaction is going on."[19]

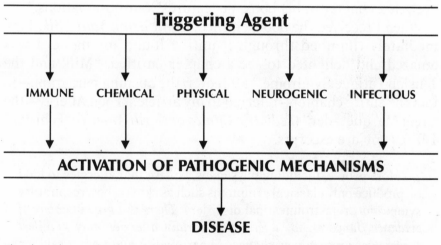

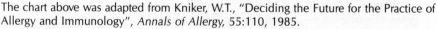

The chart above was adapted from Kniker, W.T., "Deciding the Future for the Practice of Allergy and Immunology", *Annals of Allergy*, 55:110, 1985.

In subsequent presentations at numerous medical conferences, Dr. Kniker emphasized the importance of delayed-onset adverse reactions to food. And in a chapter in, *Handbook of Food Allergies*, edited by James Breneman, M.D., he said:

"Immediate reactions to foodstuffs are often IgE-mediated, and are relatively easy to diagnose, study and document. On the other hand, delayed reactions, by their very nature, are more difficult to suspect, recognize and prove . . . A great stumbling block to the acceptance of delayed reactions to foodstuffs is the lack of epidemiological data establishing the incidence (and thereby importance) of adverse reactions to foodstuffs . . .

"When such data accumulate, it is likely that adverse reaction to ingestants will rival or surpass the importance of adverse reactions to inhalants . . . in clinical immunology and allergy [emphasis added]."[20]

Observations of Other Academicians

In the late 1970s, a friend called and said, "I'm sending you a book by Dr. Frank Oski* which I know will please and excite you. Here's why. The author is an academic pediatrician who shares some of your views about food allergies and sensitivities. Moreover, in a chapter of his book, he features your observations."

When I received the book, entitled, *Don't Drink Your Milk*, I immediately thumbed through it until I found my name. I was amazed and delighted to see a chapter entitled, "Milk and the Tension-Fatigue Syndrome." Moreover, the opening paragraph—in fact the entire chapter—referred to my article, "Food Allergy—the Great Masquerader" (*Pediatric Clinics of North America*, February 1975). Here are excerpts.

"Most people, including physicians, believe that allergies to food . . . produce only classical symptoms such as skin rashes, respiratory symptoms or gastrointestinal disorders. *There is a growing body of evidence, however, to suggest that certain allergies may manifest themselves primarily as changes in personality, emotions, or in one general sense of well being* [emphasis added].

"Dr. Crook, a pediatrician with over 20 years of experience in practice has seen over 4000 children with complaints that can be attributed to food allergies. He believes that the foods that are the

---

*Now Chairman of the Department of Pediatrics, Johns Hopkins School of Medicine.

most common offenders are milk, corn and cane sugar, and he is far from alone in his conviction."[21]

A year or two later, I came across an article by Walter W. Tunnessen, Jr.,* one of Oski's associates at the State University of New York Upstate Medical Center in Syracuse. In this article published in 1979, he presented his observations on an 8-year-old boy who was troubled by lethargy and fatigue. Yet, the boy's physical examination (except for dark circles under his eyes) was perfectly normal. So were his laboratory tests. Although Dr. Tunnessen pointed out that children with symptoms of this sort could have an emotional basis, he said:

"Before we label this child as such, consider the great masquerader food allergy . . . the proof of the pudding . . . is in some simple dietary elimination . . . a benign procedure, most often painless, not requiring hospitalization and downright inexpensive.

"The culprits I find most common are milk, chocolate and egg, although cane sugar, corn and wheat should also be considered. Removing these foods from the diet a few at a time for a week or two is all that is necessary. *Should the child improve, the eliminated foods are reintroduced . . . Relief of symptoms further supports the diagnosis* [emphasis added].

"Over the past 20 or so years, the 'voice crying in the wilderness' that has caught my attention concerning this disorder, the allergic-tension-fatigue syndrome, is that of William Crook, M.D., of Jackson, Tennessee. His article, "Food Allergy—the Great Masquerader," is worth reading and digesting . . . The manifestations of food allergy are legion.

> *I . . . had been a doubting Thomas until my son responded to dietary elimination.*

---

*Now associate chairman for Medical Education, Children's Hospital of Philadelphia (C.H.O.P.)

"I, too, had been a doubting Thomas until my son responded to dietary elimination . . . The boy presented in the case above was taken off of milk, chocolate and egg. Within a week he was a new person."[22]

Support from England

In 1987, two British academic physicians, Jonathan Brostoff and Stephen J. Challacombe, published a book, *Food Allergy and Intolerance.* Some 83 physicians and other scientists made contributions. Moreover, the book was favorably reviewed in the *Journal of the American Medical Association.* Here are comments from the preface of this book:

"As all who deal in the field will know, food allergy is an exciting, challenging, exasperating and sometimes controversial subject. Its study should be a clinical science with a diagnosis based on a combination of clinical observation to scientific investigations.

"There has been a strong tendency for the conventional physician to say that if the mechanism is not understood, then food allergy does not exist. . . . This is, of course, unacceptable. . . . *To make a diagnosis* [of food allergy] *certainly requires clinical skill, but does not necessarily need a complete understanding of a mechanism underlying the disease process or an exact understanding of the etiology . . .* [emphasis added].

"A thread running through [this book] . . . is that *the cornerstone of diagnosis of food intolerance is the removal of that food from the patient's diet, with concomitant improvement (or not) of the patient's symptoms and their reappearance on adding that food back* [emphasis added]."[23]

Support by Practicing Physicians

Countless practicing physicians have found that they can help many of their chronically ill patients by identifying and eliminating foods that are playing an important part in causing their symptoms. One such physician, my good friend, Dr. Elmer Cranton, has for over a decade used elimination/challenge diets in treating his patients with yeast-related health problems. And in a recent letter to me, he said:

> "I routinely prescribe elimination/challenge diets in all of my patients with yeast-related problems. By identifying trouble-making foods and removing them from the diet, I have decreased the patient's allergic load. Then the antifungal diet and other parts of my treatment program are much more apt to be successful."[24]

I routinely prescribe elimination/challenge diets in all of my patients with yeast-related problems.

Many other physicians who are members of the American Academy of Environmental Medicine, the American Academy of Otolaryngic Allergy, the Pan American Allergy Society and the American Holistic Medical Association, use elimination/challenge diets in helping their chronically ill patients.

So do a small but growing number of physicians who are members or fellows of the American Academy of Allergy and Immunology, the American College of Allergy and Immunology and the American Academy of Family Physicians.

One member of the latter organization, Dr. Harold Hedges,* Little Rock, Arkansas, has, for over a decade, emphasized the importance of delayed-onset hidden food sensitivities. In a comprehensive article in the November 1992, *American Family Physician,* he said:

> "The connection between food and a number of medical illnesses is clearly established. Adverse reactions to food may also be responsible for frequently recurring or chronic symptoms in patients whose medical examinations and tests are normal. In these and other patients, a well-planned and well-executed elimination diet can

---

*See also Dr. Hedges comments on the use of elimination diets in his patients with yeast-related problems in Chapter 26.

be the key to diagnosis. Specifically, use of an elimination diet might be considered when no other cause can be found for the symptoms . . .

"Many family physicians overlook the role that food and food additives play in health problems . . . Patients whose symptoms improve or clear while they're on the diet are then challenged with the omitted food, one at a time, to establish food symptoms relationships."[25]

Support in the Press

The frequency and importance of food allergies was emphasized by health columnist Jane Brody in an article in the April 29, 1990, issue of the *New York Times*, which was reprinted in the July/August 1990, issue of *The Saturday Evening Post*. Ms. Brody said:

"Millions of Americans say certain foods make them sick. Are doctors paying close enough attention?"

Brody briefly summarized the reactions of seven individuals who experienced food related symptoms. In commenting on one of these, she said:

" . . . yours truly suffered periodic attacks of abdominal pain and swelling that would last for days until dietary sleuthing revealed foods made with soybeans or dried peas as the likely cause . . . The seven of us are among the estimated 30 million Americans who experience adverse reactions to foods, reactions that most non-medical people call food allergies."

> *An estimated 30 million Americans experience adverse reactions to food.*

In discussing the controversy among physicians, Brody said:

"In researching this article I initially believed that most of the claims attacking this food or that as the cause of everything from hair loss to athlete's foot were elaborate hokum. But after looking at the medical research and learning about various people's experiences, I now wonder whether the rigid thinking of some doctors is not ill advised.

"Indeed, in dismissing symptoms that don't involve the immune system, these doctors might be doing a disservice to the health and well being of millions of Americans [emphasis added].

Certainly foods might make some people feel tired or mentally foggy.

"Perhaps a food doesn't have to affect the immune system in order to ignite a yeast infection, cause the sinuses to fill, aggravate arthritis or bring on irritable bowel syndrome. Certainly foods might make some people feel tired and mentally foggy or send some children into an orbit of hyperactivity."[26]

Comments of Jean Carper

In her nationally syndicated column which I've read from time to time, Carper talks about foods of all kinds. And in her 1993 book, *Food—Your Miracle Medicine,*[27] she lists complaints which may be food related. These include headaches, hives, asthma, eczema, irritable bowel syndrome, rheumatoid arthritis, chronic fatigue syndrome and depression. She also said that there's growing scientific recognition that these maladies are often food related.

She also told her readers that these food-induced reactions were not the usual allergies, and that scientists don't yet understand exactly why they occur. Yet, she said that they are very real and recognizing them has solved many health mysteries.

I was pleased to see that Carper cited the observations of Talal Nsouli, M.D., a Georgetown University School of Medicine allergist. I first met Nsouli when he was an allergy fellow at Georgetown over a decade ago. I've heard his scientific presentations at several conferences and I've read a number of his papers, including his observations on the relationship of food sensitivities to recurrent ear infections in children.

I've also had lunch with him and visited his office. And I have been delighted to see a young, academically trained allergist who has found that many of his difficult patients can be helped by eliminating troublemaking foods from their diet—especially wheat, milk and corn. Then, when they improve, he carries out food challenges to see if the symptoms return.

Tests for Food Allergies

During the late '80s and early '90s, a number of researchers have found that people who experience hidden or delayed-onset food allergies may often show abnormal tests. These tests include the ALCAT test, the Immuno 1 Bloodprint test and lactulose and mannitol challenge tests. You'll find information about these and other tests in Chapter 38.

REFERENCES

1. Von Pirquet, C., "Allergie," Munch Med. Wochenschr., 1906; 53:1457.
2. Speer, F., *Allergy of the Nervous System*, Charles C. Thomas, Springfield, IL, 1970.
3. Cranton, E., Personal Communication, July 1994.
4. Hunter, J.O., "Food allergy—or enterometabolic disorder?" *The Lancet*, 1991; 338:495–496.
5. Ionescu, G., As quoted by Jones, M., *Mastering Food Allergies*, Coeur d'Alene, ID, 1991.
6. Galland, L., "The Effect of Microbes on Systemic Immunity," in Jenkins, R. and Mowbray, *Post-viral Fatigue Syndrome*, John Wylie and Sons, 1991.
7. Walker, W.A., in Brostoff and Challacombe, *Food Allergy and Intolerance*, London, Balliére Tindall, Philadelphia, W.B. Saunders, 1987; pp 209–222.
8. Rowe, A.H., Sr., "Allergic Toxemia and Migraine Due to Food Allergy," California and Western Medicine, 1930; 33:785.
9. Randolph, T.G., "Allergy as a Causative Factor of the Fatigue, Irritability and Behavior Problems of Children," *J. of Ped.*, 1947; 31:560.

10. Crook, W.G., et al, "Systemic Manifestations Due to Allergy," 1961; *Pediatrics*, 27:790-799.
11. Crook, W.G., "Food Allergy-The Great Masquerader," *Ped. Clin. of N. Amer.*, 1975; 22:227–238.
12. May, C., "Food Allergy," *Ped. Clin. of N. Amer.*, 1975; 22:219–226.
13. Deamer, W.C., "Some impressions gained over a 37 year period," *Pediatrics*, 1971; 48:930.
14. Gerrard, J.W., Heiner, D.C., Ives, E.J. and Hardy, L.W., "Milk Allergy: Recognition, Natural History and Management," *Clinical Pediatrics*, 1963; 2:634.
15. Gerrard, J.W., "Familial Recurrent Rhinorrhea and Bronchitis Due to Cow's Milk," *JAMA*, 1966; 198:605.
16. Gerrard, J.W. and Esperance, M., "Nocturnal Enuresis: Studies in bladder function in normals and enuretics," *Canad. Med. Assn. J.*, 1969; 101:269.
17. Gerrard, J.W., *Food Allergies—New Perspectives*, Charles C. Thomas, Springfield, IL, 1980.
18. Gerrard, J.W., *Understanding Allergies*, Charles C. Thomas, Springfield, IL, 1973.
19. Kniker, W.T., "Deciding the Future for the Practice of Allergy and Immunology," *Annals of Allergy*, 1985; 55:102.
20. Kniker, W.T., and Rodrigues, L.M., "Non-IgE-mediated and Delayed Adverse Reactions to Foods or Additives," in *Handbook of Food Allergies*, edited by Breneman, J.C., Marcel Decker, Inc., New York and Babel, pp 125–147.
21. Oski, F., "Milk and the Tension Fatigue Syndrome" in *Don't Drink Your Milk*, Teach Services, Donivan Rd., Rt. 1, Box 182, Brushton, NY 12916.
22. Tunnessen, W.W., "An 8-Year-Old Boy with Lethargy and Fatigue," *Clini-Pearls*, 1979; July/August.
23. Brostoff, J. and Challacombe, S., *Food Allergy and Intolerance*, London, Balliére Tindall, Philadelphia, W. B. Saunders, 1987.
24. Cranton, E., Personal communication, July 1994.
25. Hedges, H.H., "The Elimination Diet As A Diagnostic Tool," *American Family Physician* (Suppl) 1992; 46:77–84.
26. Brody, J., *New York Times*, April 29, 1990.
27. Carper, J., *Food—Your Miracle Medicine*, HarperCollins, New York, 1993.

36

---◆---

Tracking Down Your Hidden Food Sensitivities

---◆---

During the past 37 years, I've seen thousands of children and adults with fatigue, headache, muscle aches, nasal congestion, irritability and other symptoms. Using elimination/challenge diets, 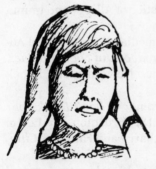 many of my patients found that foods they were eating every day were the main cause of their symptoms.

Then, in the 1980s, as I worked with patients with yeast-related health problems, I learned that *almost without exception every person with such a problem is bothered by food sensitivities.* Moreover, my observations and experiences have been confirmed by many other physicians.

To identify the foods that contribute to your symptoms, you must carefully plan and properly execute an elimination/challenge diet. Here's an edited transcript of a tape recorded visit with one of my patients which will give you specific instructions.

Q: Since I began cleaning up my house, avoiding sugar, taking anti-yeast medications and nutritional supplements, I'm a lot better. Yet, there are some days when I don't feel as good as I'd like to— and it isn't PMS. I'm wondering if some of my symptoms are food-related and I'd like to try an elimination diet. Please tell me what I'll need to do.

A: On an elimination diet you'll avoid many or all of your favorite foods. To make things easier for you, I have prepared two diets. The first one of these—a less restrictive diet—I call Diet A. Then, there's a much tougher Diet B, which I call the "Caveman Diet."

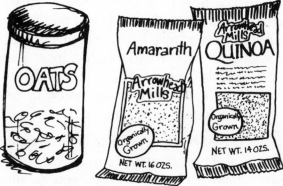

Q: I believe I'd like to try Diet A first. What foods can I eat on this diet?

A: You can eat any meats but bacon, sausage, hot dogs or luncheon meats; any vegetables but corn; any fruits but citrus. You can also eat rice, rice crackers, plain oatmeal and the grain alternatives amaranth and quinoa (obtainable from health food stores).

> *Foods you can eat include most meats,*
> *vegetables and fruits. Also rice, oats and*
> *the grain alternatives.*

Q: Anything else?

A: Yes. Nuts in their shell or unprocessed nuts of any kind.

Q: That doesn't sound too difficult, although it'll take careful planning to carry out the diet. What can I drink?

A: Water. I especially recommend bottled or filtered water.

Q: What foods do I need to eliminate?

A: Many of your favorite foods. Here's why. *The more of a food you eat, the greater your chances of developing an allergy to that* *food.* Here's a list of foods you must avoid on the diet. Milk, and all dairy products; wheat; corn, corn syrup and corn sweeteners; yeast; cane and beet sugar; orange and other citrus fruits; chocolate.

This diet also eliminates food coloring, additives and flavorings which are found in many packaged and processed foods.

If you are sensitive to foods you're eating every day, chances are you may also be sensitive to tobacco, insecticides and environmental chemicals. To gain maximum benefit from your diet detective work, do not smoke in the house or use perfumes, fumigants or other odorous chemicals.

Q: How do I get started on a diet? What do I do first?

A: Prepare menus and purchase foods you'll eat while on the diet. This requires careful planning. When you go shopping avoid commercially prepared or processed foods. Here's why. Such foods usually contain sugar, wheat, milk, corn, yeast, food coloring and other hidden ingredients that may be causing some of your symptoms.

Discuss the diet with other family members. When you're planning your diet, you'll feel less deprived if you think about the many foods you *can* eat rather than feeling frustrated because of the foods you must avoid.

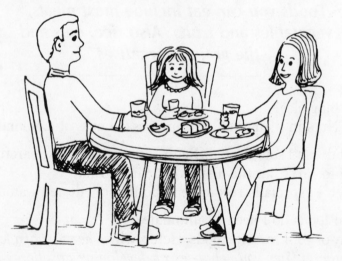

Q: Tell me more about the diet.

An elimination diet is divided into two parts.

A: The diet is divided into two parts: First you'll eliminate a number of your usual foods to see if your symptoms improve or disappear. Then, after five to ten days, when your symptoms show convincing improvement, eat the eliminated foods again—one at a time—and see which foods cause the symptoms to return.

Q: How will I know the diet is really making a difference?
A: You'll know by keeping a record of your symptoms:

> a. for three days (or more) before beginning the diet,
> b. while you're following the elimination part of the diet (five to ten days—occasionally longer),
> c. while you're eating the eliminated foods again one food per day.

You'll need, of course, to keep a detailed record of all foods you eat.

Q: How will I feel on the diet?
A: During the first two to four days of the diet, you're apt to feel irritable and hungry and you may not feel satisfied even though you fill up on the permitted foods. You may feel restless and fidgety or tired and droopy. You may also develop a headache or leg cramps.

You may be "mad" at the world because you aren't getting the foods you crave, especially sweets. You may act like a two-pack-a-day smoker who quit smoking "cold turkey." Here's why. People who suffer from hidden food allergies are often "addicted" to the foods causing their problems.*

If the foods you've avoided are causing your symptoms, you'll usually feel better by the fourth to sixth day of your diet.

Here's some good news. If the foods you've avoided are causing your symptoms, you'll usually feel better by the fourth, fifth or sixth day of the diet. Almost always, you'll improve by the tenth day. Occasionally, though, it'll take two or three weeks before your symptoms go away completely.

Q: If I improve on the diet, what do I do then? When and how will I return the foods to my diet?

A: After you're certain that you feel better and improvement has lasted for at least two days begin adding foods back to your diet—one at a time. If you're allergic to one or more of the eliminated foods, you'll usually develop symptoms when you eat the foods again.

Q: What symptoms should I look for?

A: Usually, but not always, your main symptoms will reappear. In your case, you're apt to feel more tired and depressed; and, you'll probably develop a headache or your nose will feel stopped up. However, sometimes you'll notice other symptoms, including some that had not bothered you previously—such as itching, coughing or urinary frequency.

Q: How soon will these symptoms appear after I eat a food that I'm sensitive to?

A: The symptoms will usually reappear within a few minutes to a few hours. However, sometimes you may not notice a symptom

---

*Dr. Elmer Cranton comments: "If you subsitute a nonallergic food of equal nutritional value for a frequently eaten food and feel cravings, you confirm the diagnosis of allergic addiction to that food. No matter how much you feel you need the formerly eaten food, you'll probably feel better long-term without it!"

until the next day. *If you avoid an allergy-causing food for a short period (five to seven days) you'll nearly always develop symptoms immediately when you eat the food again.* By contrast, if you avoid the food for three or more weeks, your symptoms won't return until you eat the food two or three days in a row.

Q: When I return a food to my diet, does it make any difference what form the food is in?

When you return a food to your diet, add it in pure form.

A: Yes! Yes! Yes! Add the food in pure form. For example, when you eat wheat, use pure whole wheat rather than bread since bread contains milk and other ingredients. If you're testing milk, use whole milk rather than ice cream since ice cream contains sugar, corn syrup and other ingredients.

Here are suggestions for returning foods to your diet.

Egg: Eat a soft- or hard-boiled egg (or eggs scrambled in pure safflower or sunflower oil).

Citrus: Peel an orange and eat it. You can also drink fresh-squeezed orange juice (do not use frozen or canned orange juice).

Milk: Use whole milk.

Wheat: Get 100% whole wheat from the health food store. Add water and cook for 20 to 25 minutes. Add sea salt if you wish. Eat it straight or add sliced bananas or strawberries. If you want to "wet the cereal," you can put the fruit in a blender with a little water and pour it on the cereal like milk or cream.

If you don't like hot cereals, you can use Nabisco® Shredded Wheat. However, Shredded Wheat contains the additive

BHT, which may cause symptoms. So a pure wheat product without additives is better.

Food coloring: Buy a set of McCormick's or French's dyes and colors. Put a half teaspoon of several colors in a glass. Add a teaspoon of that mixture to a glass of water and sip on it. If you show a reaction, you'll later need to test the various food dyes separately. Red seems to be the most common offender.

Chocolate: Use Baker's cooking chocolate or Hershey's cocoa powder. You can sweeten it with a little liquid saccharin (Sweeta or Fasweet). Eat the powder with a spoon or add it to water and make a chocolate-flavored drink.

Corn: Use fresh corn on the cob, pure corn syrup, grits or hominy. Eat plain popcorn. Don't use microwave popcorn because it contains other ingredients.

Sugar: Get plain cane sugar. Perhaps the easiest way to do this is to eat some sugar lumps or add the sugar to a glass of water. Do the same with beet sugar.

Q: I think I understand what you want me to do. However, a few points aren't clear. Please go over them again.

A: Okay, here they are.

1. Carefully review all your instructions. Plan ahead. Don't start your diet the week before Christmas, Thanksgiving or some other holiday—and don't start it when you're traveling or visiting friends or relatives. Ask—even beg—other family members to help you and to cooperate. Study your instructions and purchase the foods you'll need. Keep a diary of your symptoms for at least three days before you begin your diet.

   Remain on the diet until you're absolutely certain your symptoms have improved. Remember that your symptoms are apt to worsen the first 48 to 72 hours on the diet.

   Usually, you'll feel better by the fourth or fifth day although some people won't notice a significant change until they've followed the diet for seven to ten days—occasionally longer. Still other individuals with a hidden food allergy won't show a lot of improvement until they've avoided an offending food for two or three weeks. However, such people are the exception.

2. If you don't feel significantly better in 10 to 14 days,* start eating your usual foods—even "pig out." If your symptoms worsen (including your headache, fatigue, irritability or stuffiness), chances are they're food related and you'll have to do further detective work to identify the troublemakers.

3. If you improve on the diet, return the eliminated foods one at a time and see if you develop symptoms. Here's how you go about it.

   A: Add the foods you least suspect first. Save the foods you think are causing your problems until last. Remember, you're apt to be allergic to your favorite foods.

   B. If you have no idea what foods are causing your symptoms, here's a suggested order for returning foods to your diet.

1. Eggs	6. Chocolate
2. Citrus	7. Corn
3. Yeast	8. Sugar
4. Wheat	9. Milk
5. Food coloring	

4. Eat a small portion of the eliminated food for breakfast. If you show no reaction, eat more of the food for lunch and for supper and between meals too.**

5. Keep the rest of your diet the same while you're carrying out the challenges. Here's an example. Suppose you eat

---

*Your failure to improve substantially on an elimination diet may be related to other offending substances in your living and work environment (exhaust fumes, paint fumes, insecticides, sprays, carpet odors, etc.). Accordingly, before beginning your diet, clean up your environment.

**If you suffer from severe asthma, hives, or swelling, the food challenges should be supervised by a physician and carried out in his office or clinic.

wheat on the first day of your diet and show no reaction. Does this mean you can continue to eat wheat? No. Eat wheat only on the day of the challenge and don't eat it again until you've tested all the foods and the diet has been completed.

6. If you show no symptoms after adding a food the first day, add another food the second day, eating all you want—unless you show a reaction.

7. If you think you develop symptoms when you add a food but aren't certain, eat more of the food until your symptoms are obvious. But don't make yourself sick.

If you show an obvious reaction after eating a food, such as stuffiness, cough, irritability, nervousness, drowsiness, headache, stomach ache, flushing or wheezing, don't eat more of that food.

Wait until the reaction subsides (usually 24 to 48 hours) before you add another food.

If a food really bothers you, shorten the reaction by taking a teaspoon of "soda mixture" (two parts baking soda and one part potassium bicarbonate—your pharmacist can fix up this mixture for you). Or dissolve two tablets of Alka Seltzer Gold* in a glass of water and drink it. A saline cathartic such as Epsom salts will also shorten your reaction by eliminating the offending foods from your digestive tract rapidly.

Q: Thank you for those explanations. They make sense. But while we're discussing diets, let's go ahead and talk about Diet B.

A: I call Diet B the "Rare Food" or "Cave Man" Diet. On this diet you'll eliminate all the foods listed on Diet A. In addition, you must avoid beef, chicken, pork, white potato, tomato, rice, oats, coffee, tea and any food or beverage you consume more than once a week.

---

*Alka Seltzer Gold contains no aspirin.

For example, if you eat bananas and apples daily or several times a week, add them to the list of the foods you eliminate. If you snack on pecans, avoid them. But if you rarely eat a food, you need not leave it out of your diet.

Q: I can see that this is a truly comprehensive diet. Would I be able to get enough to eat?

The Cave Man Diet avoids foods you usually eat.

A: Yes. Although early on you'd probably suffer food cravings, which we've already discussed. But you can eat as much as you want of the allowed foods. So you get plenty of nutrition. My purpose in prescribing the Cave Man Diet is to avoid foods you usually eat. But to repeat—as difficult as this diet seems to be, it provides you with a variety of wholesome foods. Do you think you'll be able to carry out this Diet B?

Q: Yes—I can do anything I have to do. But let me repeat your instructions so I can be certain I understand them.

.If I feel Diet A hasn't given me the answers I'm looking for, you're suggesting I try Diet B. On this diet, I eliminate all the foods on Diet A plus pork, beef, chicken, potato, rice, oats and any food I eat more than once a week. So I'll have to eliminate twenty or more foods?

A: That's right.

Q: How about returning these foods to my diet? Do I add one food a day?

A: That's one way to do it. However, it would take you three or four weeks to complete the diet.

Q: That's a long time. And it would be hard for me to hold the line and keep from cheating. Is there another way to do Diet B in less time?

A: Yes. Carry out the elimination phase of the diet until your symptoms improve, just as we've already discussed. However, if you improve promptly (as, for example, in four or five days), you can begin returning the foods to your diet sooner. You can also shorten the period you'll have to stay on the diet by adding the foods you've eliminated four times a day.

Q: How would I do this? Please explain.

Before you add the food, make an inventory of your symptoms.

A: After your improvement is convincing and you've continued to feel better for at least 48 hours, add a single food—such as orange—for breakfast. But before you add the food, take a few minutes to make an inventory of your symptoms.*

Think about how you feel. Does your head hurt? Are you tired? Is your nose stopped up? Do you have a burning in your stomach or aching in your legs? It's important for you to "tune in" to symptoms that are present before eating the food. If you fail to do this, you're apt to blame symptoms that are already present on the food you're testing.

After you've finished your symptom inventory, eat the orange. If no new symptoms develop, wait 15 minutes and eat another orange, and then a third. If no symptoms develop, oranges aren't causing your problems.

Wait four hours, then introduce a second food (such as rice). Follow the same procedure that you followed in testing the orange. If this food causes no reaction, in another four hours try a third food (such as baked chicken). Then eat a fourth food an hour before bedtime.

So each day you'll be eating four foods. By doing this you'll

---

*Counting your pulse before and after you eat a food may also help you determine a food reaction. A pulse acceleration of six to eight beats following a food challenge is usually significant.

reduce the "adding back" phase of your diet from three weeks to seven to ten days.

Q: Would that work as well?

A: Perhaps. Such a rapid addition of foods would have several advantages. One of these would be completing Diet B in less time—two weeks rather than three more weeks. Another advantage relates to the peculiarities of a "hidden" food allergy.

Q: Could you explain?

A: I'll try. If you avoid a food you're allergic to for a week and then eat it again, it'll nearly always cause a reaction. But if you avoid it for four to six weeks, like a fire that dies down, your sensitivity to that food will decrease. And you may show little reaction when you eat it again, especially if you consume only a small amount.

Q: From what you've told me, I believe it'll be best for me to add one food four times a day. Will that be okay?

A: Yes. I feel that's the best way.

Q: Okay, now that's settled. I'd like your suggestions for getting my family to cooperate.

A: Plan the diet carefully. Discuss it with other family members ahead of time. Where possible, feature foods all the family members will eat (although they may want other foods to keep them satisfied and happy). Don't worry if your diet is limited. Even if you lose several pounds it won't hurt you and you'll soon regain them.

Q: Can I follow the diet at work?

A: Yes, if you "brown bag" it. If you're invited out to dinner, tell your host or hostess what you're doing and eat before you go or decline the invitation and ask for a raincheck.

Q: Is it best to start with Diet A? Or would you recommend Diet B first? Doing Diet B might save me time and trouble.

A: Sometimes I recommend Diet A for my patients and sometimes I recommend Diet B. It depends on how the patient feels about it and how severe and long lasting his symptoms are. However, in most patients I recommend Diet A.

Here's why. Most food-sensitive people improve on Diet A and Diet A is easier to follow than Diet B. It eliminates many of the major food troublemakers. Yet, it allows a person to eat pork, chicken, potatoes, apples and other foods which he likes but which he doesn't eat every day. And the rest of your family can eat the same diet. This makes things easier.

Q: When, why and under what circumstances should I try Diet B?

A: As I've already indicated, it depends on many different things. For example, although I've found that milk, wheat, corn, yeast, sugar, egg, chocolate and food additives are the most common troublemakers, any food can cause a reaction.

So even if you improve when you remove these foods from your diet, you may continue to show symptoms because beef, pork, chicken, apple, potato, tomato, banana, oats or other foods may be causing some of your symptoms. The only way you can tell if these foods bother you is to eliminate them from your diet and see if your symptoms improve. Then you can eat the foods again and see if your symptoms return.

Q: I think I understand. But to make sure, let me repeat your instructions. You want me to do Elimination Diet A for seven to ten days, keeping a record of my symptoms for three days before I start the diet. I continue to record my symptoms for the seven- to ten-day elimination phase of the diet. Then after I'm sure my symptoms have improved, I eat the foods again, one at a time, to see which foods bother me and which foods do not. I continue my records.

A: That's right.

Q: Suppose I complete the diet and note obvious reactions to a couple of foods, yet, there are other foods I'm not sure about—what do I do then?

A: Keep the foods that cause reactions out of your diet indefinitely. Retest the foods you're uncertain about. Here's one way you can do this. Eat the suspected food several days in a row, as for example, Friday, Saturday, Sunday, Monday and Tuesday. Eliminate the food on Wednesday, Thursday, Friday, Saturday and Sunday and then load up on the eliminated food the following Monday. If you're allergic to it, you should develop symptoms. If you show no symptoms, chances are you aren't allergic to that food.

Keep the foods that cause reactions out of your diet indefinitely. Retest the foods you're uncertain about.

Q: I think I understand; but, suppose I show a reaction when I eat wheat or egg or when I drink milk. Does this mean I'll always be allergic to these foods?

A: Yes, to some degree. Your symptoms will nearly always return if you consume as much of a food as you did before you began your diet. However, if you avoid a food you're allergic to for several months, you'll usually regain some tolerance to it. And you may not develop symptoms unless you eat it several days in a row.

Q: How do I find out?

A: By trial and error.

Q: I'm not sure I understand—please explain.

A: I'll do my best. When you avoid a food you're allergic to for several months, you'll generally lose some of your allergy to the food (like a fire that dies down).

For example, if you're bothered by a stuffed-up nose, headache and fatigue while drinking a quart of milk a day, you may be able to eat yogurt or cheese occasionally after you've eliminated milk from your diet for several months. However, suppose you eat milk-containing foods after you've avoided them for several months and show no reaction. In such a situation you may say to yourself, "The yogurt and cheese didn't bother me so maybe milk allergy isn't one of my problems. But if you start drinking milk or eating dairy products every day, within a few days or weeks some of your symptoms will return. Before you know it, you'll develop the same health problems you had before you eliminated milk.

Sometimes, though, it takes even longer for your symptoms to recur and you may not connect them to the food.

Q: I think this point is clear but why does a food bother me on some occasions and not on others. For example, I've heard of people who became congested when they drank milk in the winter but who could drink it in the summer without showing any symptoms.

A: It has to do with the "allergic load" or concomitant allergies. Along with other physicians interested in food allergy, I have found that allergic individuals may tolerate foods in the summer which they can't eat in the winter.

Part of the problem relates to chilling. Also, wintertime furnaces which stir up dust and dry out the respiratory membranes may lessen a person's resistance and make him more susceptible to wintertime infections and allergies.

In addition, during the wintertime, you spend more time indoors. Windows and doors are usually closed so there is less ventilation. Accordingly, disease-producing germs are more prevalent. Other factors include the household and office indoor air pollutants (tobacco smoke, perfumes, janitorial supplies and other odorous chemicals).

Cold weather, dust, cold germs and chemicals, plus food allergies, cause many wintertime health problems.

Q: Do other allergies, such as hay fever due to grass or bronchitis due to house dust mites or cat dander, have anything to do with the amount of an allergy-causing food I can eat?

A: Yes. The more allergy troublemakers you're exposed to, the greater are your chances of developing an allergic illness. For example, let's suppose you're allergic to milk, corn, chocolate, spring grass and house dust mites. Yet, you aren't severely allergic to any one of these substances.

Accordingly, you may play golf in the spring without being bothered by hay fever and you may be able to eat an occasional piece of cornbread or chocolate without symptoms. But if you eat a sack of popcorn, a candy bar and drink a chocolate milk shake on the same day (after cutting the grass), you may become irritable and nervous and develop nasal congestion or bronchitis.

Q: I'm beginning to understand more about hidden food allergies. But suppose I'm allergic to egg and I avoid egg for three months. Then I eat an egg for breakfast and it doesn't bother me. How will I know how much and how often I can eat egg in the future?

A: I'm glad you asked. It'll give me a chance to talk about a rotated diet. Along with many physicians interested in hidden food allergies, I've found that my allergic patients who rotate their diets usually get along well and develop fewer new food allergies.

Rotating a diet means eating a food only once every four to seven days. For example, if you're allergic to egg and after avoiding it for several months you eat an egg and it doesn't bother you, you can try eating an egg once a week and see if you tolerate it. You can do the same with other foods.

Q: Aren't some foods "kin" to each other—like chicken and egg, wheat and corn or milk and beef? Is a person who is allergic to one food more apt to become sensitive to foods in the same "family"?

> **People who are sensitive to one food in a family are more apt to be sensitive . . . to another food in the same family.**

A: The answer to both of your questions is yes. Foods are "kin" to each other. Familiar food families include the grain family, citrus family and the legume family (peas, peanuts, beans and soybeans). While there are many exceptions, people who are sensitive to one food in a family are more apt to be sensitive—or become sensitive—to another food in the family, especially if they eat a lot of it.

I've found that wheat-sensitive patients are apt to become sensitive to all other grains—especially if they eat them repeatedly or in quantity. Although I permit rice and oats on Diet A, if you find you're allergic to wheat or corn, experiment further with your diet to see if other grains cause reactions.

If you're allergic to grains, here's another suggestion. Go to your health food store and get some quinoa, amaranth and buckwheat. You can make bread and other grainlike products from these grain alternatives. Yet, they aren't "kin" to the grains.

Now for a word on milk and beef. Most milk-sensitive individuals seem to be able to eat steak and hamburger without a reaction. However, because cow's milk and beef come from the same animal, if you're allergic to milk, avoid beef for a week, then add it back and see what happens. If you're allergic to egg, limit your intake of chicken to a serving every four to seven days.

Is there anything else you'd like to know—anything at all?

Q: Nothing I can think of at the moment—my head is spinning. Do you have further suggestions?

A: Read, review and study all the instructions I've given you. When you've finished, you'll find that detecting your hidden food allergies won't be as hard as you thought it would be.

37

Immunotherapy

Such therapy stimulates or strengthens the immune system using extracts or vaccines of various kinds. For example, you may have received vaccines which help strengthen your immunity to diphtheria, tetanus, measles, polio and other diseases. *Immunotherapy* was first reported to help patients with hay fever in 1911.[1] Since that time, it has been used in treating patients bothered by allergic rhinitis (hay fever) and asthma caused by pollens, dusts and molds.

Most members of the American Academy of Allergy and Immunology (AAAI) or the American College of Allergy and Immunology (ACAI) use prick tests in determining a patient's sensitivity to various substances. Then, when such tests are positive, and they wish to hyposensitize their patients, they begin with tiny doses and gradually increase the strength of the extracts over a period of many months. However, they do not usually desensitize patients to *Candida albicans*.

Other groups of physicians interested in allergies, sensitivities and candida-related health problems use a different approach. Many of these physicians are members of the American Academy of Otolaryngic Allergy and/or the American Academy of Environmental Medicine (AAEM).

While members of these organizations may occasionally use scratch tests in studying their patients, they usually rely for diagnosis on tiny doses of extracts given intradermally (within the superficial layers of the skin) called serial-end-point titration

(SEDT). In treating their patients, although they use gradually increasing strengths of extract, the dilutions used are generally weaker than those favored by most AAAI and ACAI members. In their experience, these "optimal" or "neutralizing" doses of extract are safer and much more effective than stronger ones.

Observations of Joseph B. Miller, M.D.

During the past two decades, Dr. Miller has been the leading researcher and clinician in studying still another different type of immunotherapy* in treating patients with food and inhalant allergies and other illnesses.[2,3,4] Moreover, he's published his observations describing the relief of PMS and other progesterone related symptoms[5] and viral infections, including herpes.[6] During the past decade, Dr. Miller has found that using a similar technique, he has been able to help many patients with vaginitis and other candida-related disorders. Here are some of his comments which appeared in a recent issue of *The Allergy Letters.***

"I have a steady stream of patients referred to me by gynecologists who are unable to provide relief for their patients with intractable candida vaginitis."

Dr. Miller then described how he uses a special diet, nystatin, Sporanox and/or Diflucan. Then he states:

"After about 2 weeks, I test the patient by the intradermal neutralizing method and find the neutralizing dose of *Candida albicans* extract. I delay this test for 2 weeks in order to reduce the candida population in the colon so that there will be little or no likelihood of a systemic reaction to the test itself.

"The test is very objective. Nearly 100% of the patients neutral-

---

*Information about the methods of testing can be obtained from Dr. Miller's publications or by writing him at the Miller Center for Allergy, 5901 Airport Blvd., Mobile, AL 36608.
**Published by the International Correspondence Society Of Allergists, 5811 Outlook Drive, Shawnee Mission, KS 66202.

ized on the strongest dilution which produces a negative immediate type wheal . . . Some patients do well with one or two treatment injections a week whereas others . . . require an injection every day for the first few weeks. Each injection usually provides relief within 30 minutes.

"Some patients are so excoriated that the vulva is inflamed or ulcerated. These often require topical applications of cortisone cream for one or two days for the relief of pain and inflammation, followed for a few days in some instances by an antibiotic ointment for secondary infection and then by an antifungal cream. . . . Intravaginal medications are also sometimes needed. . . .

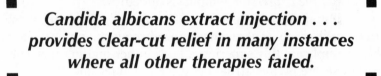

Candida albicans **extract injection . . .**
provides clear-cut relief in many instances
where all other therapies failed.

"This condition can cause terrible suffering and inability to work or perform routine duties. The condition is a clear-cut, clinical entity. The response to *Candida albicans* extract injection in neutralizing doses provides clear-cut relief in many instances where all other therapies failed."[7]

In a paper published in the *Environmental Physician* in the fall of 1994,[8] Dr. Miller summarized a four-year analysis of 50,421 consecutive tests in patients with various types of medical problems, including allergies and sensitivities to *Candida albicans*. He said that in 98.8% of the tests it was the maximum intradermally tolerated dose (MITD) that was effective in relieving symptoms in his patients.

Observations of C. Orian Truss, M.D.

In his first paper, "Tissue Injury Induced by *Candida albicans*—mental and neurologic manifestations," Dr. Truss described for the first time the favorable response of a chronically ill patient to an injection of candida extract. Here's an excerpt from his report.

"An incident that occurred in 1961 was the first indication that this organism perhaps is capable of causing disorders much more severe than conventionally attributed to it. A 40-year-old woman whom I was treating for allergic rhinitis and migraine headache, walked into the office with one of her severe headaches. It was readily apparent that she was also quite depressed, which was characteristic of the severe premenstrual symptoms that she experienced for one week each month.

"*Candida albicans* was one of her worst allergens and chronic yeast vaginitis, worse premenstrually, was a common complaint. *A small dose of candida extract relieved the headache, but the most startling result of the injection was the rapid and complete disappearance of the depression* [emphasis added].

"Her initial, unsmiling, agitated manner was suddenly replaced by a relaxed, smiling countenance. In subsequent months it was possible to duplicate this experience both in her and in other similar cases of severe premenstrual depression and tension."[9]

Further Observations by Dr. Truss

In a subsequent paper, "Restoration of Immunologic Competence to *Candida albicans*" Dr. Truss discussed diet, antifungal medications, the avoidance of antibiotics and other treatment measures. Included in the treatment program was the use of extracts of *Candida albicans*. Here are excerpts from his report.

"Injection of an extract of *Candida albicans* constitutes an attempt to strengthen the immune response to the yeast in a patient who is actively infected by the organism . . . Marked variation is exhibited among patients in the pattern of their allergic responses. It is not surprising, therefore, that in this unique situation it has proved impossible to standardize a program of injection therapy.

"The strength of the extract and the interval between injections varies not only among patients, but also in the same patient at different times of recovery."[10]

In his continuing discussion, Dr. Truss stated that he had found it "unrewarding" to steadily increase the strength of the allergy extract—a technique or method which is often successful with conventional injection therapy for inhalant allergy. He said in his experience, the use of much weaker doses in the range of 10^{*5} to 10^{*15}, were usually used in his practice and found to be effective. Yet, he emphasized that patience, time and careful re-evaluation of the patient is essential for optimal results.

Reports by Other Physicians

In a 1962 report in the *Annals of Allergy*, an Israeli physician, A. Liebeskind, described improvement in patients with candida-related health problems following the use of candida extracts. Symptoms in these patients included vulvitis, bronchitis, migraine and gastrointestinal complaints. In describing his experiences with these patients, Dr. Liebeskind said:

> "These patients were chronically ill and were treated for many years by physicians, including specialists in the various branches of medicine. They were given symptomatic treatment according to the signs and symptoms with which they presented themselves.
> "The results of this kind of symptomatic treatment proved to be a complete failure. Only by a chance subcutaneous test performed on these patients, the possibility of *C. albicans* allergy was suspected. *Subsequently, these patients were treated with hyposensitization injections of C. albicans extracts during a period of 6 to 10 months. Thirteen out of the . . . 18 patients got complete relief of their symptoms, and 5 showed a remarkable improvement.*"[11]

Reports by Hosen and Palacios in the medical literature described the effectiveness of candida immunotherapy in patients with yeast vaginitis.[12,13] In a similar report published in the *Annals of Allergy*, N. M. Kudelko, an Oregon physician, said:

> "Seventy selected patients with chronic monilia (yeast) vaginitis had unsatisfactory results from conventional treatments. After they were evaluated for an allergic diathesis, and *Candida albicans* allergens were included in their hyposensitization injections, 90% responded with good to excellent results. Gynecologists and allergists are reminded that allergy may involve the vulvovaginal tract and

that specific antiallergic therapy may be indicated in many resistant cases of chronic monilia vaginitis."[14]

In still another report, Palacios reported on the successful use of *Candida albicans* in treating persistent skin and nail problems, as well as vaginal problems.[15]

Enzyme Potentiated Desensitization

Some six or seven years ago, Belinda Dawes, a British physician, sent me an article entitled, *Enzyme Potentiated Desensitization (EPD)*.[16] In this article, Dr. McEwen told of this new method of treating allergic patients. In commenting on the article, Dr. Dawes said, "It really works. I'm excited about it."

Yet, because the special vaccine used by Dr. McEwen wasn't available in the United States, and because I was phasing down my practice, I must admit that the information slipped by and was stored away in my filing cabinet. Then, in 1990 and 1991, I heard favorable reports about the effectiveness of EPD from a handful of other physicians in England, Canada and the United States. But I didn't really become interested in this new therapy until the late spring of 1992.

At that time, I read an article by Dr. McEwen and colleagues in the May 9, 1992, issue of a major British medical journal, *The Lancet*.[17]

These investigators described their success in treating 40 children with food-induced hyperkinetic behavior using a specially prepared EPD vaccine.

I obtained further information about EPD from a pamphlet published in 1990 by Dr. McEwen. Here are excerpts:

"Since the dose of allergens needed is much smaller than that needed for conventional desensitizing injections, this treatment is also much safer."

According to Dr. McEwen, the mixture used to treat people with allergies may contain either inhalants or foods, or they may be combined. Moreover, he said that several physicians using EPD have found that it helps people with chronic fatigue syndrome, the candida related complex and related chronic health disorders.

What is EPD? According to a patient instruction booklet by W.A. Shrader, Jr., M.D.:

> "Enzyme Potentiated Desensitization (EPD) is a technique using extremely small doses of allergens in an attempt to desensitize the patient to his allergies. The doses used are the same or smaller than those employed in diagnostic skin prick testing. The enzyme, beta glucuronidase, is used to increase and alter the effects of the antigen extracts. Dr. Len McEwen pioneered the method in 1966, when he found that a single dose of grass pollen with beta glucuronidase could be as effective as a long course of conventional desensitizing injections."[18]

At this time, EPD therapy is being used by fewer than 50 physicians in the United States. Further information, including an instruction booklet, can be obtained by writing to the International EPD Society, c/o W.A. Shrader, Jr., M.D., 141 Paseo de Peralta, Santa Fe, NM 87501. (Please enclose a check for $5 to cover postage/ handling and cost of the booklet.)

REFERENCES

1. Noon, L., "Prophylactic inoculation against hay fever," *The Lancet*, 1911; 1:1572.
2. Miller, J.B., "A double-blind study of food extract injection therapy: A preliminary report." *Annals of Allergy*, March 1977; 38(3):185–191.
3. Miller, J.B., "Intradermal provocative-neutralizing food testing and subcutaneous food extract injection therapy," in *Food Allergy and Intolerance*, Brostoff, J. and Challacombe, S.J., (Ed.), London: Balliére Tindall, 1987; pp 932–946.
4. Miller, J.B., "Relief at Last! Neutralization for Food Allergy and Other Illnesses," Charles C. Thomas, Springfield, IL, 1987.
5. Miller, J.B., "Relief of Premenstrual Symptoms, Dysmenorrhea and Contraceptive Tablet Intolerance," *J. Med. Assoc., St. of Alabama*, 1974; 44:57–60.

6. Miller, J.B., "Treatment of Active Herpes Virus Infections with Influenza Virus Vaccine," *Annals of Allergy*, 1979; 42:295–305.
7. Miller, J.B., in Bishop, J.E. (Ed.), *The Allergy Letters*, 5811 Outlook Dr., Shawnee Mission, KS 66202.
8. Miller, J.B., "The Maximum Intradermally Tolerated Dose (MITD) Method of Food Allergy Testing and Immunotherapy: New Concepts," *Environmental Physician*, October 1994.
9. Truss, C.O., "Tissue Injury Induced by *Candida albicans*—Mental and Neurological Manifestations," *J. of Orthomol. Psych.*, 1978; Vol. 7 and *The Missing Diagnosis*, Birmingham, AL, p 128.
10. Truss, C.O., "Restoration of Immunological Competence to *Candida albicans*," *J. of Orthomol. Psych.*, 1980; Vol. 9 and *The Missing Diagnosis*, pp 157–159.
11. Liebeskind, A., "*Candida albicans* as an allergenic factor," *Annals of Allergy*, 1962; 20:394–396.
12. Hosen, H., "Focal Fungal Infections Treated With Immunological Therapy With Emphasis on Vaginal Monilias," *Texas Medicine*, 1971; 67:58.
13. Palacios, H.J., "Desensitization for monilia hypersensitivity," *Virginia Medical*, 1977; pp 393–394.
14. Kudelko, N.M., "Allergy and chronic monilia vaginitis," *Annals of Allergy*, 1971; 29:266.
15. Palacios, H.J., "Hypersensitivity as a cause of dermatologic and vaginal moniliasis resistant to topical therapy," *Annals of Allergy*, 1976; 37:110–113.
16. McEwen, L.M., "Enzyme Potentiated Hypodesensitization," *Annals of Allergy*, 1975; 35:98–103.
17. Egger, J., Stolla, A. and McEwen, L.M., "Control trial of hyposensitization in children with food-induced hyperkinetic syndrome," *The Lancet*, 1992; 339:1150–53.
18. Shrader, W.A., Jr., "Enzyme Potentiated Desensitization," International EPD Society, Santa Fe, NM, April 1993.

38

---◆---

Diagnostic Studies

---◆---

How does a physician make a diagnosis? How does she/he find out what's making you "sick"? There are three main methods.

- Your *history,*
- Your *physical examination*—what the physician can determine with his/her eyes, ears, and touch,
- *Tests,* including blood tests, urine tests, stool examinations, x-rays, and other more complex laboratory studies.

The Patient's History or Story

Let's talk about your history first. Many physicians feel that a patient's story provides more information than any other diagnostic method. Here are typical things your physician needs to know.

> **Many physicians feel that a patient's story provides more information than any other diagnostic method.**

When and how did your illness begin? Did your symptoms begin suddenly (like being hit by a stray bullet)? Or did they come on gradually over a period of weeks, months, or years?

A good history looks at all sorts of things, past and present. And there are dozens and dozens of pertinent things your physician needs to know about you. Here are some of them.

- What do you eat for breakfast, lunch, dinner and snack?
- Do you smoke and drink alcoholic beverages?
- What drugs or other medications do you take?
- What are your present environmental exposures at home or in your workplace?
- Are you bothered by perfumes and colognes?
- Fabric shop odors?
- Dusts or molds?
- Pollens?
- Animal danders?
- Occupational exposures?
- Your home environment—are you exposed to smoke, insecticides, gas cooking stove, or odorous carpets?
- Do you use lawn chemicals or pesticides outdoors?

To help me evaluate patients who call or write me seeking help, I have for many years said: "Write me a letter. Tell me anything and everything you'd like for me to know. You can't make it too long. Make it a story and include things you may feel aren't relevant."

I've also devised several questionnaires and history forms—including my 70-item yeast questionnaire. As you know, I assigned a high value to certain questions, especially the history of repeated or prolonged courses of broad-spectrum antibiotic drugs for respiratory, urinary, or other infections.

Other physicians, including my good friend Dr. Keith Sehnert, use additional questionnaires; one focuses on thyroid and another focuses on depression.

An Empathetic Attitude by the Physician Is Important

Questionnaires help the physician learn more about the patient's story and her concerns. No doubt about it. Yet, they should not serve as a substitute for a careful, one-on-one, private doctor/

patient discussion. *In my experience, more than anything else, people with yeast-related health problems want to be listened to by a kind, compassionate, empathetic physician.*

**People with yeast-related health problems
want to be listened to by a kind,
compassionate, empathetic physician.**

I'm reminded of information I received from two sources during my early years of pediatric practice. The first came from Dr. Barbara Korsch who, in the 1950s, ran a special Attitude Survey Clinic at Cornell Medical School. The purpose of the clinic: *finding better ways of communicating with and helping patients.*

As a part of the study, patients were asked to evaluate and grade the professionals who worked with them.

When the Cornell researchers reviewed their findings, an Italian woman physician ranked head and shoulders above all of the other physicians. As the researchers analyzed what this physician did, they learned that her ability to understand and speak English was somewhat limited. *So she looked attentively and empathetically at her patients and let them do most of the talking!*

About the same time, I took a special three-hour course at the Children's Memorial Hospital in Chicago, conducted by Dr. Jerome Schulman. The title of the course was "How to Help Your Patients in One Office Visit." Dr. Schulman gave the physicians in attendance a number of rules, including: "Listen actively." "Look at the patient." "Let the patient do 80% of the talking."

Physical Examination

A careful physical examination is important. I'm not talking only about sticking a tongue blade into your mouth and asking you to say, "Ah," or listening to your heart and lungs with a stethoscope, feeling your abdomen and carrying out other examinations. I'm also referring to the physician's overall "inspection."

How do you appear to the physician? Depressed? Cheerful? Alert? Drowsy? Agitated? Anxious? Hostile? Apathetic? And so on. All of these person-to-person evaluations add to the physician's impressions obtained from your history, detailed physical examination and the laboratory examinations, x-rays, and tests of many types.

Laboratory Examinations and Other Tests and Studies

Sometimes tests can be critically important. Here are a few examples. An x-ray of the chest of a tired patient who has been losing weight may show a tumor. An examination of the urine could show evidence of a hidden infection. Or a SMA screening blood test could show an elevated blood urea nitrogen (BUN)—an evidence of kidney failure.

So laboratory studies are often important. Take the patient who develops abdominal pain and nausea which came on 24 hours previously, and is accompanied by tenderness in the right lower part of the abdomen.

In such a patient the physician will often order a complete blood count and urinalysis. When the urinalysis is normal and the white blood count is sharply elevated, these reports, plus the findings obtained from the history and physical examination, often prompt the physician to schedule surgery. In such patients, an inflamed appendix will usually be found and removed.

But, lab tests alone aren't enough. My own daughter, Elizabeth, a few months before her fifth birthday, developed an ill-defined illness. Her symptoms included a low grade fever and abdominal pain. Several physicians examined her and her blood counts and urinalyses were normal. Then, on about the third day of her illness, her abdomen became swollen and rigid. Her problem: A ruptured appendix.

Based on this experience, plus countless others in my medical practice over the years, I never use a laboratory test alone to "make the diagnosis." A number of physicians who treat yeast-related health problems feel the same way.

How Is a Diagnosis of a Candida-Related Health Problem Made?

It is based on all three of the diagnostic steps I've just outlined. But of these three steps, history is by far the most important. And when it is combined with the response of the patient to a sugar-free special diet and antifungal medication, the diagnosis can be confirmed.

Most patients with candida-related health problems have been seen by many different physicians. One of my patients, I'll call her Harriet, said:

> "During the past year, I've seen six different doctors. I've had every test in the book and every opening in my body has been looked into. When the physicians came up empty-handed, they said 'Your symptoms are probably due to stress. Yet, you can be reassured because we don't find anything really wrong with you.'"

Harriet's story was typical of those I've heard from countless people who have written or called me. Other physicians have had similar experiences.

In March 1993 following a point-counterpoint conference at a hospital in Tarzana, California, Joan Priestley, M.D., told me about some of her experiences in studying and treating patients with yeast-related health problems. And she said:

> "When you revise your questionnaire I'd like to see you include the following question and give it a high-point score! 'In your efforts to find help, have you seen ten or more physicians?'"

Tests for Candida Albicans

Even though laboratory studies do not "make the diagnosis" of a candida-related health problem, a number of the physicians I've consulted have found that laboratory studies may help. These include:

A. Stool studies for candida and other organisms (Lab #5, 6, 8, 10 and 14).

B. Comprehensive examination of the stool (Lab #10 and 14). A number of physicians have found that such an analyses helps them study their patients with candida-related disorders and other chronic complaints. These studies evaluate digestive capacity, intestinal function and microbial status. The latter evaluation identifies predominant bacterial strains and potential pathogens. In addition, such studies provide culture and sensitivity tests for candida species.

C. Candida blood studies of various types, including measurement of candida antibodies, antigens and immune complexes (Lab #2, 4, 12, 13 and 15).

Comments of Physicians

To learn more about the experiences of practicing physicians who are knowledgeable and experienced in treating patients with yeast-related problems, I interviewed many physicians. Here are some of their comments.

Charles Resseger, D.O., Norwalk, Ohio: "I use Antibody Assay Laboratories. They do immune complexes. I've been using them for about four years. What they're measuring is not candida antibodies, which, in my opinion is worthless.

"Immune complexes contain antibody, antigen and fragments of complement. When the complexes are present in increased amounts, it means that the antigen, i.e. candida, is present in increased amounts, indicating active overgrowth. Refining the antibody technique for measuring IgG immune complexes to candida permits the detection of active candida overgrowth.

"In my experience, I've found these immune complex measurements very useful in the diagnosis of yeast overgrowth.

"I also use the Comprehensive Digestive Stool Analysis (CDSA) by Great Smokies Diagnostic Laboratory. They've bailed me out more than a few times. In addition to candida, I've also found other weird bacteria—in tremendous volumes—in the gut. I believe some of these bacteria can do just about the same thing as yeast. I'll leave them on Diflucan or Sporanox and treat them with the antibiotic."

Sidney M. Baker, M.D., Weston, Connecticut: "The mucous membrane of the digestive tract is a huge surface (about the size of a tennis court) that we expose to our environment in the form of foods and the germs that live in our digestive tract. Knowing about what's going on in the digestive tract is very helpful in assessing the health of an individual.

"I think stool analysis is a much overlooked measure in preventive medicine and is more important, in my view, than a chemistry screen for the ordinary practitioner. It really tells you a lot about what's going on in somebody's innards. I use stool analysis, permeability study, secretory IgA very frequently and think they're very informative.

"There are various mischief makers in the gut other than fungi which are probably the most important. These include various bacteria, such as Klebsiella and Proteus, that have been known to produce peculiar immune reactions with symptoms outside the digestive tract, particularly arthritis. I believe that there are many other germs, including aerobic germs and those that grow in the absence of oxygen (anaerobic germs) that we know little about currently, but are the basis of various kinds of trouble in people with chronic inflammatory disease."

James Brodsky, M.D., Chevy Chase, Maryland: "In most patients I do not rely very much on the laboratory. However, I do more stool analyses than I ever did before. Not on everyone, but in patients who may not be doing well. I use Great Smokies for the stool studies. I also ask them to do sensitivity tests to the different antifungals."

Ed Conley, D.O., Flint, Michigan: "I've been getting a lot of anti-candida antibody studies using Ed Winger's Immunodiagnostic Laboratory, Inc. or the Metametrics Lab.

"I also often do the complete digestive stool analysis with the Great Smokies Lab and I've been pleased with information I've obtained, including patients who have other organisms, including Klebsiella and Citrobacter.

"If I was ever audited for any reason the positive candida in the stools would help me stand on pretty good grounds; because candida is so controversial."

Ken Gerdes, M.D., Denver, Colorado: "The diagnosis in most patients with candida-related problems is a clinical one. Yet, if there are questions, I get studies for parasites. I usually send them to the Dowell Laboratory in Arizona.

"A stool study does not rule out candida. Frequently I'll get a stool study back that's loaded with yeasts, yet the patient doesn't look all that bad. I don't use antibody tests and to repeat, *a good history and the patient's response to diet and nystatin is the best diagnostic test.*"

Elson Haas, M.D., San Rafael, California: "I run Ed Winger's antibody studies carried out by his Immunodiagnostic Laboratories on some people—not on everybody. Here's my thinking—people who have high antibodies, I feel I have to be more careful to get rid of yeasts everywhere in their body. In such patients I'm more apt to use one of the systemic antifungals.

"I also run candida cultures and sensitivities and the comprehensive digestive stool analysis (CDSA) through Great Smokies and purged stool tests through Dowell Laboratory to assess parasites, also a common problem. These are both very helpful in evaluating the ecology, function and integrity of the GI tract."

Paul Jaconello, M.D., Toronto, Ontario: "I used Aristo Wodjani's test carried by Immuno Sciences Laboratory, Inc. What's more, I have his little machine and the test is run in my office. I've done over 500 tests now. I repeat the test after three to six months and I find the patient's candida antibody levels have often dropped indicating less immune reactivity. The test also correlates with my own clinical observations of the patient."

Michael Kwiker, D.O., Sacramento, California: "I first take a good history then I rely on the Great Smokies tests and the candida antibody test. They're both very helpful. They correlate 95% of the time to my thinking. I've also found Ed Winger's candida antibody test helpful. It helps my patients to see it on paper. It's under $100. The main thing, though, is how the patient does."

Allan Lieberman, M.D., North Charleston, South Carolina: "The best way to diagnose a yeast-related problem is through a therapeutic trial. I'd rather save the patient's money for medicine and diet."

Allen Spreen, M.D., Jacksonville, Florida: "I do the comprehensive digestive stool analysis on many of my patients. I also do the CEI test from Cerodex Lab. It puts the numbers in black and white after they've gotten real high on the questionnaire. It helps me answer the doubting Thomas. What's more, people like to see their tests to prove the clinical diagnosis."

O. Jack Woodard, M.D., Albany, Georgia: "Great Smokies Lab does tests for my patients. So I have that information up front. I have my patients send in two random stool specimens. It's very seldom I don't get a positive stool test on patients who have CRC.

"I've only seen one case of giardiasis in 200 positive stool cultures. I see Blastocystis commonly. Over half of my candida patients are affected with it. It's hard to eradicate. I also use preparations of citrus seed extract and gentian violet."

Aubrey Worrell, M.D., Pine Bluff, Arkansas: "I do a lot of work with Great Smokies. I have a lot of patients who have abnormal bacterial flora and a lot of them had candida in the stool. Yet, some patients I put on the treatment program and when they come back two weeks later, I have a lab test which shows no candida . . . yet, the patients are much better.

"So I don't let whether candida is in the stool or not influence me as to whether or not I treat them with nystatin. I also like the nystatin tablets because they get down to the colon [emphasis added]."

Tests for Food Allergies and Sensitivities

With few exceptions, people with yeast-related health problems are bothered by sensitivities to foods they're eating every day. Although the commonly used allergy scratch tests often show negative results, other tests may be helpful, including:

The ALCAT Test

This test measures changes in cell size/volume following the incubation of a blood specimen with food extracts using a specialized computer (Lab #1). Physicians who have found this test useful include internist Barbara Solomon of Baltimore, Maryland, and Douglas H. Sandberg, Professor of Pediatrics, University of Miami. In commenting on the value of this test, Dr. Sandberg stated:

> "Diagnosis and treatment of food sensitivity-related illness has been a cumbersome and imperfect process. Use of a combination of a new blood screening test, the antigen leucocyte cellular antibody test, and titration skin testing is suggested as a more efficient and effective approach to these disorders."[1]

IgG Food Sensitivity Tests (Lab #11)

During the past few years, other tests have been developed which aid in detecting hidden or delayed-onset food allergies. One such test, the Enzyme-Linked Immunosorbent Assay (ELISA), is designed to detect circulating food-specific immunoglobulin class G (IgG) antibodies.

In discussing the importance of food sensitivities and the use of this test, in an interview with Dr. James Braly, Dr. Keith Sehnert said:

> "Most of my patients come to me with what we call 'the Triad': food allergies/intolerance, candida related complex—and/or hormonal dysfunction primarily of the hypothyroid type. These three conditions are often overlooked in today's fast lane medicine. So with a careful history, examination and the help of the food specific IgG ELISA blood test, I almost always find a way to help these patients—sometimes with dramatic improvement."[2]

In October 1994, at the annual meeting of the American Academy of Environmental Medicine, Virginia Beach, Virginia, Dr. Baker presented observations that he and his colleagues had made in studying food sensitive patients.

They found a significant difference ($P = < 0.00024$) favoring the response to the avoidance of IgG reactive foods as compared to patients who followed the placebo diet. In commenting on their study, Baker acknowledged that this was a small study, and only the first pilot study. He also noted that a 12-week period is too long for compliance.

Yet, in conclusion he said:

> *"Despite negative mitigating factors, the study showed with overwhelming statistical significance, that the avoidance of IgG foods resulted in a decrease in symptom severity greater than that achieved by a placebo diet* [emphasis added]."[3]

I've had no personal experience in using the ALCAT or IgG food sensitivity tests. Moreover, these tests don't provide all the answers. Yet, they appear to help many physicians who work with patients troubled with chronic health disorders.

Tests Described at the First and Second International Symposia on Functional Medicine

In 1993 and 1994, I began to hear about lactulose and mannitol challenge tests in a discussion by Jeffrey S. Bland, Ph.D., on one of his monthly audio-tapes, *Preventive Medicine Update.*[4] Then, in June 1994, I obtained copies of syllabi presented at the International Symposia on Functional Medicine.* Here are brief excerpts from an article entitled, "Functional Assessment of Intestinal Permeability":**

> "The assessment of intestinal permeability described in a recent review article by Travis and Menzies. The most clinically applicable way of evaluating the mucosal integrity of the gastrointestinal tract is the lactulose and mannitol challenge test.
>
> "The test involves administering a solution of lactulose and mannitol, combined with glycerol, to an individual who has fasted overnight, and then collecting the urine for six hours . . .

---

*This reference to the International Symposia on Functional Medicine (1993 and 1994) barely scratched the surface of the data which was presented. To obtain information about audio-tapes and printed summaries of some of the presentations, write to HealthComm, P.O. Box 1729, Gig Harbor, WA 98335. (206) 851-3943.

**This material was excerpted from the 1993/1994 HealthComm Seminar syllabus, "Advancement in Clinical Nutrition—New Protocols for Improving Health-Functional Intestinal Problems."

"In individuals with altered gastrointestinal mucosa . . . there's increased absorption of lactulose, which is subsequently excreted in the urine . . .

"In one interesting application of this assessment protocol, patients with food allergy were evaluated by the lactulose/mannitol test and found to have an elevated lactulose-to-mannitol urinary ratio . . . Food allergy does have an adverse effect upon the gut permeability and that by proper management of food allergy, intestinal integrity may be improved."[5]

My Comments

A number of my physician consultants have found that laboratory tests help in studying patients with chronic health problems, including those which are yeast related. Such tests are especially helpful when they are carried out by a reputable laboratory and evaluated by a knowledgeable physician. *Yet, at this time, no test will give you a "yes or no" answer to your question, "Are my health problems yeast related?"*

I wish there were an inexpensive test—a blood test, stool test, skin test or other test—which (like the new pregnancy tests) would tell you and your physician—your health problems *are* or *are not* candida related.

BUT, to repeat, there are no such tests. In discussing the diagnosis of any medical disorder, I would like to again cite the editorial by Gene H. Stollerman, M.D., Professor of Medicine at Boston University entitled "The Gold Standard." In his comments, he said:

"As the insights of medical bioscience and technology increase our medical powers, I find renewed strength in my clinical skills. The medical history has become more focused and incisive as we learn better questions to ask. . . ."

In the concluding paragraph of his editorial, Dr. Stollerman said, *"Clinical experience is the gold standard on which patient care should be based."*[6]

I agree with Dr. Stollerman and with the clinicians who have found that *the patient's history and his/her favorable response to diet and antifungal medication is the best way to identify a candida-related health problem.*

I hasten to add that individuals with complex medical problems may benefit from other tests. Such tests are especially indicated in people with yeast-related disorders who continue to be sick. There are many, many tests carried out by competent laboratories which may provide critically important information and may enable the physician to structure an appropriate treatment program. In commenting on some of these tests, Sidney M. Baker said:

> "Mineral assessment is another important tool and is complicated by the fact that minerals are compartmentalized in the body in ways that make assessment of any given tissue not necessarily representative of what's going on in the whole person. Studies of blood, hair and urine, including 24-hour urinary excretion studies are often necessary to get the appropriate handle on mineral testing (Lab #7)."

Although it is beyond the scope of this discussion to describe all of the other tests which some of my physician consultants have found helpful, here are several of them.

- Tests to identify hidden nutrient deficiencies (Lab #16).
- Tests to assess the cells ability to prevent free-radical damage (Lab #16).
- Tests to study the levels of environmental pollutants in the blood and tissues (Lab #9).

Laboratories

1. **American Medical Testing Laboratories,** 1 Oakwood Blvd., Suite 130, Hollywood, FL 33020. 800–881-2685. 305–923-2990.
2. **Antibody Assay Laboratory,** 1715 E. Wilshire #715, Santa Ana, CA 92705. 800-522-2611.
3. **Atlantic Pro-Nutrients,** 4403 Vineland Rd., Suite B12, Orlando, FL 32811. 800–647-6100.
4. **Cerodex Lab,** Rt. 1 Box 32T, Washington, OK 73093. 405–288-2458.

5. **Consulting Clinical and Microbiology Laboratories,** 1020 S.W. Taylor St., Suite 855, Portland, OR 97205.

6. **Diagnos-Techs, Inc.,** 66620 S. 192nd Place, Bldg. J-104, Kenton, WA 98032.

7. **Doctors Data, Inc.,** Box 111, 170 W. Roosevelt Rd., W. Chicago, IL 60185. 800–323-2784.

8. **Dowell Lab,** 99 S. Hibert St., Mesa, AZ 85210. 602–964-7151.

9. **Enviro-Health,** 990 N. Bowser Rd., #800, Richardson, TX 75081. 214–234-5577.

10. **Great Smokies Laboratory,** 18A Regent Park Blvd., Asheville, NC 28806. 800–522-4762.

11. **Immuno Labs,** Interstate Centre, 1620 W. Oakland Park Blvd., Ft. Lauderdale, FL 33311. 800–231-2197 or 305–486-4500. Fax 305–739-6563.

12. **Immunodiagnostic Laboratory, Inc.,** 488 McCormick St., San Leandro, CA 94577. 510–635-4545.

13. **Immunosciences Lab, Inc.,** 8730 Wilshire Blvd., #305, Beverly Hills, CA 90211. 310–657-1077.

14. **Meridian Valley Clinical Laboratory,** 132nd Ave., S.E., Kent, WA 98042. 206–631-8922. FAX 206–631-8691.

15. **Metametrix Medical Research Laboratory,** 5000 Peachtree Ind. Blvd., Norcross, GA 30071. 404–446-5483.

16. **SpectraCell Laboratories, Inc.,** 515 Post Oak Blvd., Suite 830, Houston, TX 77027. 713–621-3101. 800–227-5227. Fax 713–621-3234.

REFERENCES

1. Sandberg, D.H., "Gastrointestinal Complaints Related to Diet," *International Pediatrics*, 1990; 5:21–29.

2. Sehnert, K., *Immuno Review*, Immuno Labs, 1620 W. Oakland Park Blvd., Ft. Lauderdale, FL 33311, 1993; 1:1, 5, 6

3. Baker, S.M., McDonnell, M. and Truss, C., "Double-Blind Placebo-Diet Controlled Crossover Study of IgG Food ELISA." Presented at the American Academy of Environmental Medicine Advanced Seminar, Virginia Beach, VA, October 1994.

4. *Preventive Medicine Update*, Edited by Jeffrey S. Bland, Ph.D., CEO, HealthComm, Inc., P.O. Box 1729, Gig Harbor, WA 98335. 206–851-3943.

5. Travis, S. and Menzies, I., "Intestinal Permeability: Functional Assessment and Significance," *Clinical Science*, 1992; 82:471–488 as cited by Bland, J., Syllabus, Second International Symposium on Functional Medicine, March/April 1994, Rancho Mirage, CA, HealthComm, P.O. Box 1729, Gig Harbor, WA 98335.

6. Stollerman, G.H., "The Gold Standard," *Hospital Practice*, January 30, 1985; 20:9.

PART

EIGHT

Other Topics of Interest

39

◆

Thyroid and Adrenal Hormones

◆

During my many years of pediatric practice, I spent most of my time dealing with "routine" pediatric complaints. Included were such things as diaper rashes, infections, eating disorders, sleep problems and behavior problems.

Yet, my partners and I would see uncommon—even rare—disorders. Examples included leukemia (and other forms of cancer), juvenile diabetes, meningitis, intussusception, pyloric stenosis, glycogen storage disease of the liver and Addison's Disease. And we saw enough of these relatively uncommon diseases to keep us on our toes.

Hypothyroidism

One such disorder, *hypothyroidism* (too little thyroid), I saw no more often than once every five or ten years. This condition usually developed during the early days or weeks of life. Unless it was promptly recognized and appropriately treated with supplemental thyroid, the child would fail to thrive physically or mentally.

Even less frequently, I would see a child with *hyperthyroidism* (too much thyroid). The typical youngster with this sort of problem showed many characteristic symptoms, including rapid pulse, bulging eyes, weakness and weight loss. Yet, because I saw so few children with thyroid disorders in my practice, I never developed a special interest in them.

In the early '70s, I began to see adult patients with multiple health problems. Common complaints in these patients included headache, muscle aches, fatigue, depression and chemical sensitivities. Although many of these patients improved when they avoided hidden food allergens and got rid of the odorous chemicals in their homes, a number continued to experience symptoms.

I came across a book by Broda O. Barnes, M.D., which seemed to provide a part of the answer for some of these patients. It was entitled *Hypothyroidism: The Unsuspected Illness*.[1] In this book Dr. Barnes described his success in helping many of his patients with a thyroid supplement, even though their laboratory studies showed no evidence of hypothyroidism. Although Dr. Barnes' observations seemed interesting, I did not begin using thyroid supplements in my practice.

Then in the early '80s, one of my medical colleagues who shared my interest in food and chemical sensitivities and yeast-related health problems said:

> "I've found that some of my yeast patients are low in thyroid. You ought to try Dr. Broda Barnes' basal temperature test on some of your difficult patients. As you may know, he found that when people's underarm temperature is consistently under 97.8 before they get out of bed in the morning, they're usually deficient in thyroid. Supplemental thyroid hormone will provide them with a lot of help."

> ## I was pleased and delighted by the response of many of my patients to thyroid supplements.

So I began to look for thyroid deficiency and I was pleased and delighted by the response of many of my patients to thyroid supplements. I made a brief reference to Dr. Barnes' work in the third edition of *The Yeast Connection*[2] published over eight years ago. Included also was reference to another excellent book on the subject, *Solved: The Riddle of Illness,*[3] by Stephen E. Langer, M.D., with James F. Scheer.

During the late '80s and early '90s, I gradually phased out my adult practice and devoted more of my time to children, including those with behavior and learning problems. My interest in thyroid took a back seat until I began to gather information for this book. Then in 1993 and 1994, I interviewed a number of experienced candida clinicians who said that many of their yeast patients are also troubled by hormone deficiencies.

Observations of Alan Gaby, M.D., Baltimore, Maryland

At a presentation at the annual meeting of the American Holistic Medical Association in Kansas City, March 1993, Alan Gaby, M.D., AMHA president, said:

"There are five major techniques I use in my practice: cleaning up the diet, looking at food intolerance or allergies, using nutritional supplements, treating the microbiologic aspects of illness, including *Candida albicans* or other chronic infections and, last but not least, thyroid hormone therapy, following the teachings of the late Dr. Broda Barnes.

> **Subtle hypothyroidism is an extremely common condition in western society.**

"Subtle hypothyroidism is an extremely common condition in western society . . . Although most textbooks of internal medicines say that only 3% of the population are troubled by hypothyroidism, Dr. Broda Barnes said that 40% of the population have this problem. Somebody's right and somebody's wrong. I guess it depends on how you define the disorder.

"Although hypothyroidism is not picked up by the routine laboratory tests, I base my diagnosis on the clinical condition of the patient. I agree with what I read in a veterinarian textbook which said,

'If it looks like hypothyroidism, and smells and tastes and acts like hypothyroidism, then it is hypothyroidism until proven otherwise. And you ignore the laboratory tests.' "

In his continuing discussion, Gaby said that fatigue and depression are the two most common symptoms of hypothyroidism. Other symptoms include cold hands and feet, constipation, edema (puffiness or fluid accumulation), menstrual problems, muscle aches, gastrointestinal symptoms and infertility.

Comments of Keith Sehnert, M.D., Minneapolis, Minnesota

During the past decade, this Minnesota physician has treated over 3000 patients with yeast-related disorders. To learn more about his experiences, I called him in March 1994. Here are excerpts from our interview.

"In treating my patients, I see three circles intersecting: the candida infections, the hypothyroidism and the food allergies. All cause similar symptoms. I've especially observed that people with cold hands, cold feet and chilliness, as well as fatigue, are apt to be deficient in thyroid. I prefer Armour thyroid because it has some iodine in it in addition to T_3 and T_4.

"Although the diagnosis can often be made based on the patient's symptoms and the Barnes' low basal temperature test, I also use a laboratory test. I'm not talking about the T_3, T_4 and TSH tests which usually will be reported 'within normal limits.' I also use a thyroid antibody test (FAMA) provided by Ed Winger, M.D., at Immuno-Diagnostic Laboratories, San Leandro, California.

"I've developed a 50 question hypothyroid questionnaire and when that test score is high, I can almost guarantee you that the antibody test will be high. Moreover, Dr. Winger and other immunologists I've talked to tell me that positive findings on this test precede changes in the classic T_3, T_4 and TSH. And if these people go along without thyroid supplementation for seven or eight years, the other tests will start switching."

In an interview with Marjorie Hurt Jones, R.N., entitled, "Thyroid: New Insights,"[4] Sehnert reviewed his observations and stated that many people with hypothyroidism give a history of neck injuries, while others frequently show iodine deficiencies.*

In their discussion of endocrine problems, Jones raised the question of *hypoadrenal* function in hypothyroid patients. She cited the observations of Dr. William Jefferies, and then she asked Sehnert:

> "If the adrenals actually produce inadequate hormones, then supplementing them with low (physiologic) doses of replacement therapy should produce dramatic results similar to what you see when you give supplemental thyroid . . . Right?"

In his response, Dr. Sehnert agreed and pointed out that he sometimes gives his patients an adrenal supplement. And he said:

> "It's the old balancing act. We supplement the thyroid and/or the adrenals as part of trying to restore the delicate balance of the body. When we hit both dosages just right, it's like those patients just come alive. They not only feel more energetic, they seem brighter and more interested in activities—and life in general at all levels."

Comments of Jorge Flechas, M.D., Hendersonville, North Carolina

During the past decade, Dr. Flechas has developed an interest in patients with yeast-related health problems, chronic fatigue syndrome and related disorders. Moreover, he shared his knowledge with me on several occasions. To gain an update on his observations, I called him in early 1994. Here are excerpts of what he said.

---

*In a July 1994 letter Sehnert elaborated on his thoughts about iodine deficiencies. He said in effect, "I'm seeing many more cases of hypothyroidism than I saw 30 years ago. Part of this increase is due to the decreased intake of iodized salt by most Americans. Such a reduction in iodine may depress thyroid function." Like other of my consultants, Sehnert also emphasized the overuse of antibiotics, which causes chronic yeast infections and leads in turn to many kinds of endocrine problems.

"Although I help patients with yeast-related health problems using special diets and antiyeast medication, I'm increasingly impressed with patients who develop CFS or other health problems after some type of infectious disease that seems to go on and on. They're troubled by enlarged lymph nodes and high fevers and remain sick for months.

"One thing I've looked at is the problem known as *euthyroid sick syndrome. That's the problem of the inability of the body to convert thyroid T_4 into thyroid T_3. What seems to happen is that after the infection, your thyroid simply doesn't function as well as it should.*

If you're treating a patient for yeast infections and she is not responding . . . think about hormones.

"If you're treating a patient for yeast infections and she is not responding like she should to the traditional yeast treatment, then you have to start thinking about hormones that stimulate the immune system. Number one is thyroid T_3 and the other is DHEA from the adrenal.

"I use a preparation called Thyrolar. It's a combination of thyroid T_4 and T_3. You can help a lot of people using this product."

Comments of Ken Gerdes, M.D., Denver, Colorado

This board-certified specialist in internal medicine has, for over a decade, been interested in patients with food and chemical sensitivities. Dr. Gerdes has been a leading clinician in studying and treating patients with health problems related to *Candida albicans* and thyroid dysfunction. To obtain further information, I interviewed him in the spring of 1994. Here are excerpts from our conversation.

"In my experience many people, especially women, are deficient in thyroid and may be helped by thyroid supplementation. As you know, there are several different types of these products. One of these is Thyroxin, or T_4, which is available in synthetic form in a preparation called Synthroid.

"Then there's another preparation, liothyronine, which is a synthetic preparation of T_3 called Cytomel. There are also preparations of USP Thyroid which contain a combination of T_4 and T_3.*

"In studying my own patients, I use some of the traditional thyroid tests. Yet, I feel that some of those who show normal tests may also require supplemental thyroid. Following the lead of the late Dr. Broda Barnes, I use the basal temperature. Yet, rather than having the patient take the temperature under the arm, I ask them to measure it under the tongue for five minutes . . .

"The normal temperature curve is, as you know, lowest in the morning and peaks in the mid-afternoon, then comes back down in the evening. If a patient's temperature is consistently under 97.4 or 97.6 in the morning, I often prescribe T_3 (in addition to Armour thyroid tablets), and it seems to play an important role in helping my patients get better."

Comments of Elmer Cranton, M.D., Yelm, Washington

During the past 20 years, this board-certified family physician has served as my major consultant in a number of areas, including nutrition, allergies and yeast-related health problems. During a recent interview, in discussing hypothyroidism, he said:

"A number of patients with yeast-related health problems are helped by thyroid supplements. I've used Armour thyroid for my patients for the past 20 years. It contains both T_4 and T_3. I feel it is a safe, effective product for the great majority of these patients."

---

*According to the *Physicians' Desk Reference* (1993), page 1028, "Armour Thyroid Tablets (Thyroid Tablets, USP) for oral use are natural preparations derived from porcine thyroid glands. . . . They provide 38 mcg. of levothyroxine (T_4) and 9 mcg. liothyronine (T_3) per grain of thyroid."[5]

Comments of Richard Mabray, M.D., Victoria, Texas

This board-certified obstetrician/gynecologist has studied and treated patients with yeast-related health problems for over a decade. He's also been interested in food and chemical sensitivities and hormone dysfunction. To get an update on his observations, I called him in March 1994. Here's an excerpt from our interview.

"I've always believed that thyroid and other hormone problems were an important and often underrated part of many of our patients' problems. Recently I attended a meeting of the Broda Barnes, M.D., Research Foundation, Inc., in Chicago. Since then, I've begun to feel more comfortable in aggressively addressing the thyroid issue.

> **Thyroid and other hormone problems are an important and often underrated part of our patients' problems.**

"At this meeting, the European endocrinologist, Dr. Jacques Hertoghe, explained the benefits of the 24-hour urine test instead of the blood test for thyroid we usually do. He also showed a correlation between the axillary basal body temperatures with the urine results.

"Over the next few months, I got many of my patients to do the 24-hour urine test and I was amazed to see that virtually all of my symptomatic patients were low in thyroid . . .

"As important as these findings on paper were, the aggressive correction of thyroid problems, along with attention to the adrenal cortex (Cortef) and DHEA supplementation, has simply revolutionized the lives of most of my patients.

"The cornerstone of treatment in my polysymptomatic patient is a low-sugar diet, attention to allergies and some form of antifungal medication. Equally important is the use of various hormones.

"I am amazed at how often really tough problems resolve/improve within two to three weeks. In some patients, it may take much longer to normalize the thyroid. Virtually everybody seems to improve dramatically."

Comments of Elena McHerron, Poughkeepsie, New York

Physicians do not hold a monopoly on information about health! In fact, their patients, and other people, often possess knowledge which may be more important than reports in scientific journals or medical conferences. Much of what I've learned during the past decade has come from observations of nonprofessionals like McHerron.

She has sent me medical reprints, newsletters and press clippings which have provided me with information I hadn't obtained from other sources. Because I was so impressed by her observations, I invited her to become a member of the advisory board of the International Health Foundation. In July 1994, I asked her to review what I had written about thyroid dysfunction. She said:

"I think you should give your readers more specific advice for the administration of the Barnes temperature test for thyroid deficiency. Here are my suggestions.

"With this efficient self test, people can take their basal temperature. A range of 97.8 to 98.2 is considered normal for thyroid functioning efficiently. Menstruating women should take the readings the first three days of their period. It's a good idea to do this for a week or ten days. Throw out the high and low readings and get a good average. The self-temperature test also is useful for the person who is taking supplemental thyroid hormones. It helps her to be sure she is taking an optimal dose.

"I hope you'll give Pat Puglio of the Barnes Foundation more recognition for her part in the education of lay people in doctoring their way to health. She is responsible for the connection with Dr. Hertoghe in Belgium where hormone replacement is far more advanced.

"Quoting only doctors gives them a pedestal position, something the world needs to get away from. Why not give some validation from the clients?"

Information from Patricia A. Puglio, Trumbull, Connecticut

Following up on McHerron's suggestion, I called Pat Puglio. By Federal Express she sent me a cornucopia of articles, reprints and other information about hypothyroidism. Included was one of Dr. Barnes' articles in the peer-reviewed literature published in the *Journal of the American Medical Association* over 50 years ago! Its title, "Basal Temperature vs. Basal Metabolism." Here are brief excerpts from this article which is based on Dr. Barnes' study of over 1000 patients.

"Very few patients with subnormal temperature fail to respond to thyroid therapy, both as to relief of symptoms and as to elevation in temperature . . . Preliminary observations indicate the person with subnormal body temperature is perceptibly improved in its performance, whether in industry, in the classroom or on the athletic field by bringing his body temperature up to normal."[6]

Other articles by Dr. Barnes which Pat sent me included an article on the use of thyroid supplements in treating menstrual disorders[7] and another article in the distinguished British journal, *The Lancet*, which described the prophylaxis of coronary heart disease using thyroid therapy.[8] There was also a lot of other information, including a copy of the late Dr. Barnes' curriculum vitae. In addition to his M.D. degree, he received a doctorate in physiology from the University of Chicago and taught at a number of universities.

If you'd like to know more about Dr. Barnes and his work, send your request to Patricia A. Puglio, Director, Broda A. Barnes, M.D., Research Foundation, Inc., P.O. Box 98, Trumbull, CT 06611 (203-261-2101).

Nutritional Therapy and Hypothyroidism

No chronic health problem responds to a single "magic bullet." Although thyroid supplements often help the person with fatigue, low body temperature and other symptoms, they should not be looked on as "the answer."

Christine's Story

This 35-year-old woman had taken repeated courses of anti-biotics for respiratory and urinary infections during her twenties. Then as she passed thirty, she developed many persistent and disabling symptoms, including digestive problems, PMS, fatigue, headache and depression. In 1993, following a treatment program which featured a sugar-free special diet and powdered nystatin, she showed significant improvement. Yet, fatigue and constipation continued to bother her and her morning basal temperature was low (96.6 to 97 degrees).

Although her physician considered the use of thyroid therapy, he first recommended a vegetarian diet and vitamin/mineral supplements. After being on this program for two months, Christine's temperature readings returned to normal and her fatigue and digestive symptoms no longer bothered her.

Comments of Jeffrey Bland, Ph.D., Gig Harbor, Washington

During the past decade, much of what I've learned about nutrition, preventive medicine and functional medicine has come from Dr. Bland's monthly *Preventive Medicine Update* (audiocassette). A few days before I was scheduled to send the manuscript of this book to the typesetter, I received the December 1994 issue of *PMU*.

In commenting on people with apparent thyroid deficiency, at a conference at the Broda O. Barnes, M.D., Foundation some 12 years ago, Bland proposed that dysfunctional hypothyroidism may be due to the body's inability to convert T_4 into T_3. And he suggested that zinc, copper and selenium may influence the enzyme needed to make this conversion.

He also cited a recent study carried out by researchers in the Department of Pediatrics and Child Development at a medical school in Japan. This study showed a close relationship between zinc insufficiency and the lowered activity of the enzyme needed to convert T_4 to T_3.

In his continuing discussion, Bland said that evaluating zinc, copper and selenium status in the patient with symptoms of hypothyroidism may be important in developing a proper clinical management program. He also pointed out that not all of these patients need thyroid replacement therapy; some may simply need proper mineral balancing.

Adrenal Hormones

If you're like most Americans, you've heard of cortisone, prednisone, prednisolone, Medrol, triamcinolone, dexamethasone and other related steroid drugs. These medications came into prominence over 40 years ago.

At first they were publicized as true "wonder drugs." Here's why. They would make swollen arthritic joints return to normal, blocked breathing tubes open up and severe hives and other rashes disappear within a couple of days.

But, there was another side of the coin. When these drugs were given (in customary large doses) for long periods of time, they caused serious adverse effects, including impairment of immunity and osteoporosis. And in customary large doses, these drugs also encouraged the growth of *Candida albicans*.

Cortisol

About 10 years ago, a physician friend told me that a knowledgeable and experienced physician, William McK. Jefferies, had published numerous scientific articles and a book in which he recommended small physiologic doses of cortisone acetate, or *cortisol*.

Moreover, he said that Jefferies had found that such doses were safe and effective in patients with a variety of common complaints, including rheumatoid arthritis, allergic rhinitis, chronic fatigue syndrome, asthma and diabetes.

Yet, I didn't try to look up the articles or get a copy of Jefferies' book. Like most physicians, I felt steroids were "bad guys" when given over a long period of time. Then in the fall of 1993, Elizabeth Booker, the widow of my good friend and schoolmate, Armistead Page Booker, told me more about Dr. Jefferies. She said:

"I think you'll be interested in his observations on hydrocortisone. Bill has just come back to Charlottesville to live . . . You should get in touch with him."

So I wrote to Dr. Jefferies and he sent me a copy of his 1981 book, *Safe Uses of Cortisone.*[9] Yet, somehow I did not carefully review it until Pat Puglio* sent me another copy, along with a superb 1994 paper by Dr. Jefferies entitled, "Mild Adrenocortical Deficiency, Chronic Allergies, Autoimmune Disorders and the Chronic Fatigue Syndrome: A Continuation of the Cortisone Story."

The Observations of Dr. William McK. Jefferies, Charlottesville, Virginia

In his fascinating article, which presented some of the highlights of his book, this endocrine system researcher said:

"In most endocrine disorders, varying degrees of deficiency of hormones are recognized, but deficiency of cortisol is classified only as Addison's Disease or hypopituitarism, both relatively severe and relatively rare disorders. The possibility that milder degrees of adrenocortical deficiency . . . might exist has not received much attention."

---

*In mid-October 1994, as I was putting the finishing touches on this book, I met Pat Puglio at the Annual Conference of the American Academy of Environmental Medicine, held in Virginia Beach, Virginia. I was impressed with her knowledge and her dedication in bringing Dr. Barnes' observations to both professionals and nonprofessionals.

At this same conference, I heard a number of superb presentations on *"the often overlooked important role of endocrine dysfunction in the difficult patient."* Included were two lectures by the Keynote Speaker, Jacques Hertoghe, M.D., of Antwerp, Belgium. The first of these lectures was entitled "The Insidious Role of Thyroid Dysfunction in the Difficult Patient," and, the second lecture was entitled "The Critical Role of Female Hormone Dysfunction in Difficult, Premenopausal and Postmenopausal Patients."

Other lecturers on this special day included Jonathan Wright, M.D., Richard Wilkinson, M.D., Russell Reiter, Ph.D., Mary Ann Block, D.O. and William Rea, M.D. You can obtain more information about Dr. Hertoghe's work from the Broda O. Barnes, M.D., Research Foundation and information about tapes of these various presentations by writing to the American Academy of Environmental Medicine, 4510 West 89th Street, Prairie Village, KS 66207.

> # *The possibility that milder degrees of adrenocortical deficiency . . . might exist has not received much attention.*

Jefferies pointed out that although most clinical experience in giving these drugs:

". . . has involved the administration of large pharmacologic dosages with subsequent propensity for the development of undesirable or even alarming side effects . . . Beneficial effects of small subreplacement, safe, physiologic dosages of cortisol were initially reported in 1958 in the treatment of women with ovarian dysfunction and infertility."

In his continuing discussion, Jefferies said that he had published in peer-reviewed journals observations describing his success in treating patients with ovarian dysfunction, allergies, rheumatoid arthritis and other conditions with small, safe doses of cortisol. Yet, he said:

"Still no attempts to extend or confirm these observations appeared . . . (Accordingly) a unique situation in which a normal hormone, one that is essential for life, has developed such a bad reputation that many physicians and patients are afraid to use it under any circumstances."

In a further discussion of cortisol, Jefferies said:

"Cortisol (hydrocortisone) is a normal hormone which is essential for life in humans. Its most obvious effect is to . . . provide energy and avoid hypoglycemia at times when food intake is limited, but it also helps to protect against other stresses, including the maintenance of normal immunity.
"In the treatment of adrenal deficiency in our practice, a schedule of four times daily before meals and at bedtime, has been found to have several advantages . . . Dosages of 2.5 mg. to 7.5 mg., four

times daily, are satisfactory maintenance dosages, depending upon the degree of deficiency. Therapeutic trials with such dosages of cortisol would seem to be indicated in patients with chronic fatigue syndrome.

"A noticeable improvement usually occurs within a few hours of the first dose and patients often describe the return of symptoms within a few hours of a missed dose. Occasionally, improvement is not noticed until 10 to 14 days after treatment is begun.

"Patients have been treated with this schedule of cortisol or cortisone acetate for as long as 40 years without significant problems. . . . There is . . . no reason to fear that physiologic [small] doses of cortisol will produce any of the harmful side effects of pharmacological doses [emphasis added]."

In his concluding comments, Jefferies said:

"With the evidence that at least some patients with chronic allergies, autoimmune disorders, and unexplained chronic fatigue, including the 'chronic fatigue syndrome' have mild adrenocortical deficiency, further studies of the above therapeutic approach seem indicated. Such studies will hopefully no longer be handicapped by misconceptions that have resulted largely from the unique combination of factors that have been discussed."[10]

Comments of Sidney M. Baker, Weston, Connecticut

In April 1994, this candida pioneer made the following comments about Jefferies work.

"The endocrine factor I'm most enthusiastic about is finding people described by endocrinologist Dr. William Jefferies—those with mild adrenal insufficiency. As you know, the late Dr. Hans Selye began talking about stress-related adrenal insufficiency 25 years ago after studying soldiers on the battlefield found dead from exhaustion who had no bullet holes in them.

"Jefferies, a researcher with impeccable academic credentials, came along and said in effect, *'Although you can do a lot of complicated tests to check on adrenal function, one of the easiest ways to determine adrenal insufficiency is to give a patient five to 10 mg. of hydrocortisone, four times daily for two weeks.'*

I can't believe I'm a new person.

"I've done this on a number of patients who've come back and said, 'I can't believe I'm a new person.' *In the normal person the daily output of hydrocortisone from the adrenal glands is perhaps 40 milligrams. Accordingly, if you give a tired, depressed, weak person 5, 10 or 15 milligrams and they feel like a new person, it is because they had insufficiency and now you've brought them up to normal.*

"I think Jefferies' follow-up of Selye's work and interpreting it to the medical profession in a perfectly straight-forward way is really a major contribution. I consider this approach in every patient I see with a complex chronic illness. And perhaps one time out of ten that I try it, I get a 'bull's eye.'

"In such patients, I keep them on the small dose of hydrocortisone for six months or so. Then I tell them, 'Look, you're going to run into doctors who won't believe you and they'll think this is nonsense and they'll want you to stop taking it.'

"I've found that there are certain people who can take small doses of hydrocortisone for six months and then stop it and they're fine. But there are others who are constitutionally adrenal insufficient. Such problems are especially seen in women with extra hair and acne and they may need some adrenal replacement therapy indefinitely.

"I used to do a lot of lab studies, but I no longer think they are always necessary. Incidentally, I met Jefferies several years ago and heard him talk and the lights went on in my head. His book is wonderful.

"He pointed out that some people whose lab studies show a supposedly normal adrenal profile were treated with the low dose hydrocortisone and they got better."

Further Comments by Elena McHerron

In discussing adrenal dysfunction, she said, "Pantothenic acid and vitamin C are natural extracts for assisting the adrenals . . . no prescription is necessary. I've used them for several years and they do help. Some people who write and call tell me this is all they need."

DHEA (Dehydroepiandrosterone)

I first heard DHEA discussed by Dr. Julian Whitaker at a conference of the American College of Advancement in Medicine in November 1992. I learned more about DHEA from several of my consultants and from an article by Dr. Whitaker.

Comments of Julian Whitaker, M.D., Newport Beach, California

In the February 1994 issue of his newsletter, *Health & Healing*, Dr. Julian Whitaker discussed this hormone with the big name (dehydroepiandrosterone). And he said:

> "DHEA is the 'mother' hormone produced by the adrenal gland. Your body readily converts it on demand into active hormones such as estrogen (and progesterone) . . . In addition, DHEA . . . decline signals age-related disease."

In his continuing discussion, Dr. Whitaker cited research studies by Elizabeth Barrett-Conner, M.D., of the University of California School of Medicine in San Diego who studied 5000 women. She found that those who developed breast cancer had subnormal urinary excretion of DHEA metabolites as long as nine years prior to the development of the disease.

He also cited the research studies of Eugene Roberts, M.D., who found that elderly volunteers with moderate memory loss who took DHEA supplements scored higher on two of the four measurements than those who received a placebo. And he commented:

> "DHEA blood levels are easily measured, and I often prescribe supplementation to bring a patient's blood levels up to a healthier level of 20-to-30-year olds. I am surprised at how low the blood levels of DHEA are in some patients who are ill with heart disease, diabetes or cancer. In addition, it also surprises me that so few doctors measure DHEA blood levels and prescribe supplementation . . .
>
> "There is no patent on DHEA, so no drug company is interested in promoting it as therapy. Consequently, it languishes on the shelf and many doctors are under the impression it is illegal. Though it is not

'approved' by the FDA for any specific medical condition, it is without question legal. Any doctor can prescribe it . . .

> **I've been using DHEA in my patients for some time now, with sometimes startling results.**

"*I've been using DHEA in my patients for some time now, with sometimes startling results. In fact, I cannot imagine practicing medicine without it* [emphasis added]. You do need a prescription for DHEA. For a list of DHEA references and pharmacies that compound DHEA, send a long, self-addressed stamped envelope to Phillips Publishing, Customer Service–DHEA, 7811 Montrose Rd., Potomac, MD 20854."[11]

Comments by Dr. Cranton

"DHEA supports your whole endocrine system and it's a raw material from which several steroid hormones are made. I've found it helps people with chronic health problems of many sorts. I often do a DHEA blood test to check levels and any reference lab can do the test.

"Even if people do not have a lab test, it doesn't hurt to take it. However, the lab test will help keep you from taking too much. I myself take 50 mg. time-released DHEA once a day."

Comments by Dr. Flechas

"A lot of my chronically ill patients, including those with chronic fatigue syndrome and yeast-related problems, show grossly abnormal blood DHEA levels.

"Supportive evidence for the importance of DHEA was published recently in the *American Journal of Obstetrics and Gynecology* by researchers at the University of Tennessee who found that in physiologic doses, DHEA modulates immune function in postmenopausal women."

In his continuing comments, Dr. Flechas said:

"I saw a woman recently with recurrent vaginal yeast infections. She tried everything, including Diflucan and Nizoral and Terazol vaginal creams. She was also troubled by dry skin and DHEA controls oil production of the skin.

"So we did a DHEA Sulfate level on her and the level was something like 43. (Ideally this hormone level should be 200 mcg. per dl.) So I put her on the hormone and when I saw her two months later she was much, much better. The use of Terazol was down to one day per month.

"I learned about DHEA from Dr. Guy Abraham, who was one of the original investigators. You'll find good supportive evidence in an article by Parker, 'Evidence for Adrenocortical Adaptations of Severe Illness'[12] and in the 1993 article by Dr. Peter Casson and associates from the University of Tennessee."

Additional Comments

After receiving this information from Dr. Flechas, I got a copy of the Casson article, "Oral dehydroepiandrosterone in physiologic doses modulates immune function in postmenopausal women."

These researchers carried out a randomized, double-blind crossover study of 11 patients. Some were given DHEA while others were given a placebo. In commenting on the results of their study, these investigators said:

"These findings suggest that DHEA may have immune modulatory functions . . . and most importantly enhancement of natural killer number and cell cytotoxicity . . . These data provide strong rationale for further study of DHEA replacement in adrenal androgen deficiency states, particularly in older women."[13]

I found further comments about the value of DHEA in the May 1994 newsletter of the Well Mind Association of Greater Washington, Inc. (WMAGW), 1141 Georgia Ave., Suite 326, Wheaton, MD 20902.

In a brief report entitled, "The Bright Promise of DHEA," WMAGW president and editor, John Stegmaier, commented on a

February 1994 lecture by Dr. Alan R. Gaby who cited a number of the benefits of this hormone. Included among these benefits were help for women at menopause.

DHEA was also said to "work wonders" in the elderly who were given 5 or 10 mg. a day. In such individuals, appetites returned, concentration improved and back pains abated.

It has also proved useful in people with chemical sensitivities, rheumatoid arthritis, lupus, chronic fatigue syndrome, ulcerative colitis and Crohn's disease.

REFERENCES

1. Barnes, B.O., with Dalton, L., *Hypothyroidism: The Unsuspected Illness*, Harper and Rowe, New York, 1976.
2. Crook, W.G., *The Yeast Connection*, Third Edition, Professional Books, Jackson, TN and Vintage Books, New York, 1986; p 244.
3. Langer, S.E. with Scheer, J.F., *Solved: The Riddle of Illness*, Keats Publishing, New Canaan, CT, 1984.
4. Jones, M.H., "Thyroid: New Insights," *Mastering Food Allergies*, May/June 1994, MAST Enterprises, Inc., 2614 N. 4th St., #616, Coeur d'Alene, ID 83814.
5. *Physicians' Desk Reference* (PDR), 47th Edition, "Armour Thyroid Tablets," 1993; p 1028.
6. Barnes, B.O., "Basal Temperature vs. Basal Metabolism," *JAMA*, 1942; 119:1072–74.
7. Barnes, B.O., "The Treatment of Menstrual Disorders in General Practice," *Arizona Medicine*, 1949; 6:33–34.
8. Barnes, B.O., "Prophylaxis of Ischaemic Heart Disease by Thyroid Therapy," *The Lancet*, 1959; 149–152.
9. Jefferies, W.M., *Safe Uses of Cortisone*, Charles C. Thomas, Springfield, IL, 1981.
10. Jefferies, W.M., "Mild Adrenocortical Deficiency, Chronic Allergies, Autoimmune Disorders and the Chronic Fatigue Syndrome: A Continuation of the Cortisone Story," *Medical Hypotheses*, 1994; 42:183–189.
11. Whitaker, J., *Health & Healing*, Phillips Publishing Co., Inc., 7811 Montrose Rd., Potomac, MD 20854, 1994; Vol. 4, No. 1, pp 5, 8.
12. Parker, "Evidence for Adrenocortical Adaptations of Severe Illness," *J. of Clin. Endo. and Metab.*, 1993; 60:947–952.
13. Casson, P., "Oral dehydroepiandrosterone in physiologic doses modulates immune function in postmenopausal women," *Am. J. Obstet. Gynecol.*, 1993; Vol. 169, pp 15–36.

40

---◆---

Progesterone and Estrogen Therapy

---◆---

Fools rush in where angels fear to tread!

Perhaps it *is* foolish and presumptuous for a pediatrician to talk about women's hormones. Yet, because of information I have received during the past year, I felt I could not do otherwise. My discussion will focus almost entirely on progesterone therapy.

As a pediatrician, I saw children of all ages from birth on through adolescence. But, when teenage girls developed persistent menstrual, or other problems related to their hormones, I always sought the help and consultation of a gynecologist.

Like all physicians, I knew that the ovaries produced estrogens; the level of these hormones rose rapidly, beginning at the time of menstruation; estrogens peaked in 10 to 14 days at the time of ovulation and then rapidly declined; progesterone (produced by the corpus luteum) "took over" and levels of this hormone rose rapidly, as estrogen levels declined, then fell rapidly again the week before menstruation.

Estrogen Replacement Therapy (ERT)

During my practice of pediatrics and allergy in the '50s, '60s and '70s, I had little interest in hormone-related problems in women. Then, in 1979, after learning from Dr. C. Orian Truss about the relationship of superficial yeast infections to women's health problems, I began reading articles and books about hormones.

As I dug into these materials, I realized that the female endocrine system is complex, and that gynecologists, and other physicians, held different opinions about estrogen replacement therapy (ERT).

I had known for many years that estrogens were often prescribed to control hot flashes, insomnia, vaginal dryness and other symptoms. They were also recommended by many physicians to lessen the ravages of osteoporosis and to protect the heart.

Moreover, my gynecologist brother, Angus Crook, urged my late mother to take Premarin (an estrogen) to help control her severe osteoporosis. Yet, when he made that recommendation she was in her sixties and didn't want to cope with side effects, including the possible resumption of menstruation. Many other gynecologists and family physicians during the '60s and '70s prescribed ERT.

According to Sadja Greenwood, M.D., in some middle-class areas more than half of the postmenopausal women used ERT in 1975.[1] Then, according to Greenwood, reports began to appear in the medical literature which showed that women who took ERT were found to have a five times greater chance of developing uterine cancer. So the use of estrogen declined rapidly.

Then, a few years later, new studies showed that the addition of a progestin for 12 to 14 days at the end of each 25 day course of estrogen, would protect women against uterine cancer. So physicians again began to prescribe postmenopausal hormones. Yet, the use of such hormones continues to stir up controversy.

In a 1993 booklet, *Taking Hormones and Women's Health: Choices, Risks and Benefits,* published by the National Women's Health Network (NWHN), the authors commented:

"Menopause does not automatically require 'treatment.' We are critical of the routine prescribing of hormones for healthy women because of the known risks associated with the drugs used and the lack of complete data on risks and benefits. These drugs are potent and increase the possibility of users developing some cancers and other diseases."

This booklet urged all health practitioners to be cautious about prescribing hormone replacement until the long-term effects of these drugs are known. And they said that findings must be "constantly re-evaluated." In discussing osteoporosis, they said:

> "While taking estrogen may prevent fractures in some women, it is important to note that bone loss is not the only important factor in fractures. For example, in carefully controlled studies, women with and without hip fractures were found to have similar bone densities. Other studies have found that age has a greater influence on the hip fracture than does bone density . . . Few educational efforts have emphasized that smoking and heavy drinking each independently increase the risk of fractures."[2]

Progesterone

The NWHN booklet also discussed combined hormone therapy with estrogen and a progestogen—a synthetic form of progesterone. They said that this combination is both "good and bad." In supporting this point of view, they cited studies which indicate that women using combined therapy are less likely to get endometrial cancer. Other studies, however, showed that women on combined therapy may be more prone to develop heart disease. And they said there are not adequate studies of large groups of women that can be used to verify either position.

Natural Progesterone

About the same time as I read the report from NWHN, I picked up a 1993 book entitled, *Unmasking PMS—The complete medical treatment plan* by Joseph Martorano, M.D., and Maureen Morgan, CSW, R.N., with William Fryer.[3] I was, of course, pleased to see that the authors recommended dietary changes and nystatin for women with a variety of problems, including PMS, fatigue, depression, food sensitivities, inability to concentrate and other symptoms.

In their book, they included an eight-page chapter on natural progesterone. In their discussion, they said that natural progesterone, extracted from yams or soybeans, is chemically identical to progesterone produced naturally by the body.

> **They reviewed the observations of
> Dr. Katharina Dalton, who began treating
> PMS with natural progesterone in the
> 1950s with excellent results.**

They reviewed the observations of Dr. Katharina Dalton,[4] who began treating PMS with natural progesterone in the 1950s with excellent results. They pointed out that one of the problems with natural progesterone was that effective oral forms weren't available. Accordingly, it had to be given by rectal or vaginal suppositories or solutions.

Although a number of physicians and patients used these forms of progesterone, its administration was inconvenient and led to poor compliance. Then the authors pointed out that oral micronized tablets of progesterone became available in the late 1980s. It was said to be "a giant step forward" in treating many of their patients with PMS. Over 80% of their patients who were receiving progesterone were being treated with this oral preparation. Their usual starting dose was 300 mg. of the time-released oral tablet, twice a day. Some patients needed considerably more and some considerably less.

I obtained additional information about oral progesterone from an article published by Vanderbilt University Medical Center researchers in the *American Journal of Obstetrics and Gynecology*. In this article, Joel T. Hargrove and colleagues described their experiences in studying micronized progesterone. Here are excerpts from the abstract of their study.

"The oral route of progesterone administration has long been considered impractical because of poor absorption and short biologic half-life. Recent reports suggest that micronization of progesterone enhances absorption and increases serum and tissue levels of progesterone . . . Progesterone was plain milled, micronized, plain milled in oil, micronized in oil, or micronized in enteric-coated capsules. All patients exhibited a significant increase in serum progesterone levels after oral progesterone administration . . .

"Contrary to traditional teaching, these data show that significant serum progesterone levels can be achieved by oral administration. Absorption can be significantly improved by the physical characteristics of the progesterone and the vehicle used with oral administration."[5]

In 1994 I learned more from a fascinating book, *Natural Progesterone: the Multiple Roles of a Remarkable Hormone,*[6] by John R. Lee, M.D. I obtained still further information from a discussion of natural progesterone by Dr. Lee and Jeffrey Bland, Ph.D., in the March 1994 audiocassette edition of *Preventive Medicine Update.*

In his interview with Bland, Lee tells how he became interested in natural progesterone. Although to get the whole story you'll have to read his book, here are some of the highlights. In discussing progesterone and progesterone-like substances, Lee said that they had been found in over 500 plants, including the wild yam root. And he said that he had been in practice long enough to realize that estrogen, along with calcium and vitamin D, wasn't the complete answer for osteoporosis.

Lee subsequently learned that progesterone could be given in the form of over-the-counter skin creams or patches. Using these natural progesterone products, he noted that many of his own patients felt a lot better—less breast pain and fatigue, more energy and a return of normal libido.

During his subsequent 20 years of practice, Lee noted consistent benefits in his patients from natural progesterone therapy. In his book he discusses the various functions of progesterone, which include serving as a precursor hormone for the synthesis of many other hormones, especially the sex hormones, estrogen and thyroid hormones.

Lee repeatedly emphasized the differences between *natural progesterone* and the *progestogens.* And he said that the latter hormones, such as *Provera,* while heavily advertised, can and do cause many side effects—and that such side effects are *not* caused by natural progesterone. He also said that many physicians mistakenly believe that natural progesterone may cause the same side effects as *Provera*.

Natural Progesterone and PMS

In his continuing discussion with Bland, Lee said:

> "Treatment of PMS has, in the past, included diuretics, tranquilizers, dietary changes, aerobic exercises, psychiatric counseling, thyroid supplements, acupuncture and vitamin/mineral supplements. While each may provide some symptomatic improvement, it is clear that proper treatment still eludes discovery."[7]

Then he said that he had found that natural progesterone provides significant help for premenopausal women. Symptoms, including premenstrual irritability, water retention, depression and loss of libido, would often lessen or disappear.

Yet, in his interview with Bland, Lee said that progesterone isn't a "quick fix." It is important for menstruating women to use it in such a way that it matches their normal menstrual cycle. He also said if they do not use it at the appropriate time of their cycle, they'll develop irregular bleeding. I received additional information about natural progesterone therapy from Jean Rowe, R.N., of Denver. She told me that micronized oral progesterone in a dose of 50 to 100 mg. twice daily helped many women with various health problems, including PMS.*

In her comprehensive 1994 book, *Women's Bodies, Women's Wisdom*,[8] Dr. Christiane Northrup said that natural progesterone works well with women whose major premenstrual symptom is a migraine-type headache. Although it may sometimes cause intermittent menstrual spotting, or delay the period, she said that there are no serious side effects with this hormone in usual doses.

Like Dr. Lee, Dr. Northrup emphasized the differences between natural progesterone and the synthetic progestogens. Unfortunately, many women are told that the synthetic progestins are the

---

* For more of Rowe's comments see Chapter 11.

same as progesterone. In her discussion, she also emphasized the role emotional, psychological and nutritional factors play in hormonal control.

> ## Dr. Northrup emphasized the differences between natural progesterone and the synthetic progestogens.

Natural Progesterone and the Prevention of Osteoporosis

In the early 1980s, I met Betty Kamen, Ph.D., at a health food convention. At subsequent conventions, I heard her speak on a variety of topics. I was impressed by the scope and depth of her knowledge on many different subjects. Then, several years ago on a trip to San Francisco, I had lunch with Betty and her husband, Si, and at that time she sent me articles on various subjects, including FOS, a healthy sweetener.[9]*

Then, at a health food convention in Columbus, Ohio, in March 1994, I came across her latest book, *Hormone Replacement Therapy, Yes or No?* In this fantastic book she told me a lot of things I needed to know. In the introduction of the book, Serafina Corsello, M.D., said:

> "Betty Kamen produced this most comprehensive, magnificent review of the physiology and pathology of the female reproductive cycle . . . As usual, she provides an incredible number of references which can be used by the reader for further research."[10]

Betty's books are well indexed and well documented. I was so impressed with this book that I bought a copy for each of my three daughters! In her chapter on natural progesterone, she reviews the observations of Dr. Lee. She also cites the scientific reports of Jerilynn Prior, M.D., of the Endocrinology and Metabolism Division of the University of British Columbia, who found that natural proges-

---

*See Chapter 27

terone helped prevent and treat osteoporosis. She cites the following observations of Dr. Prior which were published in the *Canadian Journal of OB/GYN* and *Women's Health Care:*

"Progesterone binds to receptors on osteoblasts, increases the rate of bone formation and remodelling when given therapeutically to oophorectomized dogs [dogs whose ovaries are removed] and slows bone loss in postmenopausal women. Progesterone acts on bone, even though estrogen activity is low or absent. Because progesterone appears to work on the osteoblasts to increase bone formation, it would complement the actions of estrogen to decrease bone resorption."[11]

Just before sending the manuscript of my book to the typesetter, I picked up the November 1994 issue of *Prevention*. In the "healthfront" section of this magazine, they cited the observations of Dr. Prior, which were published in the June 1994 issue of the *American Journal of Medicine*.[12] I obtained a copy of this report from the Jackson-Madison County General Hospital library.

Here's a summary of Dr. Prior's comments and the findings of a study carried out by her research team.

She said osteoporosis begins developing in some women in their 30s who have irregular menstrual cycles. Such women may not be ovulating and as a result there may be a lack of progesterone.

In her research study Prior gave progesterone for ten days a month, plus one gram of calcium to 61 women with menstrual cycle disturbances. As a result, the bone density in these women increased by 2%. By contrast, 14 women who were given placebo (blank) pills along with the calcium, lost 2% of their bone density during the year of the study.

I found further support for the role of natural progesterone in preventing and treating osteoporosis from Dr. Christiane Northrup's book, *Women's Bodies, Women's Wisdom*.[13] In a discussion of osteoporosis, she said that although most women start to think of bone loss only at menopause, it often begins years before. In her discussion, she cited the observations of Drs. Lee and Prior and she said that osteoporosis has been reversed in women as much as 16 years past menopause using natural progesterone in combination with other dietary factors and exercise.

Comments by Health Professionals

To learn more about hormone therapy in women, I talked to a number of health professionals, including Dr. C. Orian Truss. He told me that hormone dysfunction will often disappear following anticandida therapy. Moreover, in his book, *The Missing Diagnosis*, he said:

> "By unknown mechanisms progesterone greatly aggravates yeast growth in women . . . Also, women with chronic yeast vaginitis usually are aware that their symptoms are worse from ovulation to the next period, coinciding with the interval of increased progesterone production in the monthly cycle . . . Hormone administration not only fails to correct the problem, but indeed may aggravate it. The endocrine system is complex, and the administration of one hormone affects the function and production of the other endocrine glands . . . Rather than by attempted hormone administration, correction of these abnormalities is better left to nature."[14]

Other health professionals I talked to, including several who treat yeast-related health problems, supported the use of natural progesterone. Here's an excerpt of my conversation with Carol Jessop, M.D.

Crook: Dr. Jessop, tell me a little bit about your experiences in using natural progesterone.

Jessop: I don't know how to do it in any easy way, but I'll tell you a little bit about my experiences. Because a lot of women felt depressed and developed other symptoms following synthetic progesterone preparations, I started using natural progesterone about ten years ago. I feel it's a lot safer.

For a while I used it only in suppositories, then the Women's International Pharmacy started making it in tablets that the liver didn't break down and activate. Now they have micronized little capsules and I usually use 300 mg. twice daily.

I've found it especially helpful in women with PMS and I start it about the time a woman ovulates. I also use it in combination with estrogen in postmenopausal women. Often I use estrogen and progesterone creams mixed together that can be rubbed on the thighs or the arms. Many women prefer this rather than taking other forms of medication.

Here also are comments by George Miller, M.D., a Lewisburg, Pennsylvania, gynecologist.

"My feeling about progesterone is that as long as it does its job . . . that is protecting the lining of endometrium from estrogen overload . . . it doesn't really matter which one you use, as long as the patient's okay with it. Insofar as natural progesterone, I think you should tell women who read your book that they should individualize their treatment program with their doctor.

"Baby boomers' experiences with menopause will likely lead to more useful knowledge concerning hormones. But for those sensitive individuals who cannot tolerate the 'traditional' drugs, alternatives are genuinely needed. I look forward to the future as more research comes to the front and more is learned about how our bodies work and what we need to replace that our present environment has stolen from us. I think this segment you have put together is very good, well thought out and will be food for thought for many readers."

I also talked with a nurse practitioner (R.N.) who works with a gynecologist. She told me that, in their practice, a number of women with chronic yeast problems and endometriosis had been helped by antifungal medication and a sugar-free diet. They had found natural progesterone helped a lot of women using oral micronized progesterone at a dose of 300 mg. in the morning and 600 mg. in the evening for 14 days out of the cycle.

Yet, she said that she was disappointed that more scientific studies had not been carried out to show that natural progesterone was safer and better than the synthetics.

Progesterone Immunotherapy

One of the pioneers in using a low-dose method of immunotherapy was my long-time friend, Joseph B. Miller, M.D.* of Mobile, Alabama. In 1974, this board-certified pediatrician, allergist and immunologist published a report in the *Journal of the Alabama State Medical Association* which described the use of tiny "neutralizing" doses of progesterone. In his paper, he reported his experiences in treating women with painful menstruation, PMS, contraceptive tablet intolerance and nausea and vomiting of early pregnancy.[15]

Following Dr. Miller's lead, Wayne Konetzki** of Waukesha, Wisconsin, began to treat and help many of his patients using these tiny doses of progesterone. So did hundreds of other physicians, many of whom were fellows or members of the American Academy of Environmental Medicine*** or the American Academy of Otolaryngic Allergy.

Although Miller reported his observations in the peer-reviewed medical literature, most allergists did not use them and they have never gained wide acceptance.

My Comments

I realize that I have barely scratched the surface in discussing progesterone and estrogen therapy. Moreover, I have many more questions than answers. From what I've read and heard during the past year, supplemental natural progesterone seems to help many women with PMS and/or menopausal symptoms. It may also play an important role in preventing osteoporosis.

Obviously, natural progesterone isn't a "quick fix" and its use should be only one part of a program which includes a good diet,

---

* Dr. Miller published his observations in the peer-reviewed literature and in several books.
** For additional comments about Dr. Konetzki's observations see Chapter 12.
*** Formerly the Society of Clinical Ecology.

exercise and nutritional supplements. *Finally, it must be prescribed and monitored by your physician.**

REFERENCES

1. Greenwood, S., *Menopause Naturally*, Volcano Press, Volcano, CA 1992; p 99.
2. National Women's Health Network, Washington, DC, *"Taking Hormones and Women's Health: Choices, Risks and Benefits,"* Third Edition, 1993; pp 2–3, 6.
3. Martorano, J., *Unmasking PMS—The complete PMS medical treatment plan*, M. Evans and Company, New York, 1993.
4. Dalton, K., *The Premenstrual Syndrome and Progesterone Therapy*, Second Edition, Yearbook Publishing, Inc., Chicago, IL, 1984.
5. Hargrove, J.T., Maxson, W.S., Wentz, A.C. and Burnett, L.S., "Menopausal Hormone Replacement Therapy with Continuous Daily Oral Micronized Estradiol and Progesterone," *Am. J. of Obstet. Gynecol.*, 1989; 73:606–612.
6. Lee, J.R., *Natural Progesterone: the Multiple Roles of a Remarkable Hormone*, BLL Publishing Company, P.O. Box 2068, Sebastapol, CA 95473, 1993.
7. Lee, J.R. and Bland, J., *Preventive Medicine Update* (audiocassette), HealthComm, Inc., 5800 Soundview Dr., Gig Harbor, WA 98335 (1-800-843-9660).
8. Northrup, C., *Women's Bodies, Women's Wisdom*, Bantam Books, New York, 1994; pp 452–453.
9. Kamen, B., "FOS: A Healthful Sweetener (No Kidding!)," *Let's Live*, 1992; pp 32–34.
10. Kamen, B., *Hormone Replacement Therapy, Yes or No?* Nutrition Encounter, Box 5487, Novato, CA 94948, 1993; pp 109–124.
11. Prior, J.C., Bigna, Y., and Alojada, N., "Progesterone and the Prevention of Osteoporosis," *Canadian Journal of OB/GYN* and *Women's Health Care*, 1991; 3:181.

---

*Further information about natural progesterone can be obtained from the books by Lee, Kamen, Martorano, Northrup and from Women's Health Connection, P.O. Box 6338, Madison, WI 53716–0338.

Prescriptions for micronized oral progesterone can be obtained from a number of pharmacies, including Wellness, Health and Pharmaceuticals, 2800 S. 18th St., Birmingham, AL 35209 (1-800-227-2627); Madison Pharmacy Associates, 429 Gammon Place, P.O. Box 9641, Madison, WI 53715 (1-800-558-7046); Women's International Pharmacy, 5708 Monona Dr., Madison, WI 53716–3152 (1-800-279-5708); College Pharmacy, 833 N. Tejon St., Colorado Springs, CO (1-800-888-9358).

12. Prior, J.C., et al "Cyclic medroxyprogesterone treatment increases bone density: a controlled trial in active women with menstrual cycle disturbances," *Am. J. Med.*, 1994; 96 (6):521–530.
13. Northrup, C., *Women's Bodies, Women's Wisdom*, Bantam Books, New York, 1994; pp 452–453.
14. Truss, C.O., *The Missing Diagnosis*, P.O. Box 26508, Birmingham, AL 35226; pp 30–31.
15. Miller, J.B., "Relief of Premenstrual Symptoms, Dysmenorrhea and Contraceptive Tablet Intolerance," *J. Med. Assoc., St. of Alabama*, 1974; pp 44–57.

41

Parasites

During my many years of pediatric practice, I saw a lot of children with pinworms. As you may know, these thread-like critters live mainly in the rectum. They crawl out at night and lay microscopic-size eggs and deposit them in the folds around the anus. As a result, the child scratches his/her bottom. Then, when fingers are put in the mouth and the eggs swallowed, another crop of pinworms develop.

Although pinworms would occasionally cause more serious health problems, including appendicitis, I generally considered them a nuisance.

Also, I saw an occasional child with roundworms (*Ascaris lumbricoides*) and a few who were infested with the microscopic-size parasite, *Giardia lamblia*. Yet, to a large degree, I ignored the possible role of parasites in making my patients sick, both at that time and after I learned about yeast-related health problems.

In the mid-1980s, I began hearing more about parasites from several sources. One of these sources was Sally Harvey, R.N., who at that time staffed the hotline at the International Health Foundation. Another source of information was a discussion of parasites by Warren Levin, M.D., of New York and Jeffrey Bland, Ph.D., in *Preventive Medicine Update*.[1]

At the 1988 Candida Update Conference in Memphis, Dr. Leo Galland reported that many patients with yeast-related health problems also were infested with parasites.

In 1989, Dr. Galland and a colleague, Herman Bueno, conducted a two-year retrospective study of 218 patients who came to his clinic complaining of chronic fatigue. *Giardia* infestation was identified by rectal swab in 61 of these patients. In discussing their observations, these observers said:

> "Cure of giardiasis resulted in clearing of fatigue and related 'viral' symptoms (myalgia sweats, flu-like feeling) in 70%, fatigue in 18%, and was no benefit in 12%. This study shows that giardiasis can present with fatigue as the major manifestation accompanied by minor gastrointestinal complaints, and sometimes by myalgia (muscle aching)."[2]

In analyzing this relationship, Galland pointed out that some of the symptoms in patients with giardiasis may be related to pre-existing allergic disease. He also noted that they could be related to the effects of giardia on the nutritional status of the patient, including malabsorption, protein loss and vitamin deficiencies. In addition, parasitic infestation may also promote the proliferation of *Candida albicans.*

Another parasite, *Blastocystis hominis,* also appears to be a troublemaker. According to an article in *Practical Gastroenterology,* by Martin J. Lee, Ph.D.:

> "*Blastocystis hominis* has greater prevalence than any other parasite, but often goes undetected because of poor laboratory technique. At Great Smokies Diagnostic Laboratory, *Blastocystis* is found in 20% or more of clinical specimens. The weight of evidence supports treating it as a potential pathogen.
>
> "Together with other weak pathogens it has been reported in association with many chronic conditions, including irritable bowel, chronic fatigue and arthritic/rheumatoid complaints ... *Blastocystis* has been reported to produce gastrointestinal cramps, vomiting, sleeplessness, nausea, weight loss, lassitude, dizziness, flatus, anorexia and pruritus.
>
> "*B. hominis* may be highly variable in its pathogenicity. The organism is present in a number of healthy persons and an asymptomatic carrier state has been postulated. Many patients suffering from gastrointestinal illness have this organism as the only identifiable parasite and report clinical improvement or resolution of symptoms when *Blastocystis* is eradicated."[3]

During the past five years, I've phased out my practice and see only an occasional patient. So my knowledge of parasites and their possible importance is based on the observations of a number of my consultants.

To get an update on Dr. Galland's observations, I called him in 1993. Here are excerpts from our conversation.

Crook: Leo, what percentage of your patients do you feel have parasites to such a degree that they need to be treated?

Galland: About 30% of patients in my overall practice have parasites. Among certain groups it may approach 40%. It varies.

Crook: How do you make the diagnosis?

Galland: I examine the rectal mucus using specimens obtained by anoscopy. And I use a special stain to examine them. Yet, during the past year, I continue to do stool examinations.

Crook: What do you use in treating them?

Galland: Mainly herbal remedies, including a combination of artemisia and citrus seed extract. I especially like this product because it also is a good agent for controlling candida. But in some patients I use a mixture of antiparasitic herbs.

I was glad to receive this information from Galland, and I was especially pleased to see that he did not recommend Flagyl. Although this medication is often recommended as a "first line" anti-parasitic drug, according to the *Physicians' Desk Reference* candida overgrowth is a common side effect of Flagyl therapy.[4]

When this medication is used, nystatin and/or other antifungal medications should be given concurrently.

Still More About Parasites

In the 1970s, while a member of the advisory board of the Pritikin Foundation, I met Ann Louise Gittleman who at that time served as nutrition director of the Pritikin Longevity Center in Santa Monica, California. And our paths crossed occasionally during the next decade.

In the summer of 1992, I had a long visit with Gittleman during a trip to New Mexico. Then, in 1993, I picked up a copy of her latest book entitled, *Guess What Came to Dinner—Parasites and your health*. I was fascinated. Here's an excerpt of comments on the back cover.

> "Are you having difficulty shaking off an illness? Are you suffering from chronic fatigue? Do you have a health problem your doctor can't identify? Parasites in your body may be the cause.
>
> "If you think that parasitic diseases happen only to people in Third World countries, think again. The rate of parasitic disorders in North America is skyrocketing. An astounding one out of six people will test positive for parasites."[5]

In this comprehensive but easy-to-read-and-understand book, Gittleman told me a lot of things about parasites that I did not know. And she provides readers with just about everything they need to know about parasites, including symptoms, diagnosis, treatment and prevention. And she lists a number of laboratories which specialize in parasite testing, including:

- Great Smokies Diagnostic Laboratory, 18A Regent Park Blvd., Asheville, NC 28806. 800–522–4762.
- Consulting Clinical and Microbiological Laboratory, Inc., 1020 S. W. Taylor, #855, Portland, OR 97205. 503–222–5279.
- Lexington Professional Center, 133 E. 73rd St., New York, NY 10021. 212–988–4800.
- Meridian Valley Clinical Laboratory, 24030 132nd Ave., S.E., Kent, WA 98042. 800–234–6825.
- Parasitic Disease Consultants Laboratory, P.O. Box 616, 2177-J Flintstone Dr., Tucker, GA 30084. 404–496–1370.
- Parasitology Laboratory of Washington, Inc., 2141 K St., N.W., Suite 408, Washington, DC 20037. 202–331–0287.

Based on what I learned from Galland and Gittleman, it seems to me that if your health problems are yeast connected and you've followed your diet and taken nystatin, Diflucan or Sporanox and aren't improving, you should ask your doctor to investigate the possibility of a concurrent parasitic infestation.

REFERENCES

1. Bland, J., *Preventive Medicine Update*, P.O. Box 1729, Gig Harbor, WA, 98335.
2. Galland, L. and Bueno, J., "Advances in Laboratory Diagnosis of Intestinal Parasites," American Clinical Laboratory, 1989; pp 18–19.
3. Lee, M.J., Johnson, J.F., Baskin, W.N. and Barrie, S., "Trends in Intestinal Parasitology. Part II: Commonly Reported Parasites and Therapeutics," *Practical Gastroenterology*, 1992; Vol. 16 No. 10.
4. *Physicians' Desk Reference*, 47th Edition, Medical Economics Co., Montvale, NJ, 1993; page 2261.
5. Gittleman, A.L., *Guess What Came to Dinner—Parasites and your health*, Avery, Garden City Park, NY, 1993.

42

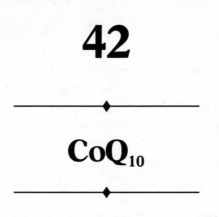

CoQ₁₀

In 1986 and 1987, I received a number of anecdotal reports by phone and by mail about a substance I'd never heard of—CoQ$_{10}$. People who wrote and called said, "You should read about CoQ$_{10}$. It helps the immune system."

Then one day, in late 1987, I picked up a book in a health food store entitled *The Miracle Nutrient, Coenzyme Q$_{10}$* by Emile G. Bliznakov, M.D. (President and Scientific Director of the Lupus Research Institute) and Gerald L. Hunt. I read the book almost from cover to cover and I was impressed. Here are some of the things I learned.

CoQ$_{10}$, also known as ubiquinone, is a nutrient that was first extracted from beef heart mitochondria by scientist F.L. Crane and his group in the United States in 1957. A great deal of the work on this substance has been carried out since that time by Dr. Karl Folkers and research colleagues at the University of Texas, Austin. It has also been researched and used extensively in Japan, where 252 commercial preparations of CoQ$_{10}$ are supplied by over 80 pharmaceutical companies. According to the authors of *The Miracle Nutrient, Coenzyme Q10*:

> "On April 14, 1986, Karl Folkers was honored with the Priestley Medal, the highest award bestowed by the American Chemical Society in recognition of superior accomplishments in chemistry and medicine. It was presented to Dr. Folkers in recognition of his work with Coenzyme Q$_{10}$, vitamin B$_6$ and B$_{12}$."

The book reviews many reports that describe the value of Coenzyme Q_{10} in people with congestive heart failure and other types of heart disease. It also discusses its effectiveness in reversing gum disease and in strengthening the immune system. Mice experiments were cited to show that CoQ_{10} boosts the performance of immune system cells, not by stimulating the production of more cells, but by inducing more energy and thus increasing the immunocompetence in the existing ones.

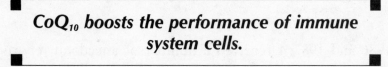

> ## CoQ_{10} boosts the performance of immune system cells.

Although, so far, research into CoQ_{10} and the immune system has received less emphasis and publicity than its role in treating heart disease, the authors of the book concluded:

> *"Our research with animal models, and the studies of other scientists, have proved conclusively that CoQ_{10} can produce a profoundly beneficial effect on the immune system* [emphasis added] . . . CoQ_{10} displays no toxic effects whatsoever . . . Clinical studies, under the auspices of the FDA, show that CoQ_{10} is much safer than many drugs presently on the market."[1]

Support for CoQ_{10}

I recommend CoQ_{10}. During the past seven years, I've used CoQ_{10} in doses of 25 mg., one to four times daily, as one part of a comprehensive program in treating my chronically ill patients with chronic fatigue, headache, PMS and other disorders. I take it myself, give it to my wife and daughters and I've also recommended it to friends. Although I can't claim that it is a magical cure which is "good for everything," here are anecdotal reports.

Bobbie's Report

One of my patients, a 46-year-old woman with recurrent asthma, sinusitis, rhinitis, fatigue, headache and other symptoms, had failed to improve on repeated courses of antibiotic drugs and bronchial dilators. Bobbie also had taken allergy extract injections for ten years. On a comprehensive treatment program which included an improved diet, vitamin and mineral supplements, small doses of nystatin for a short period of time and CoQ_{10}, she showed remarkable improvement in her health status. And, in a recent letter to me, Bobbie said:

> "I'm enjoying very good health, better than I can remember in my life. I've never gone this long without a bronchial infection since I was 12 years old. I believe CoQ_{10} has certainly contributed to my being able to stay well. I took 75 mg. a day for quite a while, but now I'm doing great on 50 mg. daily. I'm also taking the vitamin/mineral preparation Basic Preventive. Also, my mother and stepfather have been taking CoQ_{10} for over a year and have had no colds since they started taking it."

A Personal Report

Like everyone else, I would experience occasional medical problems. I'd develop a cold, sometimes followed by sinusitis, several times a year. I would also "catch a cold" whenever my wife, Betsy, had a cold—even though my diet was a good one and I took extra vitamin C and other nutritional supplements. In spite of these complaints, I've been fortunate and most of the time I've enjoyed excellent health.

In late 1987, I began taking CoQ_{10} regularly, 25 mg. twice daily. Since that time, I have experienced no respiratory infections. And I didn't develop a cold after sitting next to a woman who coughed and sneezed repeatedly during a 12-hour plane trip from Auckland, New Zealand, to Los Angeles.

A Report on CoQ_{10} and Chronic Fatigue Syndrome

In a report in their *Chronic Fatigue Syndrome Self-Care Manual*, Charles W. Lapp, M.D., and Paul R. Cheney, M.D., outlined their recommendations. These included lifestyle changes, exercise, diet, vitamins and nutritional supplements. In discussing CoQ_{10}, they said:

"This enzyme (metabolic catalyst) is thought to be involved in 95% of a cell's metabolic reactions. It has additional benefits of lowering cholesterol and blood pressure and stabilizing heart conditions. Particularly useful for improving fatigue, thought processes, muscular function and cardiac complaints. A threshold effect occurs and it may take five to six weeks for full benefit. We recommend 90–200 mg. daily (one dose or divided), for a five to six week trial. Expensive, so we discontinue if no benefit is noted in six weeks. We use sublingual form to increase its bioavailability."[2]

Reports from the Peer-reviewed Medical Literature

In an article in the *Medical Clinics of North America,* W.H. Frishman, Department of Medicine, Mt. Sinai Hospital and Medical School, New York, said:

"A biochemical rationale for using CoQ in treating certain cardiovascular diseases has been established. CoQ serves as an endogenous function as an essential cofactor in several metabolic pathways, particularly oxidative respiration . . . Its mechanism of action appears to be that of a free radical scavenger and/or direct membrane stabilizer."[3]

In a subsequent report, Frishman said:

"The substance has been used in oral form to treat various cardiovascular disorders including angina pectoris, hypertension and congestive heart failure. Its clinical importance is now being established in clinical trials worldwide."[4]

In an article published in 1992, Folkers and associates, Institute for Biomedical Research, University of Texas, Austin, said:

"Twenty years of international open and seven double blind trials established the efficacy and safety of coenzyme Q_{10} (CoQ_{10}) to treat patients in heart failure . . . After CoQ_{10}, some patients required no conventional drugs and had no limitation in lifestyle."[5]

Further Comments on CoQ$_{10}$ and Other Nonprescription Remedies

Why, if CoQ$_{10}$ and other herbal remedies are effective and safe, has the FDA removed them from the shelves of some health food stores? The reasons are multiple and complex.

In discussing this question in the preface to his fascinating book, *The Scientific Validation of Herbal Medicine*, Daniel B. Mowrey, pointed out that medical science in America is a unique combination of economic and political factors. In order for a substance to interest a pharmaceutical company, it must be effective in treating one or more health problems. In his discussion of the subject, Mowrey said:

> "Efficacy is, of course, a necessary condition. But it is not sufficient. The chemical must also be potentially profitable . . .
>
> "Medicines that cannot be patented (or otherwise made proprietary) are not economically acceptable. No matter how good a substance is, if a particular pharmaceutical firm does not have the inside track on patent rights, or if such rights are unobtainable, that firm is not going to invest millions of dollars in developing and marketing . . .
>
> "*One tactic effectively used to discredit natural products is to label them unproven*, a strategy that works well among professionals, who by virtue of their training already are predisposed to equate 'unproven' with 'ineffective,' perhaps even 'dangerous'. . .

Classifying herbs as drugs would prevent your neighborhood health food store from selling them.

"So far herbs are politically designated as foods. But there are forces that work to change all that . . . Classifying herbs as drugs would prevent your neighborhood health food store from selling them. Only pharmaceutical companies could make them and only doctors could prescribe them. But the doctor wouldn't prescribe them even if he wanted to, because the pharmaceutical company wouldn't make them.

"Why? The FDA estimates it costs over 7 million dollars to bring a new drug to market. Pharmaceutical companies put that figure close to 70 million dollars . . . Since natural substances cannot be patented, there is even less room for profit in them."[6]

In his November 1993 newsletter, *Health and Healing,* Dr. Julian Whitaker described the response of his patient, Charmaine.

"When I first met her four years ago, she was as near death as any patient I had ever seen. On a comprehensive nutritional regimen, which included large doses of CoQ_{10}, her response was almost immediate and miraculous.

"Today, Charmaine takes no heart medications at all and leads an active life. She does, however, continue to take CoQ_{10} as well as other vitamins and minerals.

"Folks, vitamins and minerals are not magic, but CoQ_{10} comes as close to a cure-all as we're likely to get and for good reasons. CoQ_{10} stabilizes and modulates the electron transfers used by all biologic systems in the extraction of energy.

"CoQ_{10} is also a potent antioxidant protecting cells from free radicals, the by-products of energy production . . . When CoQ_{10} is low, nothing in your body works well."[7]

REFERENCES

1. Bliznakov, E.G. and Hunt, G.L., *The Miracle Nutrient, Coenzyme Q$_{10}$,* Bantam Books, New York, 1987; pp 8, 64.
2. Lapp, C.W. and Cheney, P.R., *Chronic Fatigue Syndrome Self-Care Manual,* February, 1991.
3. Frishman, W.H., "Coenzyme Q$_{10}$: A New Drug for Myocardial Ischemia?" *Medical Clinics of North America,* 1988; 72(1):243–258.
4. Frishman, W.H., "Coenzyme Q$_{10}$: A New Drug for Cardiovascular Disease," *Journal of Clinical Pharmacology,* 1990; 30(7):596–608.
5. Folkers, K., Langsjoen, P. and Langsjoen, P.H., "Therapy with coenzyme Q$_{10}$ of patients in heart failure who are eligible or ineligible for a transplant," *Biochem. Biophys. Res. Commun.,* 1992; 182(1):247–253.

6. Mowrey, D.B., *The Scientific Validation of Herbal Medicine*, Cormorant Books, 1986.
7. Whitaker, J., *Health and Healing*, Phillips Publishing Company, Inc., 7811 Montrose Rd., Potomac, MD 20854.

43

Vitamin C

If you're like most North Americans, you've read and heard about double Nobel Prize winner, the late Linus Pauling, Ph.D. Twenty-five years ago Pauling wrote a book entitled *Vitamin C and the Common Cold*. Then in 1986, he published another book entitled *How to Live Longer and Feel Better*. In this book he talked about scurvy and how it killed British sailors on long ocean voyages during the 1500s, 1600s and 1700s.

Pauling also told the fascinating story of Dr. James Lind, a physician in the British navy. In the mid-1700s, Lind found that limes (and other fresh fruits) kept sailors from developing scurvy. Because his superiors didn't believe him, they ignored his observations and recommendations. And British sailors on long ocean voyages continued to suffer and die from this disease.

But in 1795 (five years after Lind died), the lime juice story spread and limes were made part of the ration on ships in the British navy. (That's how the British sailors got the name "Limeys.") Soon afterward, the scurvy "epidemic" disappeared. Yet, it wasn't until the 1930s that the Hungarian researcher, Dr. Albert Szent-Györgyi, learned why lime juice worked. *It contained vitamin C* and Györgyi received the Nobel Prize for his discoveries.

Since that time, people all over the world have consumed fruits and vegetables and scurvy (with rare exceptions) disappeared from the planet. Then, several decades ago, scientists found that individuals who did not eat plant foods could prevent scurvy by taking 45 mg. of vitamin C each day. And until recently, most members of the medical establishment have said, "Forty-five milligrams of vitamin C is all a person needs."

But, based largely on the observations of Dr. Pauling, more and more people began to take 10, 100 or 1000 times the minimal dose of vitamin C. Moreover, many scientific reports have shown that vitamin C is an important antioxidant which plays a major role in strengthening the immune system.

Robert Cathcart, M.D.

This internationally known orthopedic surgeon was troubled by a cold about every two months and constant hay fever. When he heard that Linus Pauling had said that vitamin C cured the common cold, he was ready to try anything. Cathcart started taking much larger doses of ascorbic acid powder and water, 1 tsp. (four grams) four times a day. *He was astonished to find that his symptoms of hay fever were abolished as long as he kept taking the high dosage of vitamin C.*

It was nine months before Cathcart caught another cold. Then he noticed that his symptoms were reduced for about an hour after each dose of four grams. So he began increasing his dose, both in amount and frequency. And he was astonished to find that he tolerated 50 grams/day when he had a cold. And in a couple of days the cold vanished. Yet, that much ascorbic acid would cause diarrhea if he took it when he was well.

> *Cathcart found that large doses of vitamin C helped his patients with fractures.*

Subsequently, Cathcart found that large doses of vitamin C helped his patients with fractures and other injuries heal more rapidly and with much less pain. So he began to search the literature for further information and he was surprised and delighted to find a number of reports in the medical literature dating back to the 1940s.

Included were reports by Dr. F.R. Klenner[1,2,3] who found that large doses of vitamin C helped his patients with virus pneumonia and poliomyelitis. He also read reports by Dr. Irwin Stone published in the medical literature in the 1960s and in Stone's book, *The Healing Factor: Vitamin C Against Disease*, published in 1972.[4]

So Cathcart began to give many of his patients vitamin C. He soon found that people with health problems of various sorts who took *huge* doses of Vitamin C improved more rapidly. Some 20 years ago, in a letter to the editor in the *Medical Tribune* (June 25, 1975), he reported that the "bowel-tolerance" to ascorbic acid (vitamin C) of a person with a healthy gastrointestinal tract was somewhat proportional to the toxicity of their disease.

He defined the bowel-tolerance dose as the amount of ascorbic acid tolerated orally that almost, but not quite, causes a marked loosening of the stools.[5,6]

In his further work with his patients, Cathcart found that healthy people could tolerate orally 10 to 15 grams of ascorbic acid in a 24-hour period. Yet, sick people, including those with influenza or mononucleosis, could take 200 or more grams in 24 hours.

In determining the appropriate dose, he advises his patients to begin with hourly doses of ascorbic acid powder dissolved in small amounts of water. Later, after the patient has learned to accurately estimate the proper dose, comparable doses of ascorbic acid tablets or capsules are used.

In patients with severe disease, including **AIDS** or cancer, Cathcart uses intravenous sodium ascorbate and hundreds of other physicians have followed his lead.

In a November 1994 letter to me, Cathcart said:

"In patients with yeast-related health problems, massive doses of ascorbic acid may help people regain their health. I've found that such doses help strengthen the immune system, blunt already acquired food and chemical sensitivities and reduce the symptoms of persistent viral infections.

"Here are possible mechanisms. It provides massive numbers of electrons to neutralize free radicals. Each vitamin C molecule carries two extra electrons which are lost when two free radicals are neutralized."*

My Comments

I first heard about Dr. Cathcart's observations in the early 1980s and I cited them in the first edition of *The Yeast Connection*.[7] I also referred to Norman Cousins' book, *Anatomy of an Illness*. In this book Cousins said that taking 25,000 mg. of vitamin C each day, combined with laughter therapy, played a significant role in helping him recover from a severe illness. He also described his experiences in the *New England Journal of Medicine*.[8]

In my discussion of vitamin C in *The Yeast Connection*, I also reported my experiences in helping Harvey, a 13-year-old boy with severe asthma. This youngster had been studied and treated by pediatricians, allergists and pulmonary specialists and had been hospitalized many times.

Harvey was taking regular, around-the-clock bronchial dilators and other medications. In spite of these measures, he was experiencing increasing respiratory difficulties. Out of desperation, I increased his vitamin C up to 35,000 mg. per day. His wheezing began to improve in 12 hours and cleared by the end of 48 hours, and no further injections of epinephrine were required.

By the end of the third day, his stools became loose and his vitamin C dosage was decreased to 10,000 to 15,000 mg. per day. When rechecked two weeks later, he was being continued on the same dose and his mother said that the big doses of vitamin C really made a difference.

During the past decade, many people who have written and called me have confirmed Dr. Cathcart's observations.

A Vitamin C Testimonial

In the spring of 1992, I attended a medical conference in a major city. While there I visited a former colleague (I'll call him John), a

---

*Physicians who would like copies of Dr. Cathcart's articles can obtain them by sending a business-size, stamped, self-addressed envelope to Robert F. Cathcart III, 127 2nd St., Suite 4, Los Altos, CA 94022.

graduate of Harvard Medical School and a past president of his state pediatric society.

During a previous visit, I told John of my growing interest in nutritional supplements and I sent him notes and comments about the benefits of such supplements. When he learned that Dr. Linus Pauling, the Nobel Prize winner, would be speaking at the convention, he said, "I would like to hear what he has to say."

During his presentation, Dr. Pauling, of course, talked about the benefits which could be gained by taking large doses of various nutrients and especially vitamin C.

Some weeks after the meeting, I received a letter from John. Here are excerpts.

"Let me describe the miraculous improvement in my arthritic knees since I've been on the gradually increasing doses of vitamin C . . . I'm now up to a daily intake of six grams and plan to go on up slowly until I reach 12 grams daily, unless I encounter troublesome diarrhea . . . *For the past five days I have had such a dramatic improvement in my knees that I feel like shouting from the housetops.*

"They feel as though the previous looseness has been tightened up to normal as though one would tighten the loose wobbly wheels on a cart by snuggling up the nut holding it in place. And no aches at night after walking more than usual.

"I can bend my knees almost as well as before any trouble started and can almost do a full knee bend, something unheard of last month. When I go to the grocery store, I no longer go first for the cart, using it as a walker, but can walk just as comfortably with no assistance.

"At the stores with carpet along the side of the marble floor surfaces . . . I no longer find that I want to walk on the carpet surface, because the hard surface is just as comfortable for my knees. And I no longer look for a chair to sit while Frances [not her name] spends 5 to 15 min. looking at dresses.

"I had been taking one gram of Vitamin C twice most days for the past six months, and this modest dose was sufficient so that my ophthalmologist found that the cataract in my right eye had grown almost none at all, and there was no need to make a change in the prescription for my glasses, which generally has been changed once each year for the past several years. I give credit to the Vitamin C.

"I can now walk in close to the normal upright posture, and Frances does not need to remind me to 'stand up straight.' At the health club the standard program of exercises are much easier to perform and my knees do not have the slight ache that usually goes with workout on the Lifecycle machine.

"I feel that the increased levels of Vitamin C in all of my body tissues is helping clear out some of the free radicals and is neutralizing in some fashion the prostaglandins which promote the degenerative arthritis. I like to imagine it is like a fire that burns more cleanly, with less residue, and leaves all the moving parts in better condition and healthier . . .

"I'm also taking a vitamin/mineral formula (two tablets at each meal) which contains much more than the minimum daily requirement. *And I feel much stronger and better and full of energy and ambition so that it is difficult to imagine that an 81-year-old fellow could feel any better."*

During the past two years, John made further increases in his vitamin C intake. And in October 1994, he sent me a copy of a letter he sent to Dr. Cathcart. Here are excerpts.

"I want to thank you again for getting me on the proper dose of ascorbic acid powder, which varies from 30 to 50 grams daily. I monitor my needs by following carefully the principles which you taught me.

"My degenerative arthritis in my knees and right ankle has slowed to a snail's pace and I'm able to participate in a four-day-a-week exercise program at the fitness center, including spending an hour, three times weekly, in deep water doing NO IMPACT exercise which protects my joints in a wonderful fashion.

"By following your program and taking these exercises, I like to think I'm slowing the AGING process. The cataract in my right eye which was very troublesome before I started on vitamin C is still not causing any interference with my reading. Thank goodness, because I do enjoy reading many hours each week. I will be 84 in January and expect to keep feeling peppy for many years to come. Thank you again."

REFERENCES

1. Klenner, F.R., "Virus pneumonia and its treatment with vitamin C," *J. South. Med. and Surg.*, 1948; 110:60–63.
2. Klenner, F.R., "The treatment of poliomyelitis and other virus diseases with vitamin C," *J. South. Med. and Surg.*, 1949; 111:210–214.
3. Klenner, F.R., "Observations on the dose and administration of ascorbic acid when employed beyond the range of a vitamin in human pathology," *J. App. Nutr.*, 1971; 23:61–88.
4. Stone, I., *The Healing Factor: Vitamin C Against Disease*, Grosset and Dunlap, New York, 1972.
5. Cathcart, R.F., "Vitamin C: titrating to bowel-tolerance, anascorbemia, and acute induced scurvy," *Medical Hypotheses*, 1981; 7:1359–1376.
6. Cathcart, R.F., "The third face of vitamin C," *J. of Orthomol. Med.*, 1993; 7(4):197–200.
7. Crook, W.G., *The Yeast Connection*, First Edition, Professional Books, Jackson, TN, 1983; pp 236–237.
8. Cousins, N., "Anatomy of an Illness," *N. Engl. J. Med.*, 1976; 295(26):1458–1463.

44

---◆---

Mercury/Amalgam Dental Fillings

---◆---

If your health problems are yeast connected, you'll nearly always improve if and when you:

- change your diet. This means cutting out (or sharply limiting) sugar and junk food, eating more vegetables and identifying (and avoiding) the foods that cause sensitivity reactions.
- take prescription medications, including nystatin, Nizoral, Diflucan or Sporanox. And/or take nonprescription substances, including caprylic acid products, citrus seed extract, *Lactobacillus acidophilus*, bifidobacteria (and other probiotics), garlic and/or other substances that discourage yeast proliferation in the gut.
- take nutritional supplements, including vitamins, minerals, zinc and the essential fatty acids.
- clean up your environment, especially your home and your workplace. This means avoiding tobacco smoke, perfumes, insecticides, kitchen gas stoves, laundry chemicals and other chemical pollutants.
- get adequate amounts of fresh air and sun or skylight.
- walk and take limited amounts of other exercise as your health improves.
- obtain psychological support.

But if you're doing all these things and are at a standstill, it could be because you're absorbing toxins from the mercury/silver amalgam fillings in your mouth.

Controversy About Dental Fillings

The hazards of silver/mercury fillings have been talked about by a handful of dentists during the past decade. According to those who oppose the use of these fillings, they can cause toxic reactions and play a part in making people sick. Symptoms attributed to these fillings include fatigue, headache, central nervous system dysfunction, muscle and joint pains and disturbances in other parts of the body.

An opposite point of view is expressed by the American Dental Association, which represents at least 75% of the nation's dentists. This organization continues to support the use of amalgam as a safe, effective method of tooth restoration. This controversy was brought into the public "mainstream" on CBS's "60 Minutes," December 15, 1990.

On this program, Dr. Murray J. Vimy of the University of Calgary Medical School and Alfred Zamm, M.D., of Kingston, New York, presented information on the potential and actual toxic effects of mercury/amalgam fillings. Vimy had placed silver fillings in the mouths of pregnant sheep. Three days later, mercury was found in the blood of mothers and fetuses and in the amniotic fluid. Two weeks later, it was found in other tissue samples.

> **Silver fillings were placed in the mouths of pregnant sheep. Three days later mercury was found in sheep fetuses.**

Along with their comments and presentations of scientific data were testimonials from patients whose fatigue and other chronic health problems were "turned around" following the removal of mercury/amalgam fillings.

Observations of Alfred Zamm, M.D.

During the past decade, Dr. Zamm and I have exchanged a number of letters and phone calls. He also sent me a copy of a 21-page, carefully referenced monograph entitled, "Anticandida albicans therapy: Is there ever an end to it? Dental Mercury Removal: An effective adjunct."

And, in the spring of 1994, he sent me a copy of a letter from one of his patients. Here are excerpts.

> "Today is my first Mercury Free Anniversary! I feel great! Thank you! Thank you! Thank you!
>
> "I have progressively gotten better over the years, just as you described. *No more* headaches, muscles aches, irritability, moodiness, sore throats, back pains and lack of energy . . . I still battle my yeast sensitivity and take nystatin three times a day. And if I don't watch my diet I get gassy, bloated and tired.
>
> "What thrills me most is that I'm no longer anxious or depressed or irritable (as long as I'm good on my diet). I feel at peace with myself, I think for the first time in my life! It's wonderful.
>
> "I truly appreciate your commitment and dedication to your profession and to your patients . . . Thanks so much for your invaluable care. Without it I'd still be very sick and unhappy."

Root Canals May Cause Problems

Dr. Zamm has also found that this common dental procedure plays a part in causing problems in some of his patients. One such patient was troubled by recurrent asthma, mood swings, chemical sensitivities, fatigue, blurred vision, muscle pains, hair loss and other symptoms. On a comprehensive treatment program which included diet, nystatin and the removal of teeth with root canals, the patient showed significant improvement. In commenting on why he feels root canals are unhealthy, Zamm said:

> "The 'root canal' . . . involves insertion of *cytotoxic* substances such as halogenated cyclic hydrocarbons . . . eugenol, resin and a variety of other cytotoxic . . . substances. These substances chroni-

cally leaked from these treated teeth and continued to suppress the immune system."

Further information about the toxic effects of mercury/amalgam dental fillings and root canals can be obtained from:

Alfred V. Zamm, M.D., 111 Maiden Lane, Kingston, NY 12401. Enclose a long, SASE with first-class postage.
The Environmental Dental Association (EDA), (1-800-388-8124).
Holistic Dental Digest by Jerry Mittleman, DDS. This bimonthly newsletter is published by The Once Daily, Inc. Subscription rate is $9.50/year. For a sample copy, send a long, SASE to Dr. Mittleman, 263 West End, #2A, New York, NY 10023.

Books that provide information on mercury/amalgam dental fillings include:

The Complete Guide to Mercury Toxicity from Dental Fillings, Joyal Taylor, DDS, EDA Publishing, 9974 Scripps Ranch Blvd., Suite 36, San Diego, CA 92131. $14.95 plus $3.00 shipping.
Are Your Dental Fillings Poisoning You? Guy S. Fasciana, DMD, Keats Publishing Co., 27 Pine St., New Canaan, CT 06840.
The Toxic Time Bomb, Sam Ziff, DDS, 4401 Real Court, Orlando, FL 32808.

45

Yeast-Related Drunkenness

In *The Yeast Connection*[1] I told the story of Charlie Swaart, an Arizona man, who for over a decade would become a sloppy, overbearing, hostile and sometimes even violent drunk, even though he hadn't consumed any alcohol. Moreover, on at least one occasion, Charlie was picked up for drunk driving.

Happily for Charlie, his Arizona physician learned of a report from Japan that described drunkenness caused by an overgrowth of *Candida albicans* in the digestive tract. So he placed him on nystatin and he showed significant—even dramatic—improvement. Millions of people heard about Charlie in the early and mid-1980s because his story was featured in the *Los Angeles Times* and on Charles Kuralt's TV program, "American Parade."

Charlie passed away several years ago. Although I never met him, we talked on the phone on several occasions in the 1980s. We also exchanged letters. During our conversations, Charlie pointed out that yeast-induced intoxication isn't rare. To support his point of view, he told me that he and his wife had received hundreds of telephone calls and letters from people all over the world describing yeast-related drunkenness.

A Japanese Study of Yeast-Related Drunkenness

In a 1970s article, "A Review of the Literature on Drunken Symptoms Due to Yeast in the Gastrointestinal Tract," Dr. Kazuo Iwata listed 24 reports of patients who showed "drunken syndrome" following ingestion of ordinary foods. Seventeen of the patients were males and seven were females and their ages ranged between 16 months and 75 years; most were middle-aged.

In his report, Iwata said:

"The severity of symptoms varies with each case, but the clinical pictures are characterized by occasional or frequent drunkenness or drunken feeling, which patients express as very unpleasant, frequently complicated by a variety of symptoms such as flushed face, headache, dizziness . . . sweating, fever, diarrhea, palpitation . . ."

Candida albicans was isolated in the gastric and duodenal juices of 14 of the patients and other yeasts were found in the remainder. A number of the patients gave a history of undergoing an operation of the abdomen for gastric cancer, ulcer or other diseases. And the resulting postoperative disturbances in some cases resulted in a partial blockage in the intestinal tract which slowed the passage of the contents on through the bowel.

In discussing the differential diagnosis, Iwata said:

"The differential diagnosis is essentially that of alcoholism. Patients' chief complaint is suffering occasional or frequent symptoms of acute intoxication, despite not having taken a drink of any intoxicating beverage, but they're apt to be mistrusted by doctors, especially at the initial inspection of the patients who have breath with an alcoholic odor."[2]

Stories of People With Yeast-Related Drunkenness

During the past ten years, I've received a number of calls and letters from people who said their feelings of being intoxicated were yeast related. Here are the stories of three of these individuals.

The Story of Albert

Albert (not his real name), a 26-year-old computer consultant and lease broker, called me and told me that he had been troubled by yeast-related intoxication. And because of his experiences, he said that he wanted to help bring this story into the medical mainstream. Here are excerpts from his story.

"For many years I was treated with repeated antibiotics for throat infections. I took Ceclor, Amoxicillin and many others. At the age of 20, I developed frequent heartburn, bloating and other symptoms. I then had my tonsils removed and on a limited diet I felt great. But back on an ordinary diet the bloating returned, I had constant diarrhea, I was dizzy, I couldn't make decisions, I would lie in bed all weekend and I wanted to kill myself.

"I went from doctor to doctor, including the Lahey Clinic and the Massachusetts General Hospital. I was a total wreck, had continued anxiety attacks and developed sensitivities to chemical smells of all sorts, including newspaper, tobacco, and my own deodorant."

In his continuing discussion, Albert told how he went to Dr. Carol Englander who put him on a yeast-free diet and nystatin. He showed significant improvement, but when he went off the diet and stopped the nystatin, his symptoms came back.

In the ensuing weeks, he continued to experiment with his diet and he found that a high carbohydrate diet would upset him emotionally. He would become an absolute maniac. He said:

"I was so out of control that I smashed a $350 telephone. My symptoms were such that I checked myself into a hospital. The following day I developed massive diarrhea, and by the sixth day, I was normal.

"With further experimentation I learned that after taking potatoes, sugar and fructose, I would experience the drunk-like feelings. I've now been back on the program with nystatin and diet for six weeks and I feel great."

The Story of Lucy

Lucy (not her real name), a 27-year-old woman, who had been arrested for DUI, called and begged me to help her. I told her to write me a long letter telling me more about her story.

Two days later, I received her letter which included a long history of yeast-related health problems. During infancy and early childhood she took many antibiotics for recurrent respiratory infections. She was also troubled by hyperactivity and attention deficits during her grammar school years and with vaginal yeast infections, depression and digestive problems during her teen years and on into her twenties.

I passed her story along to a lawyer who was knowledgeable in handling DUI cases. He told me that the amount of alcohol Lucy consumed wouldn't have been enough to cause an elevated blood alcohol level. So I flew to Washington and met with Lucy and her lawyer.

After reviewing Lucy's story and the details surrounding her arrest, I went to court. I was waiting to testify when the judge threw out the case because of technicalities.

I was glad that Lucy won her case. Yet, I felt like the place kicker who was ready to kick the winning field goal, but remained on the bench because the team pushed over a touchdown!

The Story of Melinda

Like Lucy, 45-year-old Melinda (not her real name) had been arrested for drunk driving and asked for my help. In reviewing her records, I learned that she had been troubled by yeast-related problems for many years. On several occasions she had responded to oral antifungal medications and a sugar-free diet.

One month prior to her arrest, Melinda suffered a compound fracture of both bones in her right leg. A day or two after her injury, she developed a severe infection; antibiotics were prescribed, which she took for the ensuing three weeks.

Three hours prior to her arrest, Melinda went to dinner with a friend. During this time she consumed two large glasses of a sugar-containing cola beverage and two eight-ounce glasses of wine. While driving home she pulled her car over to the side of the road to point out the apartment building where another friend lived.

A police officer stopped to check and make sure she wasn't having car trouble. He noticed alcohol on her breath, took her to the police station and drew her blood. Analysis by a toxicologist showed a blood alcohol level of .205.

After reviewing Melinda's story, I told her that I would help her. To obtain additional information about yeast-related drunkenness, I visited Drs. Stephen Davies and John Howard at their laboratory in London. These researchers, along with Dr. Adrian Hunnisett, published a scientific study in the *Journal of Nutritional Medicine* in 1990. In summarizing the findings of their study, these investigators said:

> "This study demonstrates that alcohol production from oral carbohydrate ingestion is not a rarity, but is remarkably common (61%) amongst patients who are chronically unwell. It also presents data to support the use of a new simple clinical test to diagnose gut fermentation that may be due to *Candida albicans* or other yeasts or bacteria, and thus identify patients who may benefit from a course of antiyeast or antibacterial therapy."

The British investigators pointed out that individuals with yeast-related health problems may have nutritional deficiencies which interfere with the metabolism of alcohol, leading to persistence of the higher levels of alcohol in the blood. And, in their continuing discussion, they said:

> "This test is well within the capability of any clinical laboratory and should prove useful in the identification of a cause of a diffuse clinical condition.
> "Further studies should be carried out, including microbiological culture of gastric and duodenal aspirates in EtOH [ethyl alcohol producers], clinical response to the appropriate antiyeast or antibacterial intervention, and on the stress on dietary micronutrient supply that EtOH production causes."[3]

Because I felt that Melinda's elevated blood alcohol level was yeast related, I flew to Wisconsin in March 1993 and testified in her behalf. Yet, my efforts, and those of her lawyer, did not meet with success. In a news article entitled "Woman Found Guilty of

Driving Drunk" summarizing the results of the trial, the reporter said, "Although a jury didn't completely buy the 'auto-brewery syndrome' defense in a drunken driving case, it didn't discount the theory . . ." He also cited the comments of the jury foreman who said that the studies presented had some credibility, but there was not enough data to prove the theory.

Melinda's case attracted the attention of lawyers throughout the U.S. and in an article in *The Champion,* published by the National Association of Criminal Defense Lawyers, entitled "A New Defense for DUI Cases: The Auto-Intoxication Syndrome," W.J. Edwards reviewed a number of articles in the medical literature which show that alcohol can be produced from ingestion of carbohydrates in people who are clinically ill. And he said:

> "Medical evidence should now be considered by the DUI practitioner. Those defending a DUI case should look more carefully at the medical history of their clients to determine if such yeast fungus could exist inside the stomach . . . Despite the jury's verdict in Wisconsin, the author believes this defense is viable. Other jurors may be persuaded to accept the effect that the common yeast has upon the human body."[4]

Laboratory Testing for Candida

How important is the production of alcohol by yeast and sugar in the intestinal tract in people with yeast-related health problems? I don't really know; yet, I hope that further research studies will be carried out.

In a recently published 36-page booklet, *The Guide to Candida and ME,* the editor and co-publisher, Lynne McTaggart, included an article entitled "New Test for Candida Growth." In her report she reviewed the studies of Drs. Hunnisett, Davies and Howard, who demonstrated that candida and other yeasts can ferment alcohol in the gut. And she said:

> "The 'Glucose Challenge Test' involves having patients who have fasted for at least three hours and abstained from alcohol for 24

hours, take five grams of glucose. Blood samples are taken before and one hour after the glucose is administered. An increase in blood alcohol over the test period is considered a positive result . . .

"Although a positive reading is not definitive proof that candida is the cause, it should raise suspicions concerning candida or other yeasts or bacteria and at least help to identify those patients who could benefit from the stringent anticandida therapy now employed.

". . . It may also be the first step toward satisfying those doctors who have labeled *Candida albicans* a phantom illness, in the absence of any laboratory test to identify its presence . . . This new test . . . simply requires a cheap and simple instrument called spectrophotometer, which is standard gear in any lab."[5]

REFERENCES

1. Crook, W.G., *The Yeast Connection*, Third Edition, Professional Books, Jackson, TN and Vintage Books, New York, 1986; pp 221–222.
2. Iwata, K., "A Review of the Literature on Drunken Symptoms Due to Yeast in the Gastrointestinal Tract," in Iwata, K., (ed), *Yeasts and Yeast-Like Microorganisms in Medical Science*, University of Tokyo Press, Tokyo, 1976; pp 260–268.
3. Hunnisett, A., Howard, J. and Davies, S., "Gut Fermentation (or the 'Auto-brewery' Syndrome): A new clinical test with initial observations and discussion of clinical and biochemical implications," *J. Nutr. Med.*, 1990; 1:33–38.
4. Edwards, W.J., ".10% Solution—A New Defense for DUI Cases: The Auto-Intoxication Syndrome," *The Champion*, 1993; 17:41–42.
5. McTaggart, L., *The Guide to Candida and ME* (first published in "What Doctor's Don't Tell You," Vol. 1, 2, 3 and 4, 1989–1994), The Wallace Press, 4 Wallace Rd., London, NI2PG.

46

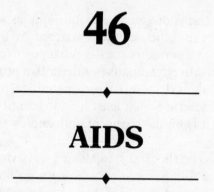

AIDS

In the third edition of *The Yeast Connection*, I cited a study in the *New England Journal of Medicine* which showed that the majority of AIDS victims developed candida infections in the mouth—just as do other patients with weakened immune systems.

I also included an interview with Dr. Alan Levin, Associate Professor of Immunology and Dermatology, University of California School of Medicine, San Francisco. He pointed out that individuals who are at risk for AIDS seem to improve when they make changes in their diet and lifestyle and take antiyeast medications. He said that this does not mean that candida causes AIDS; it means instead that the symptoms in people with weakened immune systems will improve when candida overgrowth is reduced. And he said:

> *"We must emphasize to our patients that having the candida problem does not mean they have AIDS."*

In our continuing discussion, Levin pointed out that AIDS as a disease develops because of many factors, and he said, "While I agree that the HIV virus is necessary, it takes more than this one virus to make the person sick with AIDS. And other viruses (such as the EB virus or the hepatitis virus), may contribute to a weakening of the person's immune system. And, to repeat, when the immune system is weakened, regardless of causes, candida organisms multiply."[1]

AIDS: A 1994 Update

Further Observations of Alan Levin, M.D., San Francisco, California

To learn more about the yeast connection to AIDS, I again interviewed Dr. Levin. Here are excerpts from our April 1994 conversation.

Crook: Al, tell me a little bit about what you think the role of anti-yeast medication and diet is in treating patients with AIDS. Does it make them live longer?

Levin: Yes, it does . . . Obviously, when a person's immune system becomes compromised, the first thing that happens is that candida overgrowth occurs and, also, it's well documented that the candida infection further suppresses the immune response.

  We've also found that people who have been on prophylactic Nizoral for candida are less apt to develop cryptococcal meningitis—another fungal disease which occurs commonly in people with AIDS. As you know, there are other good antifungal drugs, including Diflucan and Sporanox.

Crook: Would you treat the HIV-positive person who does *not* have AIDS with prophylactic Diflucan or nystatin?

Levin: Yes. Nystatin obviously is the most benign approach. The difficulty with the nystatin is that it doesn't get into the bloodstream, so it doesn't help those with cryptococcal meningitis.

Crook: In treating the HIV-positive patient who does not have AIDS, what dose of Diflucan would you give him prophylactically?

Levin: Between 50 and 100 mg. There are a number of different protocols. Some people seem to be able to take 50 mg. two or three times a week and obtain significant protection. The reason is that the yeast is kept under control.

  You're not fighting an acute infection. You want to keep the yeast population down so it doesn't get over the threshold. So you start out with a reasonable dose, 50 mg. a day, then you may be able to wean the patient to every second and then every third day. And you really bypass the problems with liver and blood.

Crook: Do you have a particular preference as far as the Sporanox or the Diflucan?

Levin: I personally use Diflucan more often because it seems to be a little better tolerated. But I don't have any problems with Sporanox either.

Crook: Do you use more Nizoral because it's cheaper?

Levin: Yes, but in my experience, Diflucan is a bit safer. However, you should watch each patient carefully with any of the azole drugs. I don't think that you should use these drugs without monitoring the patient because of the possibility of hepatic and other problems.

I watch every patient. On Nizoral I check them every two to three weeks and on the other drugs I check them at least every six weeks.

I do a simple chemistry panel on a reasonably regular basis. So I feel that Nizoral is perfectly okay. I don't have any real problems with it. If I monitor it carefully, I can bypass significant adverse effects.

Observations of Joan Priestley, M.D., Anchorage, Alaska

About ten years ago, Dr. Priestley, then a recent medical school graduate, stopped by my office in Tennessee. During our visit she said in effect, "Although I originally planned to become a surgeon, I became interested in other areas of medicine, including especially nutrition and yeast-related health problems."

During the next eight years, Dr. Priestley and I corresponded from time to time and in August 1992 she shared the podium with me during a lecture to a California support group, "Share, Care and Prayer."

I returned to California the following spring to talk on yeast-related illness at a "Point and Counterpoint" session at a hospital in Tarzana. Once again, Dr. Priestley provided physicians in the audience with information and support for the relationship of yeast to a diverse group of health problems.

During our conversation after the meeting, we talked about many things, including her experiences in treating patients with

AIDS. And in the summer of 1993, I called her to obtain specifics. Here are excerpts from our conversation.

Priestley: During the past several years, I've seen countless patients with AIDS, so I'm the "AIDS queen" much more than the "yeast lady." One of the first things I do is to change their diets because one of the things that gets these people into trouble is a chronically degenerative diet.

So for my initial treatment, I use the old standbys which haven't changed. My first line is the diet change, especially getting the alcohol and sugar out of the diet. I also put my patients on garlic and acidophilus.

Crook: How about the prescription antifungal medications?
Priestley: I've become a major fan of Diflucan.

Crook: To what extent do you think the program you use in a person who's HIV-positive, but doesn't have AIDS, helps?
Priestley: It helps a lot and I'll be glad to send you an update of the study of my own patients. I presented it at the Berlin AIDS Conference. It proves that this protocol can definitely keep people healthy.

Observations of Carol Jessop, M.D., El Cerrito, California

In January 1989, the late Dr. Phyllis Saifer called me and said, "Dr. Carol Jessop, a physician with impeccable academic credentials, will be talking about the yeast connection to chronic fatigue syndrome at the University of California (SF) CFS Conference in April. I know you'll be pleased with what she has to say."

I went to the conference, and I was delighted to hear her say, "Most of my patients with CFS are helped by a sugar-free, alcohol-free, special diet and antifungal medication." Since that time, I've visited with Dr. Jessop in person and on the phone on a number of occasions. Here are her comments about AIDS.

"I see a lot of patients with AIDS and 90% of them are men. But more and more women are getting AIDS. Like Al Levin, I give all of the AIDS patients in my practice antifungal drugs, whether or not they've shown local monilia infections or thrush. I keep them on Diflucan or Sporanox.

"One of my patients had had AIDS for eight years and zero T-cells for three years. He had PCP for the first time five years ago and a recurrence of PCP this last June. And people with that diagnosis don't usually live more than one year. Yet, he's on Diflucan, 200 mg. a day and a candida-free diet and he's still alive."

More About Candida and AIDS

In May 1994, Robert W. Noble, M.D., Dallas, Texas, a fellow of the American Academy of Family Physicians, sent me an article by Professor Bertrand DuPont which focused on the use of the azole drugs in treating candidiasis in patients with AIDS. Here's an excerpt.

"Oropharyngeal and esophageal candidiasis are very common in patients with HIV infection. In fact, approximately 90% of these patients will experience this form of candidiasis. Despite nearly 20 years of experience using azole antifungal agents to treat candidiasis, demonstration of *Candida albicans* resistance to therapy was rare prior to the advent of AIDS . . .

"Since 1990, however, resistance in patients with HIV infection has emerged as a growing concern."

In his continuing discussion, Professor DuPont talked about the varying sensitivities of *Candida albicans* and related fungi to the different azole drugs. Here are further excerpts from a question and answer section from the report.

Q: What is the frequency of resistance to fluconazole and should it be considered a major problem?

DuPont: Resistance is not a major problem when the total number of AIDS patients is considered. In our institution, 70 out of 1500 AIDS patients have shown resistance to fluconazole. *While it is not an overwhelming problem, it is an increasing one . . .*

Q: Such resistance seems to be related to penetration of the drug into the fungus. Would adjusting the dose solve the problem?

DuPont: Sometimes patients are seen who show resistance when taking 50 mg. of fluconazole. When the dose is raised to 100 mg., or 200 mg. in these patients, there is clearance of thrush. Several of our patients, however, were receiving up to 600 mg. of intravenous fluconazole and still had persistent thrush. So, for some patients, or some strains, there is still resistance, even with the higher dose . . .

Q: What is the best strategy for preventing resistance in patients with candidiasis?

DuPont: The patient should be started on ketoconazole. If it does not work, or if the patient cannot take ketoconazole for any reason, then fluconazole would be the next option. A higher dosage, such as 100 mg. per day, instead of 50 mg. per day, is preferred. When there is a recurrence of candidiasis after several months, it should be treated each time. If a relapse occurs when treatment is stopped after one week, then continuous therapy is indicated.[2]

REFERENCES

1. Levin, A., as quoted by Crook, W.G., *The Yeast Connection*, Third Edition, Professional Books, Jackson, TN and Vintage Books, New York, 1986; pp 326–327.
2. DuPont, B., *Candidiasis*, source unknown.

47

Free Radicals and Antioxidants

Free Radicals

Almost ten years ago, I began hearing about *free radicals* and *antioxidants*. To learn more about these topics, I consulted my good friend, Dr. Elmer Cranton, a graduate of Harvard Medical School and a past president of the American Holistic Medical Society. Dr. Cranton has published many scientific articles and several books, including his popular book, *Bypassing Bypass*,[1] which describes the relationship of free radicals to coronary heart disease and other health problems.

Although Cranton gave me a lot of information, I must confess that I still had more questions than answers. Since that time, I've read and heard a lot more about free radicals and the importance of antioxidants in controlling them.

At a health food convention in 1992, I heard a presentation dealing with these topics by David J. Lin, B.S., a summa cum laude graduate in biology and chemistry. The title of Lin's illustrated lecture was "Free Radicals Shouldn't Be Free." I was fascinated because Lin presented these topics in an easy-to-understand format. Then, in late 1993, I received a copy of his illustrated, 87-page book which provided me with additional information.

According to Lin, over 30 years ago scientists and researchers began to write and talk about free radicals. In the paragraphs that follow I'll paraphrase and excerpt some of Lin's comments. In the introduction to his book, he said:

> "Uncontrolled free radical processes may be critically involved in the cause and progression of numerous disease conditions, conditions which before seemed unrelated."

He also noted that simple nutrients, called antioxidants, are perhaps the best natural defenses against these harmful substances. According to Lin:

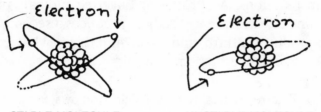

STABLE MOLECULE   UNSTABLE MOLECULE

"*Free radicals are molecules with electrons which are unpaired* [emphasis added]. Molecules are basic building blocks in nature such as oxygen, fatty acids, amino acids, glucose and DNA. Molecules are held together by electrons.

"Stable molecules have electrons that are in pairs, like a buddy system. But if a molecule has an electron which does not have a partner, it becomes unstable and reactive . . . *a free radical* [emphasis added]. It will steal an electron from a stable molecule.

"Once the stable molecule loses an electron, it becomes another free radical. This second free radical will steal an electron from a third molecule, and a destructive cycle begins. Each time a molecule loses an electron it is damaged and will damage another molecule."

Where Do They Come From?

In his continuing discussion, Lin pointed out that free radicals come from several sources.

- Our bodies are constantly making them. They help our immune system destroy bacteria and viruses. Exercise and illness also produce them. Free radicals play a number of useful functions. For one thing, they are important in producing vital hormones. They also activate enzymes.

  So free radicals are important to health. They aren't "evil." *It is only when they are produced in excessive amounts that they damage the body.*
- Tobacco smoke, pesticides, herbicides and other air pollutants also encourage the production of free radicals. One such air pollutant is ozone, which comes from vehicle exhaust.
- Chain reactions. According to Lin, free radicals produce a "domino effect." One free radical produces a second, which in turn produces a third, and so on. And this is what makes free radicals so dangerous. And he said:

"Although a free radical regains its electron by stealing it from a stable molecule, it does not regain its original form and function; it is damaged. So, it's not like passing a hot potato for someone else to worry about; it's more like a spreading fire: something that is burned is never the same again."

In his continuing discussion, Lin compares the effect of free radicals to what happens on a freeway when a tire rolls over a big 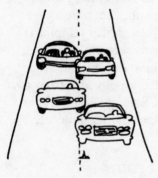 sharp nail. POW! The tire blows. The car swerves out of control and crashes into another. Then another car piles on. Then another and another, until you have a tremendous pile up. The cars represent molecules in our cells and the nail is a free radical.

Your body is composed of billions of healthy cells of all sorts; cells arranged in an orderly fashion; cells with normal membranes and layers of nuclei. Free radicals damage these cells in various ways, allowing bacteria and viruses to enter. According to Lin:

"The cells damaged by free radicals can accumulate to become full blown disease states. Just as one tiny nail on the freeway can cause a major catastrophe, so a free radical can cause and worsen serious disease conditions, including heart disease, cancer, cataracts, arthritis, Parkinson's disease and many others."

How Can We Cope with These Free Radicals?

We can, of course, make appropriate changes in our lifestyles. We can stop smoking and stop polluting our homes with toxic chemicals. We can eat foods rich in the *antioxidant* nutrients, especially fruits, vegetables, grains and nuts. These nutrients function together as a team to quench free radicals.

We can also take nutritional supplements, especially the four antioxidant nutrients—beta carotene, vitamin C, vitamin E and the trace mineral selenium.

Antioxidants

Before talking further about *antioxidants,* let's talk about "oxidants." This term comes from the word oxygen. Quoting Lin again, he said:

"Leave oils and meats outside too long and they become rancid. Rancidity involves oxidants in a process called oxidation, which is the reaction of oxygen with fatty acids and proteins to form free radicals, eventually causing spoiling."

What Is an Antioxidant?

"Anti" means against and, as I already pointed out, "oxidants" are reactive substances which take electrons from other substances—that is free radicals. *So an antioxidant fights oxidation by neutralizing free radicals which cause it.*

To recapitulate, a free radical has an unpaired electron. An antioxidant supplies the missing electron or stabilizes the free radical.

Using the analogy of the nail on the freeway again, Dr. Lin said:

"If a highway sweeper had swept the nail off the road before a car could run over it, then much damage would have been avoided . . . So antioxidants function as highway sweepers . . . averting potential devastation.

"In the body many kinds of antioxidants protect us, including enzymes, nutrients, amino acids, proteins and other biochemicals."

Antioxidants and Nutrients

These include beta carotene (pro-vitamin A), vitamin C, vitamin E and the mineral selenium. These nutrients are not made in the body, but are found in significant quantities in fruits, vegetables, grains and nuts. They function as a team to quench free radicals. Moreover, they often act in conjunction with other classes of antioxidants such as enzymes.

Beyond Free Radicals

In his concluding comments, Lin pointed out that free radicals carry out essential functions in the body. He said that they're not 'evil' and that, on the contrary, life without them would be impossible. Yet, when free radicals become excessive and uncontrolled, they can damage the body.

"Antioxidants are vital defenders against excessive free radical attacks. The role of proper nutrition in preventing disease is becoming clearer . . . Once dismissed by medical authorities as minor players in maintaining health, vitamins and minerals are beginning to be used to treat a wide variety of serious ailments. As the role of antioxidants in combating free radical pathology becomes clearer, we will hopefully be able to effectively treat diseases which have plagued us for ages."

Lin said that he feels a revolution in the concept of treating disease will soon occur and that physicians will be turning to natural safe substances, including beta carotene, vitamin C, vitamin E and selenium. He also said that there is a growing body of objective scientific evidence to substantiate the effectiveness of such therapies. Yet, he said:

> "Just as no miracle drug will ever cure all the diseases known to humankind, so no miracle nutrient will. If any lesson should be learned, it is that health depends upon much more than a simple formula. Antioxidants may help to provide many healthy benefits, but they will never replace wise diets and lifestyle."[2]

REFERENCES

1. Cranton, E. and Brecher, A., *Bypassing Bypass*, Hampton Roads Publishing Co., Second Edition, 1990; pp 59–60, 214–215, 231–232.
2. Lin, D.J., *Free Radicals and Disease Prevention*, Keats Publishing Company, New Canaan, CT, 1993. (Reprinted with permission.)

48

◆

Medicines from Plants

◆

During my years in medical school, internship and residency, I spent most of my time learning about disease; and, the therapies usually used were surgery and prescription drugs. Such drugs were most often discovered and compounded by research chemists working in the laboratories of pharmaceutical companies.

From time to time, however, I learned a little about natural remedies. One such remedy, tea made from the foxglove plant, was used by "granny women" in England in the 1700s to help people with heart disease. They knew it was effective, but they didn't know why. Over a century later, scientists learned that the *Digitalis* cardiac glycoside was the active ingredient of this plant. And today, *Digitalis* remains the drug of choice for people with weakened and failing hearts.

I also learned that orange juice prevented scurvy and that pharmaceuticals derived from the Indian plant *Rauwolfia serpentina* helped people with high blood pressure and other problems. Interestingly enough, this plant medicine had been sold in Indian bazaars for generations as a treatment for insanity.

In spite of my awareness of these plant-derived medicines, I knew little about them until the early 1980s. At that time, I was invited to give a lecture at the regional conference of the National Nutritional Food Association (NNFA). At this conference I heard about the health benefits of garlic. At subsequent conferences of NNFA and Natural Products Expositions (NPE) in the '80s and '90s, I heard about the therapeutic value of many other plant products.

Plant Medicines Enter the Scientific Mainstream

Although plant-derived medicines were rarely mentioned in medical journals or conferences in the '80s, during the mid-1990's they have received increasing attention. I found evidence of such attention in a 2½-page editorial published in the June 18, 1994, issue of the distinguished medical journal, *The Lancet*, "Pharmaceuticals from plants: great potential, few funds." Here are exerpts.

"Plants have long been a source of medicines . . . use of the herb qing hao, now a recognised source of antimalarial agents, was recorded, for haemorrhoids, in 168 BC in China. In the UK and in North America, almost 25% of the active components of currently prescribed medicines were first identified in higher plants."

In the continuing discussion of plant medicine, the editorial pointed out that as recently as 15 years ago none of the top 250 pharmaceutical companies had a research program involving higher plants. Yet, now over half of them have introduced such investigations.

"Nevertheless, support for plant-based research has been largely overlooked by the funding bodies, and investigators find it difficult to obtain grants for such projects. The National Cooperative Natural Products Drug Discovery Groups under the aegis of the National Cancer Institute in the USA represent an exception."

The editorial told of many other herbal remedies, including ginseng, echinacea, garlic and *Ginkgo biloba*. And in discussing the latter plant medication, the editorial said:

"Studies of some of these plants have yielded compounds with unique activity—e.g., ginkgolides, specific platelet activating factor antagonists that were obtained from the Chinese tree *Ginkgo biloba*. A standardized extract of ginkgo leaves is one of the most frequently prescribed medicines in Germany and is taken to alleviate cerebral ischaemia [inadequate blood flow]."

The article also stated that new test systems may reveal novel activities and compounds that could explain the traditional use of a plant previously thought to be inactive, and said:

"Thus the general immunostimulant effect of plants such as *Echinacea* species, used as a tonic and to prevent infections, was shown only with the advent of tests that could detect an increase in immune response."

Other herbal products which were favorably mentioned included artemisinin from *Artemisia annua* and flavonoids. And in the concluding paragraph, the editorial stated:

"What of the future for plant-based agents? There are many possibilities for research, but priority should be given to tropical infectious and chronic diseases for which current medications have severe drawbacks, and to the scientific appraisal of plant-based remedies that might be safer, cheaper, and less toxic items for self-medication than existing prescribable medicines. This is an area rich in ideas and flora; what is needed now is imaginative funding to match."[1]

Bioflavanols

My first knowledge of these plant-derived substances came from a six-page report by R.C. Robbins, Ph.D., published in the September 1980 issue of *Executive Health*. In this report, "On Bioflavonoids: New Findings About a Remarkable Plant Defense Against Disease," Robbins said that a possible role for bioflavonoids in human health was called to his attention by Dr. Albert Szent-Györgyi, who won the Nobel Prize for his discovery of vitamin C. In summing up his article, Robbins said:

"The evidence mounts: Bioflavonoids demonstrate a remarkable variety of activities which make them valuable.

"We now appear to have sufficient information to begin to bring these compounds into effective use in nutrition and medicine and I believe that in the closing years of the 20th century they will help to assure a higher level of human health."[2]

During the 1980s, I occasionally read or heard something about these nutritional substances, but I didn't really know much about them. Then, in June 1993, Bert Schwitters, a journalist I met in Holland, sent me an autographed copy of his brand new book, *OPC in Practice—bioflavanols and their application*. This book was written in collaboration with Professor Jack Masquelier, a distinguished French biochemist and a member of the medical faculty of Bordeaux University.

Professor Masquelier isolated a plant flavanol in 1948 and in 1951 he registered his first patent. The generic name of this flavanolic substance is "OPC," which is an abbreviation of oligomeric proanthocyanidins. Quite frankly, although the material in the book seemed interesting, I put it on my bookshelf and busied myself with other things.

In the late spring of 1994, I received a letter from Ned Turner, of Germantown, Tennessee, praising *pycnogenol*. Then, in early August 1994, I read an article on pycnogenol by Richard A. Passwater, Ph.D. A few weeks later, at the National Products Expo East in Baltimore, Nathan Keats and Norman Goldfind gave me a 108-page book by Dr. Passwater entitled, *PYCNOGENOL—The Super "Protector" Nutrient.*

Two weeks after I returned from that convention, during a telephone conversation, Walter Ward, M.D., Winston-Salem, North Carolina, expressed enthusiastic interest and support for this plant-derived substance. *I put two and two together and figured that the pycnogenol some people were talking about was, in fact, Masquelier's OPC extract described in Schwitters' book.* So I pulled the book off my shelf and read it from cover to cover. Here are some of the things I found out.

Professor Masquelier first isolated OPC from plant sources in 1947. In 1950, it entered the field of therapeutics as a vascular protector. About 30 years later (1979), Masquelier coined the term "pycnogenols" to make a clear differentiation between the non-bioavailable bioflavonoids and his bioflavanols.

In his foreword to Schwitters' book, Professor Masquelier said:

"With OPC* [pycnogenol] we finally have at our disposal a real weapon against premature aging of living structures . . . Amongst the various proposed candidates to play this role . . . OPC fulfills this condition. Used in therapeutics for 40 years, it has never provoked direct or secondary effects of a toxic nature."[3]

In a chapter in his book entitled, "The Discovery of OPC," Schwitters reviewed the history of the use of plant products. He also reviewed the observations of early researchers, including H.C. Haywarth, T. Reichstein and Albert Szent-Györgyi. He also discussed the rather complicated biochemistry which is involved in these various plant products and the terminology, including "procyanidols, procyanidines and proanthocyanidins."

What are the benefits of these plant products? Here are the comments of nutritional authority Richard A. Passwater, Ph.D.

". . . The 'superprotector nutrient' is actually more than a single nutrient. Pycnogenol (pronounced pick-nah-geh-nol) is a complex of powerful antioxidant nutrients that . . . scavenge free radicals. . . . this means that this specific mixture of nutrients can help you live better longer, stay healthier and appear more youthful. Pycnogenol can help protect you from approximately *eighty* diseases, including: heart disease, cancer, arthritis and most other non-germ diseases that are linked to the deleterious chemical action of free radicals."

In his continuing discussion of these plant-derived substances, Passwater said that they are remarkably safe nutrients that correct conditions because they strengthen capillaries, nourish the skin and balance histamine production. He said:

". . . Pycnogenol is patented. It is a registered trademark of Horphag Research Ltd. which allows the product to be used by various companies in the manufacture of food supplements.

---

*In the U.S.A. and many other countries, OPC is being marketed under the trademark "OPC-85." Both products, "OPC-85" and "Pycnogenol" fall under the protection of the U.S. Patent that describes the use of OPC as a scavenger of free radicals.

"Pycnogenol is usually sold by itself in various strengths, but it is also increasingly being used in antioxidant formulations and multiple vitamin formulations. It is available as a pure material, or mixed with fillers in capsules, or blended with binders . . . and pressed as tablets."[4]

If you'd like to know more about OPC and pycnogenol, get a copy of the Passwater and Schwitters books at your health food store.

REFERENCES

1. Editorial, "Pharmaceuticals from plants: great potential, few funds," *The Lancet*, 1994; 343:1513–1515.
2. Robbins, R.C., "On Bioflavonoids: New Findings About a Remarkable Plant Defense Against Disease and Its Dietary Transfer to Man," *Executive Health*, Pickfair Bldg., Rancho Santa Fe, CA 92067, September 1980; Vol. XVI, No. 12.
3. Schwitters, B., *OPC in Practice—bioflavanols and their application*, Alfa Omega Publishers, Rome, 1993; pp 6–7.
4. Passwater, R.A., Kandaswami, C., *Pycnogenol, the Super "Protector" Nutrient*, Keats Publishing Co., New Canaan, CT, 1994; pp 1, 108.

49

◆

Alternative Medicine

◆

In *The Yeast Connection* I talked about alternative medicine and "consumerism" and I quoted a commentary in the *New England Journal of Medicine* by John Lister. This British physician said that there seems to be an increasing dissatisfaction with certain aspects of conventional or orthodox medicine and that *one of the growth industries in contemporary Britain is alternative medicine.*

I also cited the observations of Norman Cousins, Marilyn Ferguson and John Naisbitt. Each of these well-known writers noted the growing interest of the public in diets, exercise and preventive health care.[1]

During the past decade, I've met countless people at health food conventions who've told me about "alternative" therapies. Also, hundreds—even thousands—of people who have written or called me have told me of their successful—even dramatic—response to such therapies. These have included chiropractic manipulation, acupuncture, herbal medications and other therapies which, up until recently, have been ignored or ridiculed by the medical mainstream.

But today, in the mid-1990s, alternative medicine, unlike the proverbial camel who *only* poked his nose under the tent, has moved in with its entire body. Here's evidence to support what I'm talking about.

According to a study published in the January 28, 1993, issue of the *New England Journal of Medicine*, one-third of all Americans have sought help from alternative practitioners.[2] *And most of the time they haven't told their own physicians.* Their conviction that such therapies help is documented by the money they've spent: $13.7 billion. Moreover, they've paid $10.3 billion themselves, since their private health insurance and Medicare or Medicaid doesn't cover it.

A New Book on Alternative Medicine

In a two-page article published in the *Washington Post,*[3] Margaret Mason featured the 1,068-page book, *Alternative Medicine: The Definitive Guide.* This book was put together by Burton Goldberg, a 67-year-old developer who spent almost two million dollars completing it. Mason pointed out this book should serve as a starter course for mainstream physicians to learn about alternative medicine, even though they don't have to agree with everything in the book.

More About Burton Goldberg and His Book

I received a copy of this fantastic book in early 1994. As I thumbed through it, I found many topics that interested me. Included was a discussion of the relationship of *Candida albicans* to multiple sclerosis, autism and other disorders.

Then, in September 1994, I met Goldberg at a health food convention in Baltimore and I was truly impressed by his dedication and his desire to help people. Here are excerpts from his commentary, "Why This Book Was Written."

"Two systems of health care are available in this country today: conventional Western medicine and alternative medicine. The first is the world of the American Medical Association; medical doctors who practice by the book . . . Conventional medicine is superb when it comes to surgery, emergency, and trauma.

"But there's no question that alternative medicine works better for just about everything else, especially for chronic degenerative diseases like cancer, heart disease, rheumatoid arthritis and for more common ailments such as asthma, gastrointestinal disorders, headaches and sinusitis . . .

"Alternative medicine is more cost effective over the long term. Because it emphasizes prevention and goes after causes rather than symptoms, it doesn't trap people on the merry-go-round that begins with one drug and ends up requiring them to take others to compensate for the side effects each one causes. Many alternative methods work by assisting your own body to heal itself instead of introducing strong drugs."[4]

Goldberg pointed out that it takes time for new ideas to be accepted. He also cited the story of Ignaz Semmelweiss, the Austrian physician who was ridiculed and fired from the staff of a hospital in Vienna. His offense: he asked his colleagues to wash their hands after working on cadavers before carrying out pelvic examinations! Yet, it took doctors 30 years to "catch on."

The Harassment of Physicians

During my years of practice, I've known of twentieth century American physicians who have been ridiculed and rejected by their establishment peers. One of them, Theron Randolph, a Chicago internist and allergist, was "fired" from the faculty of Northwestern University Medical School in the early 1950s because they said "his teachings were a pernicious influence on medical students."

What was Randolph's offense? Teaching his students about the importance of food sensitivities.

Even today, health professionals are being harassed because they dare to do things differently. Here are examples.

Reputable physicians in many states have been, and are, harassed by their local medical societies for prescribing nystatin, Diflucan and other antifungal medications for people with headache, fatigue, depression and other symptoms. One such physician, Jon VanCleave, D.O., Des Moines, Iowa, was harassed by Blue Cross/Blue Shield and the Iowa Board of Medical Examiners. In a November 1994 letter to me he said:

"For nearly two years I spent tens of thousands of dollars defending my treatment regimen found entirely satisfactory with my patients. My case was to come up to a hearing in their kangaroo court. I was told by several 'in the know' people that the Iowa Board of Examiners was not going to let me treat candida illnesses in Iowa, no matter how many out-of-state experts I would bring in to my defense."

> **I spent tens of thousands of dollars defending my treatment regimen found entirely satisfactory with my patients.**

Because it would have taken an additional $50,000 to proceed with the hearing, Dr. VanCleave decided to move from Iowa to Hawaii. I believed in his cause so much that I flew to Iowa and testified for him, but it was to no avail.

Here's more: Nutricology, a California company headed by Stephen A. Levine, Ph.D., a researcher with impeccable academic credentials, was raided by FDA agents in 1991. What was the reason for the raid? Levine was accused of selling "unapproved new drugs" and a restraining order was slapped on nine of his products. These included several of my favorite therapeutic agents: CoQ_{10}, flax seed oil and citrus seed extract.

Jonathan Wright, M.D., one of the best read and smartest physicians I've had the privilege of knowing, was raided by government agents. Here are excerpts from an editorial in the Monday, May 11, 1992, *Seattle Post-Intelligencer*, "FDA's Strange Raid."

"If there is any plausible excuse for the Gestapo-like tactics used in a raid on a Kent alternative-medicine clinic last week, it had better be forthcoming, and fast.

"King County Police officers, drafted by agents from the Food and Drug Administration, kicked in the door of Dr. Jonathan Wright's clinic with guns drawn and pointed at clinic employees, commanding them to 'freeze!' and put their hands in the air.

"On what grounds? Were armed terrorists believed to be getting vitamin shots in the clinic? Were naturopathic revolutionaries plotting the violent overthrow of the American Medical Association's national convention? Were crack and methamphetamine laboratories believed to be bubbling away in the back room?

"No. As far as we can tell—and it's hard to tell because neither the King County Police nor the FDA are telling anything—the justification for the U.S. District Court search warrant and raid was the allegation of unlicensed production of drugs (as in pharmaceuticals, not street drugs) at the clinic."

In continuing his discussion, the editorial writer said that there were serious questions about not only the raid's tactics, but its motivation. He pointed out that Wright had filed suit against the FDA, demanding that the agency return stocks of the dietary supplement L-tryptophan. And he said that it should be kept in mind that the holistic, dietary-oriented theories and practices of Wright and other physicians have met with resistance and disdain from many physicians. In concluding his commentary, the editorial writer said:

"It would be unconscionable if Wright were being persecuted— not to mention prosecuted—for nothing more than having the temerity to challenge the medical and regulatory powers that be. The public is owed a full and complete accounting, and soon."

To find out what had happened, I called Dr. Wright in December 1994. Here are excerpts from our conversation.

"Since the FDA kicked down the door and raided my office, they have continued a campaign of harassment. As recently as three months ago when an employee left, within 48 hours they went to her and asked, 'What went on in that clinic? What kind of things can you tell us?' Although they impaneled a grand jury in October 1992, no indictment was issued. No charges were filed. No one has made any lawsuits—nothing.

"Yet, because of the Grand Jury and all the legal activity, even with no charges filed, it has cost our legal defense fund over $200,000 and there is no end in sight. They have not let up. They have even gone to such lengths as strip-searching my wife on her way back from Taiwan. Here's why. The FDA told the customs service that she was a drug runner."

The Office of Alternative Medicine

Two years ago, in response to pressure from their constituents, the U.S. Congress created an Office of Alternative Medicine. In contrast to the billions of dollars being devoted to research on AIDS and other diseases, they allocated only $2 million to study alternative medicine.

Pediatrician Joseph Jacobs, M.D., a (then) 46-year-old physician with native American roots, was appointed to head the office. During his two-year leadership, he made friends with people in the alternative health movement. In addition, he obtained the cooperation and respect from the establishment. Yet, in the summer of 1994, he decided to pass the baton on to someone else.

Jacobs' picture and a review of his work appeared in a half-page article in the September 30, 1994, issue of *USA Today*. According to this article by Leslie Miller, one of the reasons that Jacobs decided to walk away from his historic post was the difficulty he experienced in following a middle road between two extremes of opinion.

On one side were the impatient advocates who wanted alternative medicine to be recognized overnight; on the other hand, Jacobs had to cope with what he called the "bureaucratic armada" of the National Institute of Health.

According to Miller's article, the Office of Alternative Medicine is preparing to announce a report detailing various alternative practices with recommendations for future research. It will include:

- seed grants for two centers to study alternative practices for health management, such as cancer and pain management.
- a data base on alternative therapies for health professionals and the public.
- to evaluate such subjects as herbal medicine and meditation.
- workshops to offer technological and grant-writing assistance.

In addition, an official 19-member advisory panel was named during the summer of 1994. Included on the panel will be several women's health advocates who are breast cancer survivors.

Support for Alternative Medicine

Another article by Miller, in the same issue of *USA Today,* reviewed natural remedies of all sorts, including herbal teas and chicken soup. In preparing her article, she interviewed Glen W. Geelhoed, a George Washington University professor of international medical education, and co-editor of a book entitled, *Natural Health Secrets from Around the World.*

In his comments, Geelhoed said that there are many health problems which orthodox medicine can't solve and that folk remedies may help.

He also pointed out that many times professionals and nonprofessionals learn that a particular therapy works, although the scientific proof of *why* it is effective isn't discovered until many years later.

Robert Anderson, M.D., Ph.D., Mills College, Oakland, California, also made favorable comments about alternative medicine in a letter published in the correspondence section of the *New England Journal of Medicine.*

"To be helpful to physicians who are trying to make sense of alternative medicine, the system of classification would be more useful if it differentiated with greater precision on the basis of type of treatment . . .

Dieting is a part of many healing systems, including conventional medicine.

"To illustrate as briefly as possible, in the nutritional category at least two discrete categories require very different counseling on the part of concerned physicians. One, dieting, is a part of many healing systems, including conventional medicine. A vast scientific literature provides a basis for reference essential to the concerned physician.

"The other, herbalism, is the treatment of diseases with natural substances that are ingested in large doses, often as polypharmacy.

Herbalism is almost universally based on well-enunciated, historically-derived, nonbiomedical theories of medicine that reflect centuries of clinical and cultural experience. Most physicians have little or no knowledge of herbal treatments."[5]

I found further information and support for alternative medicine in the January 1, 1995, issue of *USA Weekend*. In the sixth annual special health issue entitled, *Can Alternative Medicine Help My Headache*, many different alternative therapies were listed and discussed for treating five common ailments: headaches, arthritis, back pain, extra pounds and asthma.

The article cited the ideas and approaches of many experts, including James Gordon, M.D., of Georgetown University and Dean Ornish, M.D., and Anthony Rosner, Ph.D., Research Director of the Foundation for Chiropractic Education and Research. This issue, which was devoted entirely to alternative medicine, cited and quoted many people, including professionals and nonprofessionals. Included also were ways "not to get snookered." Some of these were: See a physician for acute conditions; look for credentials; ask for referrals; be skeptical of unrealistic claims and have realistic expectations.

Comments of Abram Hoffer, M.D., Ph.D., Victoria, B.C., Canada

This pioneer physician has carried out numerous studies which provide scientific support for the value of niacin and other micronutrients in treating patients with chronic health disorders. Through his many publications, including the *Journal of Orthomolecular Medicine,* he has provided physicians and other professionals with sound information often unobtainable elsewhere.

In a December 1994 letter to me, Dr. Hoffer wrote:

"I'm sure you're aware of the amazing turnabout toward alternative and complementary medicine. Harvard Medical School apparently has just started a new division of complementary and alternative medicine and so has Columbia University . . . For the past five years, the University of Colorado at Denver has been teaching the proper use of vitamins, etc. to their medical students.

"I do think there has been a massive shift and we are now well into the vitamins-as-treatment paradigm. The new freedom that is going to be given to American doctors will see an amazing flowering of this whole movement. You may be aware of the fact that Dr. Warren Levin has won his case and that all of the charges have been dropped. Also, the state of New York has passed legislation making it impossible to harass a doctor any more because he uses alternative treatments."

Andrew Weil, M.D., An Alternative Medicine Pioneer

This University of Arizona College of Medicine faculty member is one of the world's leading authorities on natural medicine. A best-selling author, Weil has written many books on natural medicine and related topics; including, *Health and Healing: Understanding Conventional and Alternative Medicine, Natural Health, Natural Medicine: A Comprehensive Manual for Wellness and Self-Care.* Here are excerpts from a recent article on Weil by Baynon McDowell.

"With a college major in botany, a premed interest in herbal medicine, and a medical degree from Harvard (1968), Weil has the stamp of a man who knew exactly where he was headed—to pioneer and champion the power of the body to heal itself through natural medicine."

In introducing the article, McDowell included the following quotation.

"I would like to see radical reform of medical education . . . I would like to see new kinds of institutions come into being that are somewhere between hospitals and spas that would replace many current hospitals. People would go who had chronic illness, for example, and come out knowing more about how to take care of themselves and how to use simple measures on their own. I would like to see new types of clinics in which practitioners of different systems work under the same roof. . . ." Andrew Weil, M.D.[6]

Herbal Remedies

Herbal remedies aren't all that new. What's more, during my days in medical school I learned about digitalis, the main heart medicine which was derived from the foxglove plant. Here are a few others that I know about, including some that I learned about many years ago and others I first heard about during the past decade.

Herbal Teas, Lime Juice and Vitamin C

Indians in Canada discovered that tea made from the leaves and bark of the *Arbor vitae* tree helped many members of their tribe with various complaints. In the seventeenth century, a friendly Indian passed this information to French explorer Jacques Cartier, whose soldiers in Quebec were dying of scurvy. When the soldiers drank the tea, their scurvy went away and many lives were saved. Some 75 years later, Dr. James Lind used lime juice to prevent scurvy in sailors on British ships.*

Ginkgo Biloba

This "folk remedy" from the Ginkgo tree has been used in China for a long, long time. And, a recent scientific study provides support for this therapy. Here are excerpts from a 1992 article in *The Lancet*.

"Extracts from the leaves of Ginkgo biloba . . . have been used therapeutically for centuries. Ginkgo, like ginseng, is mentioned in the traditional Chinese pharmacopoeia. . . . In Germany and France, such extracts are among the most commonly prescribed drugs."

*See Chapters 43 and 48.

The article reviewed 40 published controlled trials, most of which were conducted in Germany and France. And they found that eight trials were of good quality. They especially noted that elderly people with difficulties of concentration and memory, absent mindedness, confusion, lack of energy, depressive mood, anxiety, dizziness, tinnitus and headache were improved. And patients described in two of the trials showed "an increase in walking distance."

> "In most trials, 120 to 160 mg. a day, divided into three doses, was used . . . Treatment must be four to six weeks before positive effects can be expected. Whether beneficial effects remain when treatment is stopped is unknown. The only drawback worth mentioning is the high cost . . ."[7]

In her "Nutrition Hotline Column," which appears each month in *Better Nutrition for Today's Living*, Shari Lieberman, Ph.D., in responding to a reader who wanted to try something natural for tinnitus, said:

> "Ginkgo biloba may help this problem, as may a low-fat diet. Vitamin A, calcium, magnesium, zinc and vitamin D are very important for inner ear function, and their deficiency may be implicated in this disorder. Omega 3 fatty acids may also be useful."

Garlic

According to John Heinerman, Ph.D., in his 1994 book, *The Healing Benefits of Garlic—From Pharaohs to Pharmacists*,[8] the healing powers of garlic were mentioned by the epic poet Homer (in 850 B.C.) in his *Iliad*. It was also mentioned several places in the New Testament. It was also used by the Egyptians and the Romans.

He then cited the research studies of Benjamin Lau, M.D., Ph.D., of Loma Linda School of Medicine, who has found that aged garlic extract is effective in the prevention and treatment of cancer of the breast, stomach, bladder and skin.

He also quoted Calvin L. Thrash, M.D., Medical Director for the Uchee Pines Institute, who told him that he had seen a lady with a severe yeast problem who was troubled by multiple digestive symptoms. She had tried everything, including nystatin, and received very little help. Following dietary changes and liquid aged garlic extract, her symptoms went away.

Echinacea

I began hearing about this herb at health food conventions in the mid-1980s. I had not used it in my practice and I knew little about it. Then I began reading articles in *Let's Live, Alive* and other health food magazines which told me about the many virtues of echinacea.

In Earl Mindell's *Herb Bible,*[9] I learned that echinacea came from the purple cone flower which was used by native Americans to treat snake bite, fevers and old, stubborn wounds. Moreover, early settlers adopted the plant as a home remedy for colds and influenza. According to Mindell, word of echinacea's healing properties traveled back to Europe and studies there showed that it appears to lessen the severity of colds and flu and helps speed recovery.

In his continuing discussion, Mindell pointed out that there has been a renewed interest in echinacea in the United States because of its positive effect on the immune system. He also noted that it has been used successfully in treating candida, psoriasis and eczema.

Other Herbal Remedies

Mindell also discussed golden seal, astragalus, garlic, ginger, ginkgo, ginseng, saw palmetto, feverfew and Pau d'Arco.

This latter herbal remedy comes from the bark of two South American trees. In the third edition of *The Yeast Connection,* I mentioned its possible benefits.

During the past decade, I have continued to get reports describing the value of this tea (as a part of a yeast-control program) even though mechanisms to explain its benefits have not been documented.

A Final Word

Just as I was finishing this book and preparing to send it to the typesetter, I opened my copy of the November/December 1994 issue of *Natural Health—The guide to well-being.* It was chock-full of interesting articles. Here are several of their titles: "Grow Healthful Herbs All Winter"; "Uncommon Remedies for the Common Cold"; "Bringing Spirituality to Everyday Life."

I was especially interested in an article by Karen Baar, "The Real Options in Health Care—Consumer Guide to Alternative Health." According to her introductory paragraph:

> "Alternative treatments, both new and traditional, can empower you, reduce your need for surgery and synthetic drugs, lower your healthcare costs and generally improve your life. Here's a guide to the world of healthcare beyond doctors and hospitals."[10]

Baar's article discussed seven principles of alternative medicine. Here are several of them. Your body can heal itself; preventive medicine is better medicine; the cure and the prevention are often the same. Included in the article was a discussion of naturopathy, orthomolecular nutritional medicine, ayurveda, homeopathy and traditional Chinese medicine. If you'd like a copy of the 164-page November/December issue of this magazine, send your request and $5 to *Natural Health,* 17 Station Street, Box 1200, Brookline Village, MA 02147, Attention: Customer Service.

REFERENCES

1. Crook, W.G., *The Yeast Connection,* Third Edition, Professional Books, Jackson, TN and Vintage Books, New York, 1986; pp 264–267.
2. Eisenberg, D.M., et al, "Unconventional Medicine in the United States," *N. Engl. J. Med.,* 1993; 328:246–252.
3. Mason, M., "An Alternative Guide to Good Health," *The Washington Post,* Friday, January 28, 1994.
4. Compiled by the Burton Goldberg Group, *Alternative Medicine: The definitive guide,* Future Medicine Publishing, Inc., Puyallup, WA, 1993.

5. Anderson, R., "Physicians and Healers—Unwitting Partners in Health Care," Correspondence, *N. Engl. J. Med.,* 1992; 326:1503.
6. McDowell, B., "Andrew Weil, M.D.—Championing Integrative Medicine," *Alternative and Complementary Therapies,* Mary Ann Liebert, Inc., New York, 1994.
7. Kleijnen, J. and Knipschild, P., "Ginkgo biloba," *The Lancet,* 1992; 340:1136–1138.
8. Heinerman, J. *The Healing Benefits of Garlic—From Pharaohs to Pharmacists,* Keats Publishing, New Canaan, CT, 1994.
9. Mindell, E., *Earl Mindell's Herb Bible,* Fireside/Simon and Schuster, New York, 1992; pp 83–85.
10. Baar, K., "The Real Options in Health Care—Consumer Guide to Alternative Health," *Natural Health,* 17 Station St., Box 1200, Brookline Village, MA 02147.

50

Reducing Health Care Costs

Today, everyone is talking about health care and how much it costs. Yet, it seems to me that most of the money being spent is not for *health care*, it's for *disease care*. And billions of dollars are now being used to treat conditions that could be prevented by dietary and lifestyle changes, exercise and nutritional supplements.

The Yeast Connection and Health Care Costs

As you may have read in the preface of the first edition of *The Yeast Connection*, written over 10 years ago, I said:

> "I sincerely feel that recognition and appropriate management of yeast-connected illnesses can play a major role in what I recently referred to as the 'Coming Revolution in Medicine.'
>
> "This revolution will help physicians and their co-workers relieve much unnecessary suffering. It will also save patients, the government, business and industry (including the health insurance industry), billions of dollars."[1]

I described the story of Paige Grant Pell in Chapter 6 of this book. This Illinois professional said that she spent over $100,000 seeking help for chronic health disorders. Then, following anticandida therapy and treatment for allergies, she showed dramatic improvement.

Paige Grant Pell spent over $100,000 seeking help for chronic health disorders.

Here's another illustration sent me by Ray C. Wunderlich, M.D., of St. Petersburg, Florida. A 13-year-old boy (I'll call him Samuel) had been troubled by abdominal pain off and on for about a year. He described it as sharp and crampy and lasting about 30 minutes. The pain occurred two to three times a day and there was no relationship to food or times of stress. In addition, he felt nauseated, but no vomiting.

A complete physical examination described Samuel as a "friendly white male, in no acute distress." The details of his examination were normal. Here are excerpts of a report by a consultant who saw him:

"I think the differential here has to be inflammatory bowel disease, especially with the bleeding, the lack of weight gain over the last two years, the abdominal pain, the diarrhea. This versus the Irritable Bowel Syndrome. The laboratory studies are okay and I think this child needs an upper GI bowel follow through and a colonoscopy. We will schedule that for the same day. I will notify you of the results."

In a series of subsequent reports to the family physician, the consultant described an extensive series of diagnostic investigations and therapies. These included ultrasound examinations, endoscopies, biopsies and the antibacterial medication Azulfidine. When these didn't help, the consultant said:

"Samuel is seeing a counselor who called my office last week. The parents have given me permission to communicate with him. I discussed with the parents the possibility of using medications such as antidepressants. Also, continue the therapy as part of multimodal treatment to get him back on track.

"To get him to attend school and cover him emotionally, psycho-

logically, as well as physically . . . I think it will be helpful for him to be treated for his clinical depression [emphasis added]!"

During the next three months, Samuel continued to complain of excessive intestinal gas. He had also been seen by a psychiatrist a number of times and was diagnosed as having "school phobia."

Then through "networking," the family learned about Dr. Wunderlich's interest in yeast-related problems. Following a careful review of his history, Samuel was put on a therapeutic trial of nystatin and diet and within a few days his stomach pains, gas and school phobia vanished!

Food Sensitivities and Health Care Costs

I learned about food sensitivities many years ago from Albert Rowe, Theron Randolph and Frederic Speer and this knowledge changed my medical practice and my life. Since then, I've talked to anybody who'd listen and I've written many articles and books which emphasize the role food sensitivities play in making people sick. Although what I've had to say has often fallen on deaf ears, I've been thrilled and gratified by the response of occasional believers. Here's an example.

In 1980, Harold Hedges, an alert and inquisitive Little Rock, Arkansas, family physician, heard me talk about food sensitivities at an otolaryngology meeting at the University of Tennessee. Here are excerpts from his letter to the editor published in the *Journal of the Arkansas State Medical Society* in January 1982.

Many illnesses are caused by what we eat, drink and breathe.

"The longer I practice medicine, the more I am convinced that many illnesses are caused by what we eat, drink and breathe. I have practiced medicine since 1963 as a partner in Little Rock General Practice Clinic. I have treated many patients with obvious diseases—

diseases which can be seen by the naked eye or obviated by our sophisticated lab and x-ray examinations.

"I have also treated many patients with diseases and disorders which I could neither see with the naked eye nor specifically obviate by these same examinations. I have labeled (in good faith) these many problems as:

tension headache	fatigue syndrome	chronic sinusitis
depression	irritable bowel	nerves
anxiety	situational reactions	hypochondriasis
hyperactive child syndrome	nervous stomach	chronic recurring otitis media

"Some I even laid on the poor lowly virus. (I thank God for viruses—even if I couldn't prove it so, the patient couldn't prove me wrong!)

"The list is longer but these are just some of the more common ones. Over the years, I've had patients ask me if I thought 'something they ate' could cause their bizarre symptoms. Not really believing this, I would simply shrug my shoulders and halfheartedly agree with that possibility."

In his continuing discussion, Hedges told how he had helped dozens of his difficult patients using the elimination/challenge diets I outlined in my "picture book" *Tracking Down Hidden Food Allergy*. And he said:

"In the day of rising costs of medical care, I was really intrigued by the cost of this 'work-up,' and office call plus a diet sheet and instructions . . . *What an impact on the cost of medicine we could have if we could identify a person's chronic complaints secondary to food and inhalant reactors before being shoved into a system of testing—testing which will not disclose the culprit of their disorders* [emphasis added].

"I would suggest that each of you reading this be a 'doubting Thomas,' and don't believe any of this until seeing it work. Try it on some of your most difficult and puzzling cases; cases which have already had the usual and customary work up for that particular complaint. If you fail the first time you try these techniques, don't give it up; it certainly is not the panacea for all chronic complaints, but there are enough successes to make the extra time worthwhile. . . ."[2]

In the 11 years since Dr. Hedges published that letter in his state medical journal, he has continued to help thousands of patients using elimination diets. He has also lectured to physicians, especially family physicians, all over the United States. And in a November 1992 supplement to American Family Physician, he published an article entitled "The Elimination Diet As a Diagnostic Tool." In summarizing his observations, he said:

"Many family physicians overlook the role that food and food additives play in health problems. An elimination diet is a safe and cost effective method of evaluating adverse reactions to foods in some patients with common medical problems. Patients whose symptoms improve or clear while they are on the diet are then challenged with the omitted foods, one at a time to establish food-symptom relationships."[3]

The Yeast Connection to Food Sensitivities

At the September 1988 Candida Update Conference in Memphis, a European researcher and clinician, Gruia Ionescu, Ph.D., talked about the relationship of bacterial and fungal infections of the intestine to health problems of various types, including especially atopic eczema. And in a subsequent interview with Marjorie Hurt Jones, R.N., editor of *Mastering Food Allergies*, Dr. Ionescu said:

"We've found approximately half of our allergics have a problem with candida overgrowth in their gut. And many people diagnosed with candida infections exhibit intolerances to food also . . . In our clinic in West Germany we focus our attention on improving the health of the gut . . . especially its lining, the intestinal mucosal. Here's an overview of our rationale:

"When the gut contains an overgrowth of candida, the lining becomes very inflamed . . . and less efficient at handling food. Because the walls are more permeable, they start to leak . . .

"We have found that the best diet in the world will not give the patient adequate nourishment if he has abnormal bowel flora. In healthy people, beneficial bacteria predominate in the delicate balance of organisms. They prevent the pathogenic bacteria yeast fungi or mold from running rampant."[4]

In discussing food sensitivities with Sidney Baker in June 1993, he said:

"If all you know about a person is that they have unreasonable sensitivities to things, the odds are that they have a yeast problem behind it. Many of the patients I see who are sensitive to a lot of things are out of balance biochemically. Their digestive function is disturbed, or they have a chronic infection and adrenal insufficiencies, or they've had an invasive life event.

"These are some of the main categories I think of, yet the yeast problem is by far the most frequent, just in terms of overall incidence."

Anticandida Therapy and Health Care Costs

In a presentation at the American Academy of Environmental Medicine in October 1993, George E. Shambaugh, Jr., reviewed his observations on 67 of his patients, and he said:

"Every one of these patients reported substantial improvement a year or more after beginning the treatment program. This program included anticandida therapy, allergy testing with an emphasis on mold allergies, and candida immunotherapy.

"The average amount of money these patients had spent before coming to my office was over $4000. For a comprehensive program of evaluation and therapy, including medication, tests and vaccines, the average cost in my office was $1654.13 . . .

"Recognition and proper management of the candida related complex is indeed both cost effective and successful. It puts an end to expensive laboratory tests and fruitless examinations by physicians who not only refuse to recognize this syndrome, but angrily reject the suggestion that it is relevant . . ."

Dr. Shambaugh also cited the article by Dr. Arnold Relman, the (then) editor of the *New England Journal of Medicine*, who in a 1988 editorial, "Assessment and Accountability of Medical Care," said:

> "We can no longer afford to provide health care without knowing more about its successes and failures."[5]

Better Nutrition Can Reduce the Cost of Health Care

In the September 1994 issue of *Better Nutrition*, Frank Murray, in an editorial, "Ways to Decrease Our Oversized Health-Care Bill," cited a Florida physician, who, writing in the June 2, 1994, issue of *Medical Tribune* said:

> "In order for a health-care reform package to be truly successful, there needs to be more sources of preventive medicine techniques. Prevention is not just mammograms, CAT-scans and Pap smears."

The editorial pointed out that medical students and graduate physicians should have training in preventive medicine and health-maintenance techniques. In addition to correcting dangerous life-styles, such as poor dietary habits, physicians need to pay closer attention to the use of alternative medical practitioners such as chiropractors, acupuncturists, nutritionists, etc., rather than a broad surgery-only, or prescription drug-only approach to disease.

Murray also cited the comments of the late Linus Pauling published in the October 15, 1993, issue of the *Los Angeles Times*, in which Pauling said that, "It's time the government finally caught up with a large and rapidly growing body of scientific research on nutrition."

In citing additional comments by Pauling, Murray said:

> "In 1954, when he received his first Nobel Prize, much was unknown about the role of vitamins in promoting and preserving

health. Now, some forty years later, science has painted a relatively detailed picture of the important role of vitamins in preventing illness, but 'government regulators at the FDA remain locked in a Cold War against vitamins, when they could be encouraging education about preventing the common cold and other maladies.'

"After more than two decades and countless new studies, the FDA remains at odds with many in the scientific community regarding beneficial claims on vitamins' role in preventing cancer, heart disease and birth defects, among others.

In concluding his editorial, Murray quoted this comment by Pauling.

"As a scientific investigator, I am interested in ongoing research on medical problems, including determining as reliably as possible the values of optimum intakes of vitamins and other nutrients."[6]

REFERENCES

1. Crook, W.G., *The Yeast Connection*, First Edition, Professional Books, Jackson, TN, 1983; p vi.
2. Hedges, H., Letter to the Editor, *J. Ark. St. Med. Assoc.*, January 1982; 78(2).
3. Hedges, H., "The Elimination Diet as a Diagnostic Tool," *American Family Physician*, November 1992 Supplement.
4. Ionescu, G., as quoted by Jones, M.H., *Mastering Food Allergies*, 2615 N. 4th St., #616, Coeur d'Alene, ID 83814.
5. Relman, A., "Assessment and Accountability of Medical Care," Editorial, *N. Engl. J. Med.*, 1988.
6. Murray, F., "Ways to Decrease Our Oversized Health-Care Bill," *Better Nutrition*, September, 1994; p 6.

51

More About the Candida Controversy

During the past decade the relationship of superficial yeast infections to chronic illness has, to a large extent, been ignored—even ridiculed by most physicians. Here are examples of what I'm talking about.

In a report on what they call the "Candidiasis Hypersensitivity Syndrome," approved by the Executive Committee of the American Academy of Allergy and Immunology (AAAI), a number of statements were made, including:

1. The concept is speculative and unproven.
2. The basic elements of the syndrome could apply to almost all sick patients at some time.
3. There's no published proof that *Candida albicans* is responsible for the syndrome.[1]

The American College of Allergy and Immunology (ACAI) made an identical "proposed position statement." The Committee on Scientific Affairs of the American Medical Association (AMA) published shorter, but similar, negative opinions about the role candida may contribute to a diverse group of health disorders.

In response to the statements by AAAI and ACAI, I prepared a nine-page report answering their various negative statements point by point. I also responded to the comments of the Committee on Scientific Affairs of the AMA. Although I was a member of all three of these organizations, they did not reply. And they gave no indication that they would like additional information, or would like to hear "the other side of the coin."

Paula's Story

This 33-year-old woman gave a history of her active personal and professional life—very active. She worked ten hours a day, ran 15 miles a week, developed pimples and was put on tetracycline, which she took for 18 months (between the ages of 27 and 29). After taking this antibiotic for several months, she began to develop concentration problems, anxiety, fatigue, depression and other symptoms.

She saw a number of physicians who said, "your problems are caused by stress." Yet, Paula's symptoms were so disabling that she had to give up her job and she stayed in bed most of every day.

Then, she found a physician who put her on nystatin, a sugar-free diet and nutritional supplements. Here are excerpts from a recent letter she sent me.

"Thank you so much for writing your book. And thank the International Health Foundation for putting me in touch with the doctor who helped me. Rather than feeling like a limp wash cloth, I'm now back to 95% of where I started from. I have 10 to 14 hours of energy each day, although I do still get tired in the late afternoon and evening.

"I'm writing you first to give you a progress report and next to send a small check with this letter for you to turn over to the International Health Foundation. I strongly believe in your efforts, so you can count me as an annual contributor.

"Next, I want to tell you that *I have been appalled, even embittered, by the lack of knowledge and resistance of doctors in this university medical center community* about the relationship of superficial yeast infections to chronic illness. I realize that doctors and scientists are taught to believe in reliable information gathered in controlled studies and I suspect that malpractice litigation has strengthened that tendency.

"But common sense should prevail when you and other doctors have gathered volumes of information that has returned so many chronic sufferers back to normal lives. It is truly beyond my comprehension why this information is so submerged. I would like to help raise the level of awareness, understanding and acceptance in this city. I go to church with the university's associate director for patient care services. I plan to meet with her and explore the reasons why there is such a deficit of acceptance and what would be needed to correct it.

"I think that a good place to start would be with the nurses and physician assistants who work with health insurance companies. It would be in the best interest of the company to embrace this therapy because it is less expensive in both the short run, and in the long run. I also thought of these allied health workers for another reason. It would help them make their case before congressional committees on how their skills could be used to heal patients and reduce overall health-care costs.

"In my opinion, most traditional doctors are close-minded due to the way they've been educated and also due to the horribly litiginous environment in America."

Encouraging Signs of Change

I'm happy to report that things are changing and more "establishment" physicians are becoming interested. Here's evidence of such interest.

In February 1993, I was invited to participate in a POINT-COUNTERPOINT discussion, entitled, "The Yeast Connection—Allergy or Fallacy?" It was one of a series in the Department of Medical Education Tarzana Regional Medical Center, Tarzana, California. In my presentation I provided those in attendance with supporting documentation. William B. Klaustermeyer, M.D., Professor of Medicine, UCLA, presented an opposing point of view.

A month later, I made a similar presentation to physicians in the Departments of Obstetrics and Gynecology of the East Memphis Baptist Hospital. Then, in October 1993, I served as chairman of a four-hour workshop in New Orleans.*

---

*See also Chapter 20.

In preparing for these presentations, I sought help and consultation from many knowledgeable and experienced physicians whose comments are cited in various parts of this book.

The Comments of George F. Kroker, M.D.,* La Crosse, Wisconsin

This statement is so comprehensive, and yet so succinct, that in my opinion, "it says it all." *I sincerely hope that it will be carefully read and digested, not only by skeptical physicians, but also by people who feel their health problems are yeast related.*

"I'm writing in response to your request for my impressions in treating Candida Related Complex. As you know, I am a university trained, board-certified physician. I treated my first patient with this illness in late 1978 after I had missed this diagnosis in one of my patients and learned more about it from Dr. Orian Truss in Birmingham, Alabama.

"I became intrigued as to why this illness had such diverse manifestations; as you know, I subsequently reviewed the classical literature on Candida-related pathology and contributed a chapter on this subject to an allergy textbook.[2]

"I have treated several thousand patients with this illness over the last 14 years. I have arrived at the following clinical impressions over that time:

1. *Candida-related complex cannot be treated successfully without simultaneous attention to a sugar and yeast-free diet* [emphasis added].
2. *Candida-related complex often is associated with other illnesses, most notably mold allergy, chemical sensitivities, autoimmune thyroiditis, and food intolerances. Unless these illnesses are screened for, the treatment for Candida (antifungal medicine and diet) may completely fail to ameliorate the patients symptoms. I cannot overemphasize the importance of the "total load" in dealing with these patients. This makes it hard to set up a study* [emphasis added].

---

*Diplomate, National Board of Medical Examiners; Diplomate, American Board of Internal Medicine.

3. Candida-related complex seems to be a chronic and relapsing illness in many patients. Patients may have a remission in illness and need no antifungal medication and be more lenient on their diet, only to relapse and have a return to illness with stress, dietary overindulgence, antibiotics, etc.

   Candida-related complex seems to coexist frequently in patients with premenstrual syndrome and also in patients with chronic fatigue syndrome. Treating the Candida illness seems to often improve both of these other problems.

4. Unfortunately, Candida remains a disease in search of a laboratory test for diagnosis. *The best test remains the history and a one-month trial of antifungal medication and diet* [emphasis added]. I have tried to utilize antibody assays, cultures, etc., and they all fall short of diagnostic certainty."

REFERENCES

1. The Practice Standards Committee, American Academy of Allergy and Immunology, "Candida Hypersensitivity Syndrome," *J. Allergy Clin. Immunol.*, 1986; 78:271–273.
2. Kroker, G.F., "Chronic Candidiasis and Allergy," in Brostoff, J. and Challacombe, S., *Food Allergy and Intolerance*, Balliére Tindall, Eastbourne, England, and W.B. Saunders, Philadelphia, PA, 1987; pp 850–870.

PART

NINE

---◆---

Appendices

---◆---

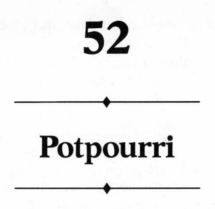

52

Potpourri

The information in this book comes from many sources. These included professionals I interviewed and nonprofessionals who wrote me. I also read hundreds of articles in professional and lay journals and reviewed dozens of books. *Each day, I learned things that I hadn't known before.*

As I worked to complete the book, my good friend and typesetter, John Adams said, "Billy, if you want your book to be published, stop making additions." He even sent my secretary a FAX which said "break Dr. Crook's pencil!" But as I sorted through the mountain of papers in my office, I found more material which I felt would interest and help my readers. Here it is.

More About Yeast-Related Problems

Celiac Sprue and The Yeast Connection During the '60s and '70s, I began to read and hear more about celiac sprue (CS), a relatively uncommon inherited disorder which affects digestive metabolism. It manifests itself principally as an inability of the small bowel to digest and absorb gluten-containing foods.

In the early '80s, I began to correspond with Lloyd Rosenvold, M.D., of Hope, Idaho, who described a possible relationship between gluten intolerance, yeast overgrowth in the intestinal tract and multiple sclerosis. In a letter to me, Dr. Rosenvold told me that several members of his wife's extended family had been troubled by multiple sclerosis. They improved significantly when given nystatin, along with a gluten-free diet. And I included his comments in the third edition of *The Yeast Connection*.[1]

Dr. Rosenvold published further observations in a 1992 book, *Can a Gluten-Free Diet Help? How?* In a chapter entitled, "When Celiac Meets Candida," Rosenvold said:

> "I believe in *some* cases (maybe even many cases) the presence of celiac sprue, which is secondary to gluten intolerance offers a fertile . . . culture medium for the propagation of yeast organisms. In any case of intestinal yeast infection the possibility of a concomitant CS should be considered until it can be confidently ruled out. . .
>
> "How are CS and yeast infections connected, if they are? I'll briefly state my simple concept. The putrefactive processes in the bowel, incidental to the maldigestion and malabsorption present as a result of the CS, furnishes . . . an ideal culture medium for the propagation of *Candida albicans*. . . .
>
> "Physicians often fail to recognize that there may be a distinct interaction between CS and intestinal yeast infection. Actually, the CS makes chronic yeast infection possible by furnishing the habitat and culture medium for the candida yeasts.[2]

Halitosis   Could bad breath be yeast connected? According to Dr. Martin Zwerling and associates, the answer is "yes." In a report in a peer-reviewed medical journal, these professionals told of their success in helping 70 out of 79 patients, including 15 with halitosis. Here's an excerpt from their article.

> "It was thought possibly that candida could also ferment foods in the stomach and cause halitosis [bad breath]. In a busy ENT practice it is not difficult to find patients with intractable bad breath, most of whom have had their tonsils and teeth removed, along with assorted abdominal organs, in unsuccessful attempts for relief.
>
> "Fifteen patients with halitosis were placed on the therapeutic trial (avoidance of sugar and foods rich in yeast and mold, elimination of antibiotics, steroids and birth control pills . . . and nystatin and/or ketoconazole).
>
> "Within 24 to 48 hours all 15 patients reported marked improvement in their breath odor and this was confirmed by their families

and the examining physician. This is the first report of the use of antiyeast treatment in halitosis."[3]

Golf Champion JoAnne Carner's Story   In a cover story article in the January 1988 issue of *Golf Digest*, JoAnne Carner told how yeast infections took a toll on her body and her golf game. Here are excerpts from her report.

"My doctor diagnosed the illness as caused by *Candida albicans*, a yeast infection. I'd been vulnerable to colds and bronchitis for a long time, but never understood why. I just accepted it as the way things were. The first time I noticed something was drastically wrong was when I was playing with Arnold Palmer in the Mazda Tournament in Jamaica in December 1985.

"My arms were aching and I was tired all the time. Over the next four months I had bronchitis twice and tonsillitis twice. The antibiotics I was taking were killing the good bacteria in my system, as well as the bad bacteria. When that happens, yeasts start to take over and slowly work on your immune system. I was feeling weak and run down.

"In a tournament, trying to walk up any little hill would kill me. Some of the other women players had to help me. I could barely make 18 holes, then I would go back to my room and collapse.

"Because of the infection, I had a dry mouth all the time. I couldn't wait to get to the water fountain. I could drink nine glasses of water and still feel dry in the mouth. Dry and bloaty. I was weighing more than I had ever weighed in my life. I didn't like the way I felt or looked."

In her report, Carner described the diet she went on which included the avoidance of milk, sugar, yeast and fruit. She said the diet helped her lose weight and that her golf game improved. And she said:

"It's amazing how many people have written me about my illness and weight loss. Apparently *Candida albicans* infections are quite common in women. It's not that serious a thing, only when it sweeps throughout your system because of antibiotics. One woman wrote that she had the same dry mouth that I had. She said she was suck-ing on candy all the time because her mouth felt terrible.

"I wrote back that she was actually contributing to the affliction because it feeds on sugar. If you have any questions, pick up a book entitled *The Yeast Connection* by Dr. William G. Crook."

Spouses Need Treatment Too   Candida, like other microorga-nisms, can be transmitted from person to person through intimate contact, including sexual relations. Although a sexual partner with a strong immune system may not seem to be bothered by yeast problems, most physicians feel that partners should be treated. Here are the comments of Geraldine Donaldson, M.D., Livermore, California.

"I treat the spouse—I insist upon it. And I insist upon them being on treatment for at least a month . . . even if they don't have symp-toms. If they have jock itch or nail fungus infections, I will treat them longer.

"Although a man may show no obvious signs of yeast or other fungus infections, he's apt to reinfect his wife. I've found that quite often. I usually try very, very hard to talk the husband into going into treatment for a month anyway. If he is uncircumcised, I usually rec-ommend an antifungal cream underneath the foreskin.

"I put them on the full treatment program with oral antifungals and I try to get them to follow the diet. I tell them if they don't follow the diet the treatment won't be effective."

Endocrine Disturbances in Women with Yeast Infections   Some 15 years ago, researchers at the Medical University of South Caro-lina described endocrine abnormalities in women with chronic vaginal candidiasis. Here are excerpts from an abstract of their report.

"Seventeen of thirty patients with chronic vaginal candidiasis (CVC) of at least five years duration had varying degrees of men-strual problems and defective T-lymphocyte function; eight devel-oped amenorrhea. In a group of 40 CVC patients, titers of autoantibodies to ovary, thymocytes, a T-cell line . . . and a B-cell line, were significantly higher than those in 45 normal females . . .

"Significant correlations were found between anti-Candida, anti-ovarian, and anti-thymocyte antibody titers . . . The results suggest the presence of one or more cross reactive antigens on ovarian follicle, T-lymphocytes (especially the helper cell subpopulation), and Candida."[4]

Headaches and Candida Albicans   In an article in the Fall 1992 issue of the *Journal of Advancement in Medicine,* Gunnar Heuser, M.D., and colleagues presented their findings on studying 17 patients with recurrent classic or common migraine. Those selected met the following criteria:

- A classic or common migraine of more than two years duration, with at least two attacks of headache per month.
- All had shown resistance to well-established treatment modalities for migraine headache.

In addition, recurrent vaginal yeast infections and food sensitivities were frequently observed in this patient population. The patients were instructed to keep a diary of their headaches and the medications used. They were also started on a restricted diet and given acidophilus supplements.

Four weeks after initiation of the restricted diet, the patients were placed on oral nystatin. All patients in the group were found to have elevated blood titers of candida antigen, antibodies and immune complexes. Patients who complied with the diet and the outlined treatment program showed a decrease in headaches and in candida titers.

Noncompliant patients continued to have headaches and elevated titers. Asymptomatic controls showed small fluctuations of titers, but these were in a range much lower than the experimental symptomatic group. Based on their observations, these investigators concluded that, "Some vascular headaches have candidiasis as a trigger and respond to appropriate treatment."[5]

Nystatin Helps Acne   In a letter to the editor in the May 1989 issue of the *Journal of the American Academy of Dermatology,* H.L. Newbold, M.D., said:

"By chance I've discovered that powdered oral nystatin shows promise as a valuable drug for the treatment of acne vulgaris. I would like to pass along information gathered so that others can follow-up with more extensive trials. Also, the following observations may give new insights into the pathogenesis of acne and lead to more effective treatments."

In his case report, Dr. Newbold told of his experiences in treating a 44-year-old man who was troubled by marked chemical sensitivities. The patient was given testosterone enanthate injections which reduced his sensitivities. However, as a side effect, acne developed.

In an attempt to further reduce his patient's sensitivity, Dr. Newbold gave him a therapeutic trial of powdered oral nystatin (1/2 tsp.) in water, six times daily. The nystatin did nothing to lessen his sensitivities, but his acne disappeared. Twice the nystatin was withdrawn. Each time the acne flared and cleared again with the return of the nystatin.

Digestive Problems and Garlic   Some 25 years ago, Calvin Thrash, M.D., and Agatha Thrash, M.D., founded the Uchee Pines Institute for Health and Education as a ministry of the Seventh Day Adventist Church. (30 Uchee Pines Rd., #31, Seale, AL 36875–5703.) Although I have never met Calvin and Agatha, we have exchanged many letters. Here are excerpts from a letter by Dr. Calvin Thrash.

"I saw a 45-year-old lady with a severe yeast problem—almost unable to eat anything, lots of gas, bloating, discomfort, poor digestion, etc. She has tried everything, including nystatin, with minimal help. I told her to take the liquid Kyolic, three teaspoons, three times a day, along with diet, and some other suggestions. She called me three months later to say that within two weeks her symptoms were all gone.

"She also told me that she had familial hypercholesterolemia [elevated cholesterol] with it usually running around 350 in spite of being a total vegetarian . . . At the end of the two months on Kyolic she had her cholesterol checked again and it had dropped to 220. She said it has not been that low in her adult life."

Chronic Urticaria (Hives) Some years ago, I read a paper by a prominent allergist who said that he would rather see a tiger walk into his office than a patient with chronic urticaria. He felt this way because finding the cause of this disorder is often impossible. Prednisone, a steroid medication, which is often given to relieve symptoms may bring on other problems, especially if it is given for many weeks or months.

In my own practice of allergy in the '60s and '70s, I saw a few patients with chronic hives. In one of them, an elimination diet enabled a hidden troublemaker (yellow food color) to be identified and eliminated, and the hives went away. Yet, the other patients continued to suffer from welts, itching and swelling for many months—even years.

In *The Yeast Connection,* I told the story of Robert, a refrigeration technician with severe hives and a frightening swelling in his throat.[6] Because Robert gave a history of receiving multiple courses of antibiotic drugs, I prescribed nystatin and a sugar-free diet. Within a few weeks, Robert was able to stop the prednisone and periodic injections of epinephrine were no longer necessary.

For a period of 12 years, I did not see Robert as a patient, and I often wondered how he was getting along. Then, in early 1994, Robert's wife stopped me on the street. She told me that he took nystatin and followed his diet for a year and his hives never returned. During the past several years, I've seen two other patients with chronic hives who have responded to a sugar-free diet and antiyeast medications.

Do antiyeast medications cure hives? Absolutely not. Yet, if a person with this disorder gives a history of repeated or prolonged courses of antibiotic drugs, a sugar-free special diet and antifungal medication is certainly worth a try.

Lyme Disease (LD) and The Yeast Connection During the past few years, a strange and often puzzling infectious disease has received national attention. It first appeared in the town of Lyme,

Connecticut. It is caused by a microorganism, *Borrelia burgdorferi*, and is transmitted to humans through the bite of infected ticks.

The disease occurs in several stages. Initially there's a flu-like illness which is often associated with a red, expanding rash. Weeks to months later, neurologic or cardiac symptoms develop.

Broad-spectrum antibiotics have been found effective in treating patients with LD, especially when given during the acute stage. Yet, in spite of such treatment, many patients with this illness continue to experience problems. In a report in the *Pediatric Clinics of North America*, University of Pennsylvania researchers said:

> "At this time there is no evidence to suggest that many months of antibiotic treatment are better than the current standard therapy and may actually be harmful. . . . Some manifestations [of LD] are the result of persistent infection, whereas other symptoms are a consequence of immunologic changes secondary to the infection. Most disease manifestations are not specific to this illness. . . . the illness is overdiagnosed and overtreated."[7]

During the past several years, I've received copies of *Lyme & Disease Update (LDU)*, a nationwide monthly publication. In almost every issue, I read the reports and letters from people with LD who continued to experience problems even though they had taken long-term courses of antibiotics.

One such story published in the October 1994 issue told of a 26-year-old man with LD who had been taking antibiotics for many months but who "kept getting sicker." His story prompted me to respond. Here is an excerpt from my letter published in the December 1994 *LDU:*

> "I'm writing to urge all Lyme disease sufferers who take antibiotics to take antiyeast medications along with the antibiotics. Here's why. *While antibiotics are controlling the microorganisms that cause Lyme disease, they knock out friendly germs in the intestinal tract. As a result, a whole cascade of problems develops, including a weakening of the immune system* . . . [emphasis added]."[8]

Yeast-Related Autism   Because I have received so many phone calls and letters from the parents of children with yeast-related autism during the past several years, I have encouraged parents to make their children's stories known to medical leaders. Here's one such letter by a Wisconsin mother.

American Academy of Pediatrics
141 N. W. Point Blvd.
Elk Grove Village, IL 60007

To Whom It May Concern:

I'm writing as a parent of a 3-year-old boy diagnosed with pervasive developmental disorder and/or autism. Our son met normal developmental milestones until approximately 20 months of age. At that point he started to lose speech and regress socially. He was treated for many episodes of otitis media from age seven months and on . . . At the age of 2 years, 8 months, he received the diagnosis of pervasive developmental disorder.

One treatment has appeared to significantly improve my son's condition. The drug Diflucan brought about impressive changes in his mental abilities and behavior. These included: eye contact, attention, decreased stereotypical behaviors, listening, play and communication.

While this treatment may not be standard in the treatment of autistic disorders, I implore you to acknowledge the anecdotal reports of such improvements and seriously consider further study of candidiasis and autism.

The diagnosis of autism is devastating to families. We need all the hope and help we can get. I'm not saying that antiyeast medications and dietary changes would be effective for all autistic children. Yet, even if such a treatment helped only a small percentage of these persons, I believe it should be explored.

Sincerely,

Beverly Brown (not her name)

More on Yeasts in the Stools During the past decade, Elizabeth Naugle of College Station, Texas, has made extensive searches of the American and German medical literature. Although it would take another book to discuss all of the articles she sent me, I found many of them interesting and informative. Here's an abstract from one of the articles which described the findings of Italian researchers.

> "The authors report that 20 patients in whom a large number of dead or severely damaged yeast cells, supposedly *Candida albicans*, were the possible cause of chronic recurrent diarrhea and abdominal cramps.
>
> "It is suggested that the presence of large numbers of these microorganisms in stools may be considered among the possible etiologies of diarrhea in the irritable bowel syndrome.
>
> "The possible source of these yeast-like cells, the causes of cell damage and the mechanisms by which these organisms may induce diarrhea should be investigated."[9]

In commenting on this article, Naugle said, "It helps explain the paradox of negative stool cultures in patients with yeast-related health problems because dead cells can't be cultured."

Head Clearing Effect of Diflucan Recently Ray C. Wunderlich, Jr., M.D., St. Petersburg, Florida, wrote me about some of his experiences in treating his patients with antifungal medications. Here's an excerpt.

> "I've had about ten patients who had various chronic illnesses ranging from arthritis to seizures to MS to gastrointestinal disorders. Upon treatment with Diflucan, 200 mg. a day, a decisive head clearing occurred. In other words, foggy thinking, brain-fag [exhaustion] or spaciness remitted.
>
> "Several of these patients had MS. One is an entertainer who travels across the world. None had 'classic' symptoms/signs to suggest candidiasis. Upon discontinuing treatment, symptoms usually recur. The longest duration of treatment so far is two years. Why would anyone choose such an expensive placebo?"

Single Dose Treatment for Acute Vaginitis   Eight hundred and seventy women with vaginitis were enrolled in a study. Approximately three-fourths of the women had acute vaginitis (less than four episodes per year). Half of the women were given a single 150 mg. tablet of Diflucan, and the other half were treated with daily intravaginal medication for seven days. The cure rate in each group of patients was almost identical.[10]

More About Nutrition and Nutritional Supplements

Suggestions for Obtaining Safer Foods   In an article in the Fall 1993 issue of the newsletter published by the Nutrition for Optimal Health Association, *NOHA News*, editor Marjorie Fisher discussed the hazards of pesticides found on and in many of the foods we eat every day. Here is an excerpt.

> "No pesticide is 'safe' because pesticides are, by their very nature, designed to be biologically active and kill various kinds of organisms . . . A very large proportion of all the pesticides used today are neurotoxic, and many are expressly designed to disrupt nerve function."

In her continuing discussion, Fisher cited the comments of Joan Gussow, Professor of Nutrition and Education at Columbia University, who said that consumers have become so fixated on fat, cholesterol, fiber, antioxidants and other parts of food, that they've lost sight of what's going on in the food supply. In discussing what to do about pesticides in the food, Fisher said:

> "We can greatly reduce our own and our family's exposure to pesticides by buying organic food. These purchases help society at large, as well as ourselves directly. By creating a demand for the products of the organic farmers, their distributors and the stores selling their products, we're helping those committed to no pesticide use. (Including no insecticides, herbicides, nor fungicides.)
>
> "We should, of course, be alert to false claims and deceptive actions. For example, the regular grocery store that advertises a

small section of 'organic' produce, although they have contaminated the entire store by employing exterminators.

"Even with a tiny plot of land we can grow a great deal of our own food organically. . . . From our own garden it can be a delight to eat fresh herbs, vegetables and fruits at the peak of their ripeness and wonderful flavor."

If these excerpts interest you and you'd like a copy of this eight-page newsletter and other information, send a long, stamped (2 stamps), self-addressed envelope and a donation of $2.00 to NOHA, P.O. Box 380, Winnetka, IL 60093.

Why Many of Us Do Not Eat Things That Are Good for Us Why do most of us eat too few foods that are good for us and too many foods that aren't? There are a number of reasons which you are familiar with. Here are some of them.

Few of us have gardens, or orchards; we eat on the run; we eat and enjoy ice cream, butter, thick steaks, fried chicken, hamburgers, french fried potatoes and other high fat foods. We've also been brainwashed by advertisements from companies that make processed foods that are loaded with sugar and partially hydrogenated fats.

Here's still another reason. *Physicians have been given little information about nutrition during medical school and residency training.* And few articles in the medical literature or programs at postgraduate conferences have emphasized the importance of truly good diets. Although in the 1990s changes are being made, physicians continue to receive more information about treating disease than about preventing it through optimal nutrition.

In the January/February 1994 issue of the *Nutrition Action Healthletter*, on a page entitled, "Just the Facts," appeared these comments:

- Amount spent in 1993 by the National Cancer Institute to promote its "5-A-Day for Better Health" campaign, which encourages people to eat more fruits and vegetables: $400,000.
- Amount spent in 1992 by Kellogg™ to promote Froot Loops® cereal: $13 million.

- Amount spent in 1992 by Kellogg™ to promote Frosted Flakes®: $34 million.
- Minimum number of daily servings of fruits and vegetables recommended by the National Cancer Institute: 5.
- Percentage of general and family practitioners who say they eat at least 5 servings of fruits and vegetables every day: 20 . . .
- Price the farmer received for the potatoes in a 16-oz. bag of potato chips that sells for $1.92: 24¢
- Price received for the corn in an 18-oz. box of corn flakes that sells for $1.77: 9¢
- Price received for the wheat in a 1 lb. loaf of bread that sells for 75¢: 4¢
- Number of schools out of 545 surveyed that served lunches averaging less than 30 percent of calories from fat: 5.
- Number that served lunches averaging less than 10 percent of calories from saturated fat: 1.[11]

More About Probiotics   Elizabeth Naugle recently sent me information about *Saccharomyces boulardii,* a probiotic organism which belongs to the brewer's yeast family. Researchers who studied mice with weakened immune systems found that by giving oral preparations of this probiotic, that *Candida albicans* did not translocate (spread) from the intestinal tract to deeper tissues.

This probiotic is available in the form of "lactic yeast tablets." According to information I received, one of these tablets with each meal will help re-establish the normal bacteria in the intestinal tract. Although I've had no personal experience in using this product, it sounds like a valuable addition to the probiotic team. It may be available in some health food stores. For more information you can call 1–800-545-9960.

For a copy of Naugle's essay, "Altered Bowel Ecology: Candida and dysbacteriosis" (with references from the international medical and scientific literature), write to the Candida Research Information Foundation (CRIF), P.O. Drawer JF, College Station, TX 77841–5146. Please enclose a donation of $5.00.

Too Much Iron Can Cause Problems   You do not need an iron supplement unless you're losing a lot of blood during your menstrual periods, or you've had a surgical operation accompanied by extensive blood loss.

According to Dr. Elmer Cranton, "Iron is so potentially dangerous that I recommend blood testing before prescribing it for anyone. Too much iron can shorten your life." In a presentation at a health conference in Atlanta several years ago, Dr. Cranton said that physicians should assess iron status carefully in adult patients. He recommended the serum ferritin test, and said that the levels should be under 100. He also said:

> "You'll be a lot healthier if you're between 50 and 70 if you periodically donate blood. A study was made several years ago of people in this age group who donated blood on a regular basis and others who did not. *The death rate of those who donated blood was half of that observed in those who did not.*"

Cranton also sent me a copy of a front page article by David Stipp from the Tuesday, September 8, 1992, issue of the *Wall Street Journal* entitled, "Heart Attack Study Adds to the Cautions About Iron in the Diet—Evidence rises that nutrients long seen as beneficial could often be harmful."

In his report, Stipp focused especially on a study published in *Circulation* (a journal of the American Heart Association) which suggested iron levels have a closer association with heart attacks than any other risk factor except for smoking. He also cited the observations of a young South Carolina physician, Jerome Sullivan.

This physician became interested in finding the answer to these questions: *"Why is heart disease much less frequent in women than in men before middle age?"* and *"Why do just as many women as men in the late '50s, '60s and '70s develop heart disease?"* The apparent cause: Women get rid of some of the unneeded iron through menstruation up until menopause.

Why does iron cause trouble? Although all the answers aren't known, it may have to do with free radicals and iron appears to increase free radical damage. (You'll find a discussion of free radicals and antioxidants in Chapter 47.)

More Support for Vitamin Supplements   During the last decade, I've read a number of reports about vitamins by Jack Challem, a nationally known science and technology writer. His articles have appeared in many publications, including *Bestways, Health News and Review, EastWest, Natural Health, Let's Live* and the *Journal of Orthomolecular Medicine.*

And for the past two years, I've subscribed to his newsletter, *The Nutrition Reporter.** Recently, Challem sent me a copy of his 55-page booklet, *Getting the Most Out of Your Vitamins and Minerals.*[12] I was impressed with what I read, including the many references from the peer-reviewed literature. Here's an example of what I'm talking about.

Challem cited two major studies which were reported at the November 1992 meeting of the American Heart Association. One of these studies, "The Nurses' Health Study," followed 87,245 women, ages 34 to 59, who were free of heart disease when the study began in 1980. In discussing this study, he referred to the observations of Meir Stampfer, M.D., an associate professor at the Harvard School of Public Health. In citing Stampfer's findings, he said:

> "After adjusting for age, smoking, obesity, exercise, and other risk factors, Stampfer and his colleagues found that the nurses taking vitamin E supplements had only two-thirds (64 percent) the risk of cardiovascular disease, compared with those not taking the vitamin supplement. Women who took vitamin E for more than two years had an even lower risk of developing heart disease, only 54 percent."

Nutritional Supplements and People Power   During the early 1990s, and even before, a number of people in the nutritional food industry were harassed by U.S. Government agents. And on several occasions, health food stores were raided, and supplements, including *Ginkgo biloba* and CoQ_{10}, were pulled off the shelves. The reason: the safety and the efficacy of these substances were said to be unproven.

Soon it became apparent to consumers and industry leaders

---

*P.O. Box 5505, Aloha, OR 97006–5505.

that even more restrictive laws were on the drawing board. So many, many people, including several members of the U.S. Congress, sprang into action. And they were successful, as you'll see from this excerpt from the October 25, 1994, statement by President Bill Clinton:

> "Today I am pleased to sign S.784, the 'Dietary Supplement Health and Education Act of 1994.' After several years of intense efforts, manufacturers, experts in nutrition, and legislators, acting in a conscientious alliance with consumers at the grassroots level, have moved successfully to bring common sense to the treatment of dietary supplements under regulation and law."

President Clinton cited the work of Senators Orrin Hatch and Tom Harkin, Congressman Bill Richardson and other legislators. And he said that the passage of this legislation speaks of their determination and he appreciated their work. In his continuing discussion, he said:

> "But most important, (this legislation) speaks to the diligence with which an unofficial army of nutritionally conscious people work democratically to change the laws in an area deeply important to them. In an era of greater consciousness among people about the impact of what they eat or how they live, indeed how long they live, it is appropriate that we have finally reformed the way the Government treats consumers and these supplements in a way that encourages good health."

In spite of the passage of this law, some people are still concerned. And according to a December 29, 1994, Associated Press report, some supplement makers feel the law still gives the FDA too much authority over vitamins, herbs and other supplements. If you have comments or suggestions, write to Nutritional Health Alliance, P.O. Box 25317, Washington, DC 20007. FAX #703-359-9343.

More About Linus Pauling In an editorial in the September 8, 1994, issue of *Medical Tribune*, "The sage of vitamin C is remembered," Nicholas K. Zittell paid tribute to Dr. Linus C. Pauling who died of cancer at the age of 93. Zittell pointed out that Pauling was the only person ever to have won two unshared Nobel Prizes. He summarized some of Pauling's work as a brilliant chemist and also as a compassionate political activist who worked to uphold self-evident truths. About 25 years ago, Pauling coined the term "ortho-molecular." He used the term to convey the idea that many chronic health disorders could be corrected by "straightening" the concentrations of various nutrients in the body.

Zittell also cited the work of those who supported him, including Arthur M. Sackler, M.D., publisher and founder of *Medical Tribune,* who said at the time of Pauling's controversy with the Mayo Clinic about vitamin C and cancer, "Linus, whom I have admired for four decades and known for two, has spent more time trying to convey some simple concepts in nutrition than he spent earning the Nobel Prize in Chemistry—or the Nobel Prize for Peace." In his continuing discussion, Zittell said:

> "Ten years later Dr. Pauling's perseverance is downright prescient—an emerging body of evidence (some of it, ironically, published in Dr. Pauling's old nemesis, *The New England Journal of Medicine*) suggests that vitamins A, C, E and beta carotene may reduce the incidence of heart disease and cancer. This is more than 30 years after he asked the Food and Nutrition Board to increase the recommended dietary allowances for vitamins and minerals."

And he quoted further comments of Dr. Sackler, who said, "The message of Linus Pauling is simple, clear and direct. We can reduce the toll of cancer and cardiovascular diseases, we can retard degenerative processes, we can correct many mental disorders and much mental retardation. And we can do all this—now—if we get (his) findings and message to the public. For generations to come, people the world over will be indebted to this great scientist for helping make their world a better place and their lives longer, fuller and happier."

A New Form of Vitamin C During the past decade, researchers in the United States and Scandinavia have studied Ester-C,* a new patented form of vitamin C. In studies carried out in the Department of Pharmacology at the University of Mississippi, Ester-C and L-ascorbic acid (plain vitamin C) was given to two groups of rats. In analyzing their observations, the investigators concluded, "These results support the hypothesis that Ester-C is absorbed more readily and excreted less rapidly than L-ascorbic acid."[13]

In a subsequent human clinical study, other researchers compared Ester-C with ascorbic acid in 12 men, ages 27 to 45. Here's a brief summary of their findings: "Ester-C produced higher WBC levels, was excreted less in the urine, and was associated with lower urinary oxalate output than L-ascorbic acid."[14]

In another animal study, a Norwegian veterinarian found that C-Flex (Ester-C labeled for animals) provided symptomatic relief of chronic joint problems, while a group given a placebo preparation showed no improvement. In still another study in rats, Ester-C was found to be 4 to 5 times more potent or effective than ascorbic acid in preventing scurvy.[15]

Vitamin B_{12} If you're bothered by fatigue, high doses of vitamin B_{12} may help you. I base that statement on my own limited experience in treating a few patients, plus reports by others that injections of this safe, inexpensive vitamin are often highly effective.

In the Fall 1993 issue of the *CFIDS Chronicle*, Charles W. Lapp, M.D., and Paul R. Cheney, M.D., Ph.D., in discussing vitamin B_{12} said:

> "The Cheney Clinic received more inquiries about the use of high dose cyanocobalamin (B_{12}) than perhaps any other Chronic Fatigue Syndrome (CFS) therapy. Physicians are particularly incredulous that such a simple and time worn medication could possibly be helpful. Nevertheless, informal polls show that the majority of CFS pa-

---

*This product can be found in most health food stores and further information about it can be obtained from Inter-Cal Corp., 421 Miller Valley Rd., Prescott, AZ 86301. 602-445-8063.

tients improve with vitamin B_{12}. Furthermore, this drug is safe, inexpensive and easy to administer . . .

"Justification (for the use of B_{12}) was based on articles (*NEJM*, 1988; 318:1720–28. *NEJM*, 1988; 318:26), which reported that 28% of patients with neuropsychiatric abnormalities (including paresthesia, sensory loss, ataxia, dementia and psychiatric disorder) responded to therapeutic doses of B_{12}, even though there was no evidence of anemia or macrocytosis."[16]

In their continuing discussion, Lapp and Cheney stated that some 50 to 80% of their patients improved with this simple therapy. The vitamin B_{12}, given in doses of 2500 to 5000 mcgs., is administered by injection every 2 to 3 days. In some patients they have given large doses daily for long periods of time without side effects.

Here's more. For over 20 years, H.L. Newbold, M.D., a New York physician, has been writing and talking about the beneficial effects of vitamin B_{12} injections in the treatment of fatigue, backache, depression, poor memory and other health problems. You'll find further information in his 1991 book.[17]

I found further support for the value of B_{12} in a report[18] by Damien Downing. He cited a study which showed that severe psychological symptoms could be caused by vitamin B_{12} deficiency. Other descriptions of the value of vitamin B_{12} in combating physical and mental symptoms are scattered throughout literature.[19,20,21]

Magnesium   Many people, especially women, take calcium supplements in the hope of preventing osteoporosis and other disorders. Calcium is important—but magnesium is of equal or greater importance.

In the early 1980s, after learning about candida-related disorders, I asked Dr. Sidney M. Baker about magnesium. Here are a few of his comments, "Magnesium deficiency is widespread. The average daily need for magnesium in adults is between 500 and 1000 mgs. and a lot of people simply aren't taking that much. For my patients I recommend oral magnesium chloride."[22]

A year or two later, as I was working to update and expand *The*

Yeast Connection, I learned more about magnesium from Leo Galland, M.D. Like Baker, he pointed out that magnesium deficiency occurs more often than generally recognized. In discussing magnesium, he said:

> "The richest sources of magnesium are also the richest dietary sources of essential fatty acids . . . seed foods (including the whole grains, nuts and beans) and seafoods. Other foods which are relatively rich in magnesium include buckwheat, baking chocolate, cotton seed, tea, whole wheat, collard greens, parsley and other leafy green vegetables. Magnesium is also plentiful in seafood, meats and fruit. What's more, you can protect your magnesium storers by avoiding the 'magnesium wasters'; saturated fats and soft drinks, especially those containing caffeine."[23]

During the past several years, I've learned a lot about magnesium from preventive medicine specialist Alan Gaby, M.D. In discussing magnesium in an editorial in the *Journal of Advancement in Medicine* several years ago, Gaby said, "Properly administered magnesium is entirely free of adverse side effects. Equally important, its cost is negligible."[24]

In his superb 1994 book, *Preventing and Reversing Osteoporosis—Every Woman's Essential Guide,* Gaby includes a seven-page chapter entitled, "Magnesium: the mineral that 'does it all.'" In discussing the therapeutic uses of magnesium, Gaby cited its importance in helping people with heart attacks, asthma, chronic fatigue, depression, fibromyalgia, hypoglycemia, PMS and other disorders. In discussing magnesium and osteoporosis, he said:

> "As much as 50% of all magnesium in the body is found in the bones. It should not be surprising, therefore, that studies have demonstrated a role for magnesium in the prevention and treatment of osteoporosis."

Gaby also cited the research of Dr. Guy E. Abraham, who conducted a trial of magnesium therapy in 26 postmenopausal women. All the women were taking either estrogen alone or estrogen plus a progestogen. All the women were given dietary advice, including: avoiding processed foods; limiting protein intake; emphasizing vegetable protein over animal protein; limiting the consumption of refined salt, sugar, alcohol, coffee, tea, chocolate and tobacco.

Each participant was also offered a daily supplement containing vitamins, 500 mg. of calcium (citrate), 600 mg. of magnesium (oxide) and other minerals. Nineteen of the women took a supplement, while six chose not to.

Bone density studies were then carried out eight to nine months after treatment was begun. In the women who did not take the supplement, the average bone density increased slightly by 0.7%. In those who did take the supplement, the results were dramatically better—an average increase in bone density of 11%.

In his continuing discussion, Gaby, like Galland, stressed the importance of diet. And he pointed out that 80% of the magnesium is lost when whole grains are refined to make flour, and he said:

"Because this nutrient is so critical in so many different ways and because supplementation is safe and inexpensive, I advise nearly all of my patients to take a magnesium supplement or a multiple vitamin and mineral formula that contains magnesium . . . It should be noted that many of the one-tablet-per-day vitamin/mineral supplements contain very little magnesium. Multiple-nutrient supplements that contain enough magnesium are generally those that recommend between three and six tablets per day."[25]

Gaby also pointed out that too much magnesium may cause loose bowels in some people and that individuals with renal failure should not take magnesium without medical supervision.

New scientific studies show that magnesium plays an important role in people with asthma, bronchitis and other airway diseases. According to Jeffrey Bland, Ph.D., individuals with these lung problems are helped by a daily intake of 400 to 600 mg. of magnesium.[26]

Enzymes   About ten years ago, I attended a seminar on food allergies and sensitivities conducted by Dr. William T. Kniker, Professor of Pediatrics and Head of the Department of Allergy and Immunology at the University of Texas (San Antonio).

In his discussion, Dr. Kniker described the various manifestations he'd seen in patients with food allergies and sensitivities. And he said that avoiding the troublemaking food was the best way a person could control symptoms. Yet, he said that in some patients he had found pancreatic enzymes useful.

I had heard little or no discussion of this enzyme treatment until the summer of 1993 when Michael McCann, M.D., Parma, Ohio, described his use of a pancreatic enzyme supplement in patients with multiple food allergies at the Food Allergy Symposium in Denver.*

In an abstract of his presentation, Dr. McCann pointed out that the treatment of food allergies in adults has generally been limited to avoidance and the use of drugs such as antihistamines, epinephrin and cortisone. He then described his experiences in treating a 37-year-old woman with lifelong eczema, intermittent diarrhea and weight loss.

Her prior treatment consisted of avoidance of foods which were known to cause allergic reactions, intermittent corticosteroids, antihistamines and oral cromolyn. *Yet, the treatment was only partially successful and she continued to be bothered by both skin rashes and digestive symptoms.*

This patient was given two to four capsules of a pancreatic enzyme supplement (25,000 u protease/per capsule) before each meal. *She showed a complete clinical remission and resolution of eczema for the first time in her adult life. She was also able to discontinue all other drugs.*

Dr. McCann concluded that breaking up the allergens in food proteins by the pancreatic supplement, lessened the absorption of large allergenic food particles (polypeptides) and, thereby, decreased the symptoms in food allergic patients.

I reported Dr. McCann's observations in the September 1993 newsletter of the International Health Foundation and I asked for

---

*Sponsored by the American College of Allergy and Immunology.

feedback from other physicians. In January 1994, I received a letter from R.W. Noble, M.D. Here are excerpts.

"I've used the enzyme Pancrease frequently, and at times Pan-Five, for people with food allergies and have been pleased with their response. Many of these patients were troubled with digestive upsets, such as excessive gas. It also relieved these symptoms as well.

"What is the mechanism? It seems to me that people with these reactions are absorbing incompletely digested products. These reactions may resemble the reactions of people with lactose intolerance who are helped by the administration of lactose.

"Although I've used these enzymes primarily for digestive complaints, several of my patients have reported that they felt better and showed improvement in other food-induced symptoms while taking these enzymes."

In February 1994, I received a further report from Dr. McCann, who said:

"In general, Pancrease only helps food sensitive patients who show significantly positive skin tests. It does not seem to work in patients with negative skin tests and other kinds of food intolerance. I've obtained my best results in patients with chronic eczema who have multiple positive skin tests . . . 3+ or more.

"There are lots of these patients around and dermatologists mostly ignore diet history and skin testing. You have to look at a patient's whole diet, and sometimes you'll run into oddball sensitivities, such as vanilla, white potato and rice. But, Pancrease really works routinely in food allergic patients! Almost all of them."

More On Rotation Diets   Rotating your diet isn't easy. Yet, if you're bothered by food sensitivities, a rotated diet is important. To obtain further information and help, I suggest the following resources:

Natalie Golos and Frances Golos' book, *If This is Tuesday, It Must be Chicken*, Keats Publishing, New Canaan, CT, 1983. I've known Natalie for almost 20 years and have been a dinner guest in her home. She is a knowledgeable authority of food and chemical sensitivities and a member of the American Academy of Environmental Medicine.

Sondra K. Lewis' 1995 book, *Allergy and Candida Cooking—Rotational Style*, Canary Connect Publications, P.O. Box 5317, Coralville, IA 52241–0317. In introducing her chapter on rotated diets, Sondra said that the rotation of foods accomplishes the following three main goals:

1. It helps you maintain your tolerance to the foods you can eat now, greatly lessening your chances of becoming allergic to other foods.
2. Helps in the treatment of current food allergies.
3. Aids you in identifying foods that could be causing your problems.

This book is loaded with information, including helpful hints, meal planning for each day and 200 pages of recipes.

Nicolette M. Dumke's book, *Allergy Cooking With Ease*, Starburst Publishers, P.O. Box 4123, Lancaster, PA 17604, 1992. I liked this book so much that, with the help of my colleague, Nell Sellers, I wrote the foreword. Nicki Dumke's book isn't only a recipe book, it encourages people to enjoy family, friends, work and recreation.

Sally Rockwell's *Cooking With Candida Cookbook* (revised), P.O. Box 13056, Seattle, WA. I've known Sally for over a decade. She is a knowledgeable nutritionist who, through her lectures, newsletters and books, has helped many people with food allergies and yeast-related health problems.

Donna Gates and Lynn Schatz, *The Body Ecology Diet: Recovering Your Health and Re-Building Your Immunity*, BED Publications, Atlanta, GA, 1993.

You can also learn more about rotated diets, food sources, grain and grain alternatives and other information from *The Yeast Connection Cookbook*, Professional Books, 1989. In commenting on this book, George and Leslie Kroker said:

"We think one of the most outstanding features of this book is the emphasis on diversification of foods. A wide variety of foods not only offers optimal nutrition, but lessens the likelihood of new food sensitivities from developing in the future."

You'll also find help from Mary Beth Hughes' fascinating computer program that creates individual diets for allergic patients. It's called the AllerDiet Program. Here is what it contains:

- a complete list of foods, families and special combinations to select from on the menu;
- a diet created with a list of foods to avoid, including close relative and common sources;
- an eating list—foods you can eat;
- a patient education section showing the foods you may be sensitive to;
- a four-day rotated diversified diet;
- recipes and substitutes for critical foods like egg, milk and wheat;
- hidden food facts, eating out tips, food preparations and combining guidelines.

To get further information about this special program, write to AllerDiet, 4903 Creek Shadows, Kingwood, TX 77339. 713–360-6655 and FAX# 713–360-6551. You'll also find additional information about rotated diets in these newsletters:

Mastering Food Allergies, edited by Marjorie Jones, MAST Enterprises, Inc., 2614 N. 4th St., #616, Coeur d'Alene, ID 83814. (6 issues a year, back issues are available),

Canary Connect News, edited by Sondra K. Lewis and Lonnett Dietrich Blakely. Canary Connect Publications, P.O. Box 5317, Coralville, IA 52241–0317. 319–351-2371.

More About Vegetables   In October 1994, I spoke at the National Nutritional Health Association Annual Conference at St. Charles, Illinois. My topic was "The Yeast Connection: What's New?" After my presentation, I visited the exhibits and did a lot of networking. During my rounds, I picked up a copy of *Better Nutrition*, an informative journal which I've read and admired on many occasions. An article in the September 1994 issue entitled, "Meatless Meals," discussed the health benefits of vegetarian diets. Here's an excerpt.

"Although it is generally not known, vegetarians consume a wider range of foods than non-vegetarians. A typical vegetarian diet contains vegetables, fruits, beans, soybeans, nuts, nutbutters, whole grains, such as breads, pasta, rice and hot and cold cereals, and various ethnic favorites. . .

"Soybeans, a mainstay of many vegetarian diets, contain high amounts of protein, iron, B-complex vitamins and trace minerals. By 1995, the soybean market is expected to reach almost $1.4 billion annually . . ."

Then I stopped by the Better Burger* exhibit. Rather than being made from meat, the burgers contained a wide variety of natural foods. Here's a list of the ingredients. Fresh organic vegetables: carrots, onions, spinach, parsley, zucchini, celery, potatoes and split peas. Other ingredients included brown rice, oat and rye flour, sunflower and sesame seeds, tamari and herbs, fresh garlic, walnuts and almonds.

I also talked with Sue Moody, the president of the Midwest division of the Natural Nutritional Food Association (NNFA). During our conversation, I asked her about her grandchildren. In replying, she said:

"Our grandchildren, from ages nine months to ten years, are never sick. They almost never have to go to a doctor. We live on a farm and give them lots of fruits and vegetables. Their good diet helps keep them healthy."

What I Eat   I've written and talked so much about nutrition in my hometown that when I eat away from home I see many eyes looking at what I put on my plate. And I must admit that I sometimes "cheat"—especially if no one's looking.

---

*For more information about the Better Burger, write to Doug Bryan, Rt. 9 N.W., Twin Maples Plaza, Saugerties, New York 12477.

Yet, as each year passes, I eat a much better diet. It features more vegetables (including beans of all kinds), fruits and whole grains. I occasionally eat fish, although I worry about where it comes from. I occasionally eat chicken, especially if I'm invited out to dinner and my hostess serves it. Yet, after seeing those TV specials about today's birds raised in "chicken hotels" and contaminated with salmonella, I'm no longer a chicken enthusiast.

On rare occasions, I'll even eat a burger. (I've always liked them.) So I was delighted when I learned that one of the new fast food "eateries" in my hometown served meat-free Gardenburgers. My wife, Betsy, and I occasionally eat well-cooked eggs. They're loaded with all sorts of good nutrients and micronutrients and I don't worry about them elevating our cholesterols.

If you'd like to know more about what to eat, and what not to eat, and how to prepare your foods, you'll find lots of information in these books:

The Yeast Connection Cookbook, Crook, W.G. and Jones, M.H., Professional Books, Jackson, TN, 1989.

Staying Healthy with Nutrition, Haas, N.M., Celestial Arts Publishing, P.O. Box 7327, Berkeley, CA 94707, 1992.

The Food Pharmacy to Good Eating—with more than 200 health recipes, Carper, J., Bantam Books, New York, NY, 1991.

Food—Your Miracle Medicine—How Food Can Prevent and Cure over 100 Symptoms and Problems. Carper, J., HarperCollins Publishers, New York, NY, 1993.

Food For Life, Barnard, N., Harmony Books, P.O. Box 7327, Berkeley, CA 94707, 1993.

Jane Brody's Good Food Book, Brody, J., Bantam Books, New York, NY, 1987.

More About Good Fats   During the past decade, I've learned a lot from articles I've read in newsletters, including the *Health Hunter Newsletter* published by The Center for the Improvement of Human Functioning, Inc., 3100 N. Hillside Ave., Wichita, KS 37219.

I was especially impressed by the lead article in the June 1994 issue by Donald R. Davis, Ph.D., "The good fat: Omega 3." For many years, Dr. Davis worked with the late Roger Williams, Ph.D., of the University of Texas in Austin.

Williams discovered two of the B vitamins (folic acid and pantothenic acid) and believed in supplementing the diet with an "insurance" vitamin/mineral formula. Yet, he was an even stronger advocate of eating wholesome, unprocessed foods from a wide variety of sources.

In his article, Davis said that the essential Omega 3 dietary fat comes from a variety of sources, including walnuts, flax seeds and their oils (not hydrogenated) and in small amounts from other nuts, vegetables, greens and algae.

Other Helpful Information

The Importance of Touch   In his book, *Touching, The Human Significance of the Skin*, Ashley Montagu told of experiments in rats that showed:

> "The more handling and petting rats received, the better they did in laboratory situations . . . Equally remarkable was the influence of gentle handling upon behavioral development. And such handling produced gentle, unexcitable animals."[27]

In the March 1994 issue of *Hippocrates*, appeared a segment entitled, "Healing Hands." According to the article, scientific studies during the past decade show that physical contact may prevent people from getting sick as often and can speed recovery when they do.

I read more about the importance of touch in an article in the July 1994 issue of *Health Confidential*, "Important: Get Your Daily Dose of Touch. Yes . . . Touch" by Tiffany Field, Ph.D., of the University of Miami School of Medicine. Here are excerpts.

> "Human touch has remarkable restorative effects on the body. It reduces anxiety, stress and depression. It promotes relaxation and relieves pain. It fosters sound sleep, bolsters the immune system and enhances productivity. And—it feels great."

In discussing the biochemistry of touch, Field said that when you are deprived of touch, stress hormones are produced that can make you feel jittery and weaken your immune system. In discussing methods of touch, she said that family members can exchange massages.

She also recommended massage therapists. To find a licensed massage therapist, check the Yellow Pages under "massage therapy schools," or contact the American Massage Therapy Association, 820 Davis St., Suite 100, Evanston, IL 60201, 708–864-0123.

In the concluding sentence of her article, Field said:

> "Fortunately, the growing influence of Eastern cultures and the rise of alternative medicine are making touch more acceptable in our culture. I believe that the day is coming when massage and other forms of touch will become a part of mainstream medicine in America."[28]

Hugging   In a chapter of their book, *Chicken Soup for the Soul—101 Stories to Open the Heart and Rekindle the Spirit,* the authors, Jack Canfield and Mark Victor Hansen, talked about hugging. Included was the following piece sent to them by one of their seminar graduates:

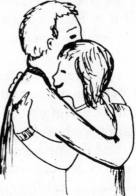

> "Hugging is healthy. It helps the body's immune system, it helps keep you healthier, it cures depression, it reduces stress, it induces sleep, it's invigorating, it's rejuvenating, it has no unpleasant side effect and hugging is nothing less than a miracle drug.
> "Hugging is all natural. It is organic, naturally sweet, no pesticides, no preservatives, no artificial ingredients and 100 percent wholesome.
> "Hugging is practically perfect. There are no moveable parts, no batteries to wear out, no periodic checkups, low energy consumption, high energy yield, inflation proof, nonfattening, no monthly payments, no insurance requirements, theft-proof, nontaxable, nonpolluting and, of course, fully returnable."[29] (Source unknown.)

Acupuncture   Several thousand years ago, the Chinese discovered that when certain points on the body were pressed, punctured or heated, that symptoms of many types would go away. The beneficial effects were thought to be due to the release of energy blocks in the meridians. As the art developed, practitioners found that such therapies not only alleviated pain, but also influenced the functioning of internal organs and body systems.

In the late '80s, while on a trip to the Orient, I developed sharp pains in my lower back. I could hardly stand up to walk. So I called a young Chinese physician I had met a couple of days earlier. He came over to my hotel and while other members of my tour group looked on with fascination, he inserted and twisted acupuncture needles in my lower back. By the following morning, I was much improved and by the next day my pain had disappeared.

According to an article in the November 1993 issue of *Cincinnati*,[30] countless Americans now undergo acupuncture from some 6500 licensed practitioners. Complaints which have been helped by acupuncture include asthma, PMS, depression, arthritis, headaches, neck pain, stiffness and sexual dysfunction.

I found further information about acupuncture in the December 1994 issue of *Prevention*.[31] Reporter Sharon Stocker told of her visit to Patrick J. LaRiccia, M.D., Director of the Hospital of the University of Pennsylvania's Acupuncture Pain Clinic in Philadelphia.

In her report, Stocker said that Harvard, Yale, UCLA, the University of Maryland and other leading medical schools are all investigating acupuncture as a potential adjunctive treatment for a variety of health problems.

She also provided readers with a number of tips, including: Do not rely on acupuncture to treat serious illnesses without seeing a physician; ask for disposable needles; get a referral to a physician acupuncturist. You can obtain the names of physicians from the American Academy of Medical Acupuncture (AAMA) (1-800-521-AAMA). Or, you can write to the Academy at 5820 Wilshire Blvd., Suite 500, Los Angeles, CA 90036.

Acupressure Massage In discussing acupressure and other types of oriental bodywork in the book, *Alternative Medicine—The Definitive Guide,*[32] the authors said that whereas acupuncture uses needles, acupressure uses the pressure of the fingers and hands. Moreover, acupressure is the older of the two techniques. It has been found to be an effective technique which people can use to relieve the pain and discomfort of headaches and other disorders.

In her *PMS Self-Help Book,*[33] Dr. Susan Lark includes a 24-page illustrated discussion of acupressure massage which she recommends for women with PMS. And she said that she has used acupressure on patients in her practice with pneumonia, viral infections, headaches, muscle strains and other problems. In many of these patients, it worked when nothing else seemed to be effective.

You can do acupressure either on yourself or it can be done by a friend. Your hands should be clean and your nails trimmed and the room should be warm and quiet. Pressure should be applied slowly with the tips or balls of the fingers and held at the point of discomfort for one to three minutes.

Strength Training According to an article by Jane E. Brody in the January/February 1995 *Saturday Evening Post,* strength training is an important part of any physical fitness program. It can lower your total cholesterol, increase your good cholesterol and lessen your chances of developing heart disease. It can also reduce your risk of developing back problems and joint problems and give you more self-confidence.

What is "strength training"? It is the process of building muscle power by lifting weights or working against resistance. Special equipment, like the Nautilus or Universal machines, have been designed to help you accomplish this training. Yet, Brody says that most of the recommended exercises can be done with nothing fancier than a few full cans from your supermarket, or plastic bottles filled with water or sand.

I found a further discussion of these methods of strengthening your body and improving your quality of life in a 1994 book, *Age Erasers for Women*.[34] In a chapter entitled, "Resistance Training," the authors cited the observations and recommendations of a number of exercise physiologists, including Alan Mikesky, Ph.D., and Miriam E. Nelson, Ph.D.

Detailed instructions were given for women who wanted to get started. Here are some of them. First, go to your physician for a checkup. Then, get help from a physical therapist, exercise physiologist or other experienced person. Start out with light weights, gradually increase, keep at it and do lifts you like.

It's never too late to start. Research studies at Tufts University cited by Dr. Mikesky showed that people in their 90s showed significant strength gains following weight training.

Al Gore, A Defender of the Environment   Whether you're a Democrat or a Republican, I urge you to read Al's 1992 book, *Earth in the Balance*. As you may know, Al is convinced that "the engines of human civilization have brought us to the brink of catastrophe, even though some politicians and business leaders think the threat isn't real."

In his book, Al tells us that the threat *is* real. Using the latest research he demonstrates that the quality of our air, water and soil is at grave risk.

During the past several years, as I've talked to various groups, I've said, "Al Gore is a personal friend of mine who will never forget me. Here's why. When he was 11 years old, I stitched up a laceration on his head and the local anesthetic didn't work! But he doesn't hold it against me."

I didn't see Al again until he became a Congressman and made regular visits to Jackson. I nearly always went to the local courthouse to participate in his rap sessions with his West Tennessee constituents. I also paid a visit to the Gore home in Arlington when Al was in the Senate and to his parents' home in Carthage. I kept up with Al—and with Tipper—for other reasons.

Al was always an advocate of good nutrition and preventive medicine. When his son was gravely injured and was hospitalized at Johns Hopkins, Al called me on the phone and asked, "What vitamins and/or other nutritional supplements do you recommend for young Al?"

Tipper has also supported me in my efforts to bring "the yeast connection" into the medical mainstream. For six years she served as a member of the Advisory Board of the International Health Foundation. My final "Gore connection" is Al's uncle, Judge Whit LaFon, who is my best golf and gin rummy buddy.

In this book, I've expressed my concerns about the increasing incidence of health problems which affect people of all ages and both sexes. These include breast cancer and endometriosis in adults and behavior and learning problems in children. I feel that these, and other problems, are related to the chemical pollution of our environment.

If we expect our children and grandchildren to enjoy a truly good life, all of us need to heed the recommendations Al Gore makes in his book.

Pesticides and Breast Cancer   A number of scientific studies show that women who are exposed to DDT and other chemicals are much more apt to develop breast cancer than other women. Evidence of this relationship was cited on a national television program in early 1994. Women in one Long Island community, which was sprayed intensively with DDT in the 1950s and early 1960s, showed an incidence of breast cancer four times greater than women in another Long Island community of comparable size which wasn't sprayed.

Although DDT has been banned in the United States, it is widely used in other countries and should be a cause of concern to all of us. Moreover, such concern was eloquently expressed by David Perlmutter, a Naples, Florida, neurologist. In a letter to the editor, published in the April 20, 1994, issue of the Journal of the American Medical Association (Vol. 271), Perlmutter expressed concern over the pesticides in imported fruits and vegetables. Here are excerpts from his letter.

"Breast cancer, which now affects one in eight American women, must truly be regarded as a modern epidemic. This year 180,000 American women will be diagnosed as having this disease and a third of them will die of it . . . Recent evidence strongly supports the relationship between tissue levels of organochlorines (like DDT) and the incidence of breast cancer . . .

"The U.S. government, hoping to stimulate the American economy, stands poised to approve the General Agreement on Tariffs and Trade (GATT). To stimulate worldwide agricultural trade, the GATT rules could allow substantial levels of pesticide residues on U.S. import produce. *Levels of DDT 5000% higher than current U.S. standards will be permitted on imported peaches and bananas, with similar deregulation affecting grapes, strawberries, broccoli and carrots* [emphasis added].

"While recognizing the importance of national economics, this agreement, which affects safety standards of imported produce, demonstrates that the health of American women is not a primary concern."

Hormone Copycats   I first heard that dioxin and other chemicals could affect hormones from Mary Lou Ballweg of the Endometriosis Association in 1993 (see Chapter 12). A short time later, George Miller, a Lewisburg, Pennsylvania, gynecologist, told me about Theo Colburn, Ph.D., and the work of the National Wildlife Federation. So I wrote to Dr. Colburn and she sent me additional information about the adverse effects of dioxin, PCBs, mercury, cadmium and dozens of other common chemicals.

Then, in the spring of 1994, I saw reports in major magazines and on national TV describing the frightening effect of these chemicals on humans and animals.

Some of the most disturbing evidence has come from wildlife, including alligators, fish, turtles and birds. Yet, the same chemicals which are affecting animals, also are affecting humans. Breast cancer now strikes one woman in nine and endometriosis and other autoimmune diseases are increasing. Then, in December 1994, just as I was completing the final section of this book,

Giovanna Medina and Pat Connolly* sent me a summary of the April 4, 1994, monograph, "Hormone Copycats," published by the National Wildlife Federation—Great Lakes Natural Resource Center. Here is an excerpt.

"No component of the chain of life is safe . . . from minute 'water fleas' in backyard ponds to polar bears at the north end of the globe . . . Slowly, we are waking from a state of denial. Hormone copycats are ubiquitous in pesticides, building materials, consumer products and environmental pollutants, largely beyond our individual control.

"The reality of what is happening in the environment and the personal cost of pollution are dawning on us. These are not someone elses' problems . . ."

To obtain a copy of the 61-page report, "Hormone Copycats," send $6 to National Wildlife Federation, Great Lakes Natural Resource Center, 506 E. Liberty St., Ann Arbor, MI 48104. FAX 313–769-1449.

Menopause In July 1994, Penelope Young Andrade, a professional who specializes in psychotherapeutic approaches which integrate body, feelings, mind and spirit, sent me a fascinating packet of material which included a copy of the speech she had given at a menopause symposium and a seven-page paper entitled, "One Woman's Menopause Discoveries."

In these papers she discusses the multiple causes of menopausal symptoms, including diet, hormonal changes, spiritual and energetic changes and yeast-related problems. Here are excerpts from her comments.

"Watch out for yeast. Candidiasis loves menopause. If you have been eating too many refined carbohydrates, fermented foods . . . and you have vaginal and bladder symptoms (or depression, diges-

---

*The Price Pottenger Nutrition Foundation, P.O. Box 2614, La Mesa, CA 91943–2614. 619–575-7763.

tive difficulties, headaches, dizziness, weakness, irritability, heart palpitations, muscle pains, panic attacks, anxiety, sudden anger, sleep disturbances, weight gain) that have not responded to other treatment, consider a candidiasis diagnosis . . . For me the yeast connection was an important piece of the puzzle in successfully negotiating my menopause journey.

"After I was willing to see that I had yeast, *I realized my body and psyche had been trying to alert me* to that for over a year. I had ignored this because the antiyeast diet . . . is quite restrictive . . . There is a new antifungal drug, Diflucan (fluconazole) available now which is very effective *IN CONJUNCTION WITH THE DIET* . . . This is a prescription item and needs to be regulated by a physician. It is a strong medicine. I found I could not tolerate it for more than a week at a time even in a small dose (50 mg. twice per day). A week or two will give you a jump start on yeast management.

"For the long run, I have discovered the wonders of homeopathy. I have been using hydrastis in conjunction with a total homeopathic program with great results. I find I can control my yeast and ameliorate other menopause symptoms with a much less restrictive diet as the homeopathy helps to bring my total organism into balance."

Does Your Stomach Burn? During the past decade, countless people who experience burning in the upper part of their abdomens have taken medications, such as Tagamet and Zantac. Although these medicines lessen acid secretion and relieve symptoms, recent research studies appear to provide better answers.

The research I'm talking about shows that the eradication of a microorganism, *Helicobacter pylori,* may often solve the problem.

Credit for finding the answer goes to Barry Marshall, M.D., a young Australian/American physician. This exciting story was summarized by Cory SerVaas, M.D., recently in the September/October 1994, *Saturday Evening Post* and in the *Saturday Evening Post Health Update Newsletter.* Here are excerpts.

"One of the most innovative young minds in medicine today was the honored guest at the Third Annual Saturday Evening Ball. By now, scientists the world over are applauding Dr. Barry Marshall for finding the cause of, and better yet, the cure for gastric ulcers.

"Dr. Marshall's discovery that the bacterium *Helicobacter pylori* causes gastritis and gastric ulcers, has had a dramatic impact on millions of lives. By taking a prescription of Flagyl, tetracycline and Pepto-Bismol, more than 80 percent of ulcer patients are cured and freed from a lifetime of taking Tagamet and Zantac. This is great news for the many sufferers of gastritis and stomach ulcers."[35]

Dr. Marshall's discovery is exciting. I was especially interested in reading the *Saturday Evening Post* report for several reasons. First, I was pleased and proud because Dr. Marshall is a member of the faculty of the University of Virginia School of Medicine (my alma mater). Then, I was privileged to enjoy a one-on-one dinner with him at a conference in New York two years ago when he presented his findings to a group of physicians.

I haven't heard of any adverse effects of the three medications being used to combat the *Helicobacter pylori* infections. Yet, since tetracycline and Flagyl encourage the growth of *Candida albicans* in the digestive tract, adding nystatin and a probiotic to the treatment program is an option worth considering.

Constipation   Many people with candida-related health problems are troubled by digestive symptoms, including abdominal pain, bloating and diarrhea. Such symptoms are often labeled "irritable bowel syndrome" (IBS). Yet, constipation can also be a common and frustrating symptom. And sometimes it continues in spite of laxatives and dietary changes.

In an article in *Alive*, "Constipation can be the culprit," Zoltan P. Rona, M.D., M.Sc., a Toronto physician, said:

"Constipation may be a feature of irritable bowel syndrome, food allergy, diverticulosis, abdominal infection, dehydration, bowel obstruction, long periods of immobility, stress and depression.

"The first thing to do about constipation is to increase your water intake to at least eight large glasses of spring water per day. Avoid coffee and regular tea. Diluted fruit juices are fine. Increase your consumption of high fiber foods such as whole grain breads, pastas and cereals, vegetables, legumes, fruits, seeds and nuts.

"Eliminate your intake of refined carbohydrate foods such as sweets, chocolates, cakes, white flour products, white rice and other processed foods. They are constipating."

In his continuing discussion, Rona pointed out that milk is a common cause of constipation, especially in children, and that lack of exercise also plays a role. And he said:

"As a word of caution, remember that each case has to be assessed on an individual basis and special medical or nutritional tests may be necessary to decide on the optimal treatment. One such test is the comprehensive digestive and stool analysis (CDSA). . . ."[36]

Rona also cited the observations of Dr. Leo Galland who has found that many people with chronic digestive symptoms (including constipation) harbor the parasite *Giardia lamblia,* and that natural herbal remedies, including probiotics and citrus seed extracts, may help.

Artificial Lighting   Fluorescent light may be contributing to your health problems, especially if you work in a windowless office or building and spend little time outdoors.

Research in a new field called photobiology studies how light interacts with life. It also shows how ordinary fluorescent lighting may play a part in causing health problems in adults and children. Natural sunlight—or skylight—even when the sun isn't shining, contains all the colors of the rainbow. Yet, most artificial lighting contains only a few colors.

During the past decade, a number of observers have reported on the benefits of bright lights in treating *Seasonal Affective Disorder (SAD)*, a term applied to people who become depressed during the winter months. In one of these studies published in the *Journal of Women's Health*,[37] Gabrielle M. Cerda, M.D., and Barbara L. Parry, M.D., Department of Psychiatry, University of California, San Diego School of Medicine, found that light therapy significantly reduced the symptoms of depression in women with PMS.

How and why does broad spectrum light help? From what I've read, it affects the pineal gland's secretion of a hormone that regulates the human biological clock. *To get the benefits of light, you should spend at least a half hour a day outside in natural light and obtain special broad spectrum lights for your home and office.* These lights, which fit into standard fluorescent fixtures, can be purchased at garden supply stores, hardware stores, some lighting departments and health food stores.

Water During the 1980s and early 1990s, numerous reports have appeared in newspapers, magazines and on TV describing contaminated public water supplies in many communities. And in a December 1993 cover story article published in *Health Confidential,* Richard P. Maas, Ph.D., associate professor of environmental studies, University of North Carolina, Asheville, said:

> "Americans are concerned about their drinking water . . . and rightly so. Roughly 20% of households have dangerous levels of lead in their tap water . . . And the once sporadic cases of bacterial and industrial chemical contamination seem to be occurring with increasing frequency.
> "Yet despite the real and ever-growing threat, there are effective ways to protect yourself and your family."

In his continuing discussion, Maas pointed out that the biggest threat in water comes from lead. It can cause a variety of serious health problems ranging from brain damage in children to kidney damage, high blood pressure and brittle bones in adults.

Where does the lead come from? The most common sources are lead-containing pipes or plumbing fixtures in your home or, much less commonly, from lead pipes in the municipal water system. To protect yourself, Maas made the following suggestions.

• Purge your water faucet for one minute in the morning before you drink. Since lead leeches into the water much more rapidly than previously thought, you'll need to purge it again if it's been more than a few minutes since the last time you drew water. To save time and water, keep a gallon pitcher of water from a purged tap in your refrigerator.

- Have your water tested. Unless you have had your water tested, you do not know whether you need to be purging the faucet or whether the purging is effective.

    Your local water utility may provide you with a free test kit. Such kits are also available from other sources, including:

Suburban Water Testing Lab
3600 Kutztown Rd.
Temple, PA 19560
800-433-6595 ($35)

Clean Water Lead Testing
29½ Page Ave.
Asheville, NC 28801
704-251-0518 ($17)

National Testing Laboratories
6555 Wilson Mills Rd.
Cleveland, OH 44143
800-458-3330 ($35)

- You can also purchase a water purification system. There are several types, including cation-exchange filters, reverse osmosis filters and distillation units. Costs range from less than $200 to $400. Another safe option, according to Maas, is bottled water. And he said:

"We've tested a variety of brands . . . choose bottled *spring* water over bottled water from a municipal water supply. Even better *distilled* water. It's cheaper than spring water and should be absolutely free of lead or almost any other impurities."[38]

What Is Health Care?　　What is health? What is health care? In my opinion, too often, people in the government and in the press and media talk about "health care," when they are really talking about "disease care." The same situation seems to hold true in Canada. In her January 1994 editorial, Rhody Lake, editor of *Alive,* the Canadian Journal of Health and Nutrition, discussed this issue.

She cited an article on the health care industry which was illustrated with a hypodermic needle being injected into something called "health care funding." And she asked, "Is this what 'health' has come to mean (anno domini 1994)? Drugs and a hypodermic needle?"

In her discussion, Lake said that the Canadian pharmaceutical market had expanded from $7.3 billion in 1988 to more than $10 billion in 1991. And that spending on prescribed drugs increases by 10% each year. In discussing the health of Canadians, she said:

> "As new antibiotics come on the market, the bacteria they're sup-posed to kill become immune to them. . . . All types of cancers are on the increase. Heart disease is still the number one killer despite drugs and biotech. Diabetes is escalating . . .
>
> "There is another saner, safer, more effective, less costly way to go for the *health* of Canadians. It's simple and it works. Even the U.S. National Cancer Institute recognizes the preventative and curative properties of diet and lifestyle."[39]

Medical Research: What Should You Believe?   This was the title of the cover story of the October 1994 *People's Medical Society Newsletter*. The article said that often reports in medical journals which are discussed in the press and media provide consumers with conflicting advice. As an example, they cited a Finnish study which found that beta carotene supplements did not reduce the risk of lung cancer. Yet, many other reports show that taking beta carotene and other supplements make you less likely to develop health problems of various sorts.

In their discussion, my good friend Charles B. Inlander and his editorial staff describe scientific misconduct and fraud, which has been reported on a number of occasions. While they said that such episodes are uncommon, they do occur.

The article also pointed out that there can be flaws in the design, differences in the overall health of study participants and differences in the way data is analyzed. In summarizing their thoughts about medical research, the article said:

> "The bottom line is that medical research is not perfect . . . When it comes to medical research, what should you believe?
>
> "Not everything. Not nothing. You should evaluate each study for its individual merits, take it as food for thought. But don't make rash medical decisions or change your lifestyle solely because of a single study."[40]

A similar point of view was expressed by Cynthia Crossen, a reporter and editor at the *Wall Street Journal*. In her 1994 book, *Tainted Truth,* Crossen points out that many studies and surveys today which seem to be objective are designed with a certain outcome in mind.

Indoor Plants Absorb Pollutants   Research I've read about in the past several years show that healthy indoor plants may absorb many indoor air pollutants. One report stated that two healthy growing plants (about two feet high in a 10 x 10 room) will absorb and destroy most polluted substances. Plants do this through the leaves, soil and roots. The beneficial microorganisms in the soil do their part in breaking down the gasses.

Electromagnetism   During the past decade, Robert O. Becker, M.D., has studied the known or suspected hazards from microwaves, electric appliances, power lines and video display terminals. If these topics interest you, get a copy of his 1985 book (co-authored by Gary Selden), *The Body Electric—Electromagnetism and the Foundation of Life* (William Morrow, New York) or his 1992 book, *Cross Currents* (J.P. Tarcher).

Eliminating Toxic Chemicals from Your Body   Formaldehyde, trichlorethylene, pesticides and other toxic chemicals may play a part in making you sick. The presence of these toxins can now be determined by laboratory studies. If high levels are found, detoxification can be carried out.

For more information about "detox" programs, write to William Rea, M.D., 8345 Walnut Hill Lane, Suite 205, Dallas, TX 75231 or Allan Lieberman, M.D., Center for Ecological Medicine, 7510 Northforest Dr., North Charleston, SC 29418.

Headaches and the Herb Feverfew   In the January 1, 1995, issue of *USA Weekend,* Jim Duke, Ph.D., a leading expert on herbs, cited a report in the Harvard Medical School Letter which said that eating feverfew leaves has become a familiar method for preventing migraine attacks in modern England. You can obtain more information about feverfew and other herbs from the American Botanical Council, P.O. Box 201660, Austin, TX 78720; Fax #512-331-1924.

Take Charge of Your Emotions During the past ten years I've subscribed to *Insight,* a monthly Nightingale-Conant (NC) audiocassette program.* Featured on one side of each tape are the practical and inspirational messages of the late Earl Nightingale. On the other side there are helpful discussions by business leaders, psychologists and other professionals and nonprofessionals.

I stashed away dozens of these tapes in a drawer and I often pick one at random to listen to again as I drive to the office, the airport or the golf course. In December 1994, I pulled out a tape by psychologist and best-selling author, Wayne Dyer.

On this tape, Wayne told an amazing personal story. He and his two young siblings were abandoned by their father when Wayne was only three years old. He never met his father and held many negative feelings toward him.

In the early 1970s, Wayne decided to look for his father. Following a search through hospital records in New Orleans, he found that his father died there and was buried in Biloxi, Mississippi. He then went to Biloxi and stood by the side of his father's grave. He forgave his father for all of the terrible things he had done to his family and to others, and he said that this forgiveness has played a major role in his life since that time.

In commenting on this experience, Wayne said in effect:

> *"No one can depress you. No one can make you anxious. No one can hurt your feelings. No one can make you anything other than what you allow inside. If you have love inside, you should fill up with it. And the only way to do this is to forgive everybody.*
>
> "I've adopted this approach with every human being I've ever had any conflict with . . . even a minor one. I send them gifts and tell them about any wonderful or loving thing I remember about them.
>
> "The more you do of this, the better. *If you don't believe that what goes around comes around, the next time you see somebody down,*

---

*For more information write to Nightingale-Conant Corporation, 7300 North Lehigh Ave., Niles, IL 60714. 1–800-323-5552.

smile at them . . . just say hello and be friendly toward them and you'll be delighted to see what happens."

UltraClear and UltraClear Sustain These powdered nutritional products* are designed to provide nutritional support to patients with dietary needs related to: hepatic detoxification, chronic fatigue syndrome, arthralgia and myalgia, food allergies, chemical sensitivities and other chronic health disorders.

Ingredients include rice protein concentrate, rice syrup solids, medium chain triglycerides, calcium citrate, magnesium citrate and therapeutic levels of many antioxidant nutrients. They contain no dairy, lactose, gluten, wheat, yeast, soy, egg, artificial coloring or animal products.

A number of clinicians I've talked to, including Dr. Leo Galland, use these products in studying patients with suspected food sensitivities.

To learn more about UltraClear and its companion product, UltraClear Sustain, I interviewed Nick Nonas, M.D., Denver, Colorado. Here is an excerpt of his comments.

"I've had some very interesting experiences with UltraClear Sustain in candidiasis. I've found it especially useful in patients who are troubled by *gas, bloating, diarrhea, nausea and other gastrointestinal symptoms*. UltraClear Sustain contains two ingredients that I feel are critical in controlling candida nutritionally.

"One is inulin from Jerusalem artichoke. It furnishes nutrients that the gastrointestinal cells need for regeneration. The second of these ingredients is FOS, which dramatically increases the activity of the probiotics, including *Lactobacillus acidophilus* and *bifidus*.

"In my experience, taking UltraClear Sustain along with the probiotics helps lessen the irritation often found in the gastrointestinal tract. And I've had several people following this program who have been able to get their candida under control without any nystatin.

"I use the product in addition to the candida control diet which

---

*Information about these products can be obtained from HealthComm International, Inc., 5800 Soundview Drive, Gig Harbor, WA 98335.

avoids yeasty foods, dairy products, sugar and the glutinous grains. UltraClear Sustain comes in a can that lasts about a week or so. I start with a small dose and gradually increase it over the course of two weeks. It usually helps rather quickly and it can work in two or three weeks. Most people don't need to take it for more than a month or two."

Looking for an Alternate Health Practitioner   In 1991, the editors of *Let's Live Magazine* published a Health Care Survey. And in November 1991, they published results. They found that at least 43% of the respondents would consider seeing an alternative medicine doctor, or are planning to consult one in the near future. In their continuing discussion, they said:

"How do people find these doctors? Well, more are found by the most reliable form of advertising . . . referrals and word of mouth . . . If you're interested in contacting a naturopathic or homeopathic doctor in your area, here are a few sources:

"Call the American Association of Naturopathic Physicians in Seattle, Washington, 206–323-7610. Leave your name and complete address and they will send you a list of naturopathic doctors in your area.

"Write to the National Center for Homeopathy, 801 N. Fairfax St., Suite 306, Alexandria, VA 22314; 703–548-7790."

In July 1994, *Let's Live* published another survey which showed that their readers were concerned with better health and better living. Then, in January 1995, they published the results of their survey. Here are a few of their findings.

"Almost half of the readers who responded to the survey were between 25 and 45; 36% have one to three years of college education and 18% have an advanced degree; 46% are semi-vegetarians and 75% are nonsmokers; most readers (41%) work out regularly at least three times a week; 74% take more than one supplement every day; 31% frequently use some form of alternative medicine.

"Overall, *Let's Live* readers are well-rounded in their approaches to natural health. Keep up the good work!"

On January 1, 1995, the entire issue of *USA Weekend* was devoted to alternative medicine. Included was a listing of organizations which provide additional information. Here are several of them.

Center for Mind/Body Medicine, 1110 Camino del Mar, Suite G, Del Mar, CA 92014; 619–794-2425.
Center for Mind/Body Medicine, 5225 Connecticut Ave., N.S., Suite 414, Washington, DC 20015; 202–966-7338.
American Massage Therapy Association, 820 Davis St., Suite 100, Evanston, IL 60201.
American Foundation of Traditional Chinese Medicine, 505 Beach St., San Francisco, CA 94133; 415–776-0502.

Castor Oil Packs   In the mid-1980s, I received a letter from an Arizona woman who told me that castor oil packs had helped her overcome digestive and skin problems. They had been prescribed by her physician, Gladys McGarey, M.D. Although I've never used them, I've learned from various sources that these packs have been used therapeutically in India, China, Persia, Egypt, Greece and Rome, as well as the Americas.

What is the value of these packs? They're said to increase eliminations from the gastrointestinal tract, relieve pain, reduce inflammation, improve lymphatic circulation and draw acids and infection out of the body.

Castor oil packs are made by saturating folded four-ply wool or cotton flannel with cold-pressed castor oil. You may purchase the oil at a health food store, or order it by calling 1-800-468-7313.

These packs are then placed directly on the skin of your lower abdomen and covered with a piece of plastic. Then cover the pack with a hot water bottle or a heating pad. You then recline for an hour with the packs in place. In discussing these packs in her book, *Women's Bodies, Women's Wisdom,* Dr. Christiane Northrup said that preliminary studies done at the George Washington School of Medicine indicate that they improve immune system functioning.

Autism, Exciting New Findings An informal conference on autism* was held in Dallas, Texas, in late January 1995. Participants included clinicians and researchers from major medical centers.

Several speakers reported the favorable response of many autistic children to a treatment program which featured dietary changes, nutritional supplements (especially vitamin B_6 and magnesium) and antifungal medications.

One conference participant from a major teaching hospital presented clinical and laboratory studies which showed autism may be yeast related. Here's a brief summary of his observations. *Fungal metabolites were found in the urine of all 18 of the autistic children who were studied.* Over 75% of these children gave a history of frequent infections which had been treated with antibiotics.

Following treatment with oral antifungal medications (nystatin, Nizoral, or Diflucan) for seven days, laboratory findings returned to normal and the children showed significant improvement.

REFERENCES

1. Crook, W.G., *The Yeast Connection*, Third Edition, Professional Books, Jackson, TN and Vintage Books, New York, 1986; pp 293–294.
2. Rosenvold, L., *Can A Gluten-Free Diet Help? How?* Keats Publishing, New Canaan, CT, 1992; pp 28–32.
3. Zwerling, M.H., Owens, K.N., Ruth, N.H., "Think Yeast—The Expanding Spectrum of Candidiasis," *J. South Carolina Med. Assoc.*, 1984; 80:454–456.
4. Mathur, S., et al, "Anti-ovarian and Anti-lymphocyte Antibodies in Patients with Chronic Vaginal Candidiasis," *J. Reprod. Immunol.*, 1980; 2:247–262.
5. Hueser, G., Hueser, S., Rahimian, P. and Vojdani, A., *J. of Advan. in Med.*, 1992; 5:177–188.
6. Crook, W.G., *The Yeast Connection*, Third Edition, Professional Books, Jackson, TN and Vintage Books, New York, 1986; p 186.

*This conference was sponsored by the Autism Research Institute, 4182 Adams Ave., San Diego, CA 92116.

7. Ostrov, B.E. and Athreya, B.H., "Lyme Disease, Difficulties in Diagnosis and Management," *Ped. Clin. of N. Amer.*, 1991; 38(3):535–553.
8. Crook, W.G., "Antiyeast Medications Recommended" in *Lyme and Disease Update*, 1511 N. Stockwell Rd., P.O. Box 15711–0711, Evansville, IN 47716.
9. Caselli, M., "Dead Fecal Yeasts and Chronic Diarrhea," *Digestion*, 1988; 41:142–148.
10. Package insert, Pfizer-Roerig, Division of Pfizer, Inc., New York, NY 10017.
11. *Nutrition Action Healthletter*, January/February 1994, Center for Science in the Public Interest, 1875 Connecticut Ave., Washington, DC 20009–5728.
12. Challem, J., *Getting the Most Out of Your Vitamins and Minerals*, Keats Publishing Company, New Canaan, CT, 1993; p 27.
13. Bush, M.J. and Verlangieri, A.J., "An Acute Study on the Relative Gastro-intestinal Absorption of a Novel Form of Calcium Ascorbate," Research Communications in *Chemical Pathology and Pharmacology*, Vol. 57, No. 1, July, 1987.
14. Wright, J.W. and Suen, R.M., "A Human Clinical Study Ester-C vs. L-ascorbic Acid," *International Clinical Nutrition Review*, Vol. 10, No. 1, January 1990.
15. Verlangieri, A.J., et al., *Life Sciences*, 1991; 48:2275–2281.
16. Lapp, C.W., Cheney, P.R., *CFIDS Chronicle*, Fall 1993, Published by the CFIDS Association of America, Inc., P.O. Box 220398, Charlotte, NC 28222–0398. 800–442-3437. FAX, 704–365-9755.
17. Newbold, H.L., *Dr. Newbold's Type A/Type B Weight Loss Book*, Keats Publishing Company, New Canaan, CT, 1991.
18. Downing, D., *Journal of Nutritional Medicine*, P.O. Box 3AP, London, W1A 3AP, 1990.
19. Holmes, J.M., *British Medical Journal*, 1956; 2:1394–1398.
20. Ellis and associates, *British J. of Nut.*, 1973; 30:277–283.
21. Lindenbaum, J., et al, "Neuropsychiatric Disorders Caused By Cobalamin (Vitamin B_{12}) Deficiency in the Absence of Anaemia or Macrocytosis," *N. Engl. J. Med.*, 1988; 318:1720–1728.
22. Baker, S.M., personal communication, May 1985.
23. Galland, L., in Crook, W.G., *The Yeast Connection*, Third Edition, Professional Books, Jackson, TN and Vintage Books, New York, 1986; pp 364–366.
24. Gaby, A.R., Editorial, *J. of Advan. in Med.*, 1988; 1:179–181.
25. Gaby, A.R., *Preventing and Reversing Osteoporosis*, Prima Publishing, P.O. Box 1260BK, Rocklin, CA 95677, 1994. 916-786-0426; pp 39–45.
26. Bland, J., *Preventive Medicine Update* (audiocassette), HealthComm International, P.O. Box 1729, Gig Harbor, WA 98335, December, 1994.

27. Montagu, A., *Touching, The Human Significance of the Skin*, Harper & Row, New York, 1972; pp 15–16.
28. Field, T. *Health Confidential*, July 1994, 55 Railroad Avenue, Greenwich, CT 06830.
29. Canfield, J. and Hansen, M.V., *Chicken Soup for the Soul.* Health Communications, Inc., Deerfield Beach, FL, 1993, pp 16–18.
30. Hines, K., "Making Their Point," *Cincinnati,* 1993; 27(2):63–64.
31. Stocker, S., "Conquer Chronic Pain and More with Acupuncture," *Prevention,* December 1994; pp 76–79.
32. The Burton Goldberg Group, *Alternative Medicine—The Definitive Guide,* Future Medicine Publishing, Inc., Puyallup, WA 1994; p 110.
33. Lark, S.M., *PMS Self-Help Book,* Celestial Arts, Berkeley, CA, 1984; pp 165–188.
34. Editors of Prevention Magazine Health Books, *Age Erasers for Women,* Rodale Press, Emmaus, PA, 1994; pp 591–595.
35. SerVaas, C., "Search for the Cure Continues," *The Saturday Evening Post,* September/October 1994 and *Saturday Evening Post Health Update Newsletter,* Summer 1994, The Saturday Evening Post Society, 1100 Waterway Blvd., Indianapolis, IN 46202.
36. Rona, Z.P. in *Alive* —Canadian Journal of Health and Nutrition, Burnaby, B.C., Canada, 1993; issue 127.
37. Cerda, G.M. and Parry, B.L., "The Effects of Bright Light Therapy on Symptoms of Depression, Anxiety, and Hibernation in Patients with Premenstrual Syndrome," *Journal of Women's Health,* 1994; 3(1):5–15.
38. Maas, R.P., *Health Confidential,* 55 Railroad Ave., Greenwich, CT 06830, December 1993.
39. Lake, R., *Alive*—Canadian Journal of Health and Nutrition, Burnaby, B.C., Canada, January 1994; Issue 137:4–5.
40. *The People's Medical Society Newsletter,* October 1994, Vol. 13 No. 5, 462 Walnut St., Allentown, PA 18102.

Other Sources of Information

Professional Organizations

Many physicians and other professionals interested in yeast-related health problems are members of one or more of the organizations listed below. You may be able to obtain the names of professionals in your area who are members of these organizations by writing to them. Enclosing a stamped, self-addressed envelope would expedite their response.

American Academy of
  Environmental Medicine
  (AAEM)
4510 W. 89th Street
Prairie Village, KS 66207
FAX #913-341-3625

American College of
  Advancement in Medicine
23121 Verdugo Dr., #204
Laguna Hills, CA 92653
FAX #714-455-9679

American Association of
  Naturopathic Physicians
2366 E. Lake Ave. East,
  Suite 322
Seattle, WA 98102
FAX #206-323-7610

American Holistic Medical
  Association
4101 Lake Boone Trail,
  Suite 201
Raleigh, NC 27607
FAX #919-787-4916

Pan American Allergy Society
P.O. Box 947
Fredericksburg, TX 78624
FAX #210-997-8625

See also my comments on pages 77–79.

Lay Organizations and Support Groups

A number of lay organizations and support groups in the United States, Canada, England and other countries provide information and help for people with chronic health disorders. These include multiple chemical sensitivity syndrome (MCSS), chronic fatigue syndrome (CFS/CFIDS), fibromyalgia syndrome (FMS) and many others.

By writing to these organizations you may be able to obtain information that may help you. Many are nonprofit organizations and are staffed in part by volunteers. In writing enclose a stamped, self-addressed envelope. A small donation to help cover costs would also be appreciated.

Autism Research Institute
4182 Adams St.
San Diego, CA 92116
Bernard Rimland, Ph.D.
FAX #301-588-2454

Broda O. Barnes, M.D.,
    Research Foundation, Inc.
Patricia A. Puglio, Director
P.O. Box 98
Trumbull, CT 06611
Phone and FAX
    #203-261-2101

CFIDS Association of
    America, Inc.
P.O. Box 220398
Charlotte, NC 28222–0398
800-44-CFIDS
FAX #704-365-9755

Endometriosis Association
Mary Lou Ballweg
8585 N. 76th Place
Milwaukee, WI 53223
Phone #414-355-2200
FAX #414-355-6065

Fibromyalgia Network
Kristen Thorson
P.O. Box 31750
Tucson, AZ 85751–1750
Phone #602-290-5508
FAX #602-290-5550

Human Ecology Action
  League (HEAL)
P.O. Box 49126
Atlanta, GA 30033
Phone #404-248-1898

Hyperactivity Helpline
P.O. Box 10085
Arlington, VA 30359
Phone #703-524-5566

New York HEAL
506 E. 84th St.
New York, NY 10028
Phone #212-517-5937

Partners in Health
Director, Margaret Corbin,
  M.A.
7 Portsmouth Terrace
Rochester, NY 14607
Phone #716-473-5400

Price-Pottenger Nutrition
  Foundation
P.O. Box 2614
La Mesa, CA 91943–2614
Phone #619-574-7763
FAX #619-574-1314

National Vulvodynia
  Association
P.O. Box 9309
Silver Spring, MD 29016–9309
Phone #301-460-6407

The Well Mind Association of
  Greater Washington, Inc.
1141 Georgia Ave., Suite 326
Wheaton, MD 20902
Phone #301-949-8282

Newsletters and Magazines

Alive—Canadian Journal of Health and Nutrition, published 11
  times a year. 7436 Fraser Park Dr., Burnaby, B.C., Canada, V5J
  5B9. $24.50 (Canada).
Allergy Alert, Sally Rockwell, Editor, P.O. Box 31065, Seattle, WA
  98103. 206-547-1814. $18/6 issues a year. Also available from this
  source are books, tapes and telephone counseling.
Allergy Hotline, published monthly by Hotline Printing and Publishing, P.O. Box 161132, Altamont Springs, FL 32716. $35/year.

Better Nutrition for Today's Living, published monthly by Communication Channels, Inc., 6151 Powers Ferry Rd., N.W., Atlanta, GA 30339. Available in most health food stores. 404-955-2500.

Bottom Line Personal, Board Room, Inc., 55 Railroad Ave., Greenwich, CT 06830. Published 24 times a year. $49/year.

Canary News—Newsletter of the Chicago-area Environmental Illness/ Multiple Chemical Sensitivity (EI/MCS) Support Group, 1304 Judson Ave., Evanston, IL 60201. $15/year.

CFIDS Chronicle, published by the CFIDS Association of America, Inc., P.O. Box 220398, Charlotte, NC 28222–0398. $30/year (includes membership and 4 issues).

DAMS (Dental Amalgam Mercury Syndrome), published by DAMS, Inc., 725–9 Tramway Lane, NE, Albuquerque, NM 87122–1601. $20/year (includes membership).

Delicious Magazine, 1301 Spruce St., Boulder, CO 80302. 303-939-8440. $24/year. Published monthly.

Earl Mindell's *Your Guide to Healthier Living*, Phillips Publishing, Inc., 7811 Montrose Rd., Potomac, MD 20854. $39.95/year.

Earl Mindell's *Joy of Health*, published monthly by Phillips Publishing, Inc., 7811 Montrose Rd., Potomac, MD 20854. $69/year.

Ecological Health Organization and Action Coalition (ECHO), P.O. Box 281116, East Hartford, CT 06128–1116. $10/year. Published quarterly.

Emphasis—Your Health, a health journal by Uchee Pines Institute for Health and Education, 30 Uchee Pines Rd., #31, Seale, AL 36875–5703. (A donation of $5 or more is requested.)

The Energyseeker, Newsletter of CFIDS Awareness and Support Services, Karen Lee Moyer-Horejs, R.N., Editor, 23732 Hillhurst Dr., #9, Laguna Niguel, CA 92677. $18/year, 11 issues.

Fibromyalgia Network, newsletter for fibromyalgia syndrome/ chronic fatigue syndrome patients. Published quarterly, $15.

Dr. Julian Whitaker's *Health & Healing—Tomorrow's Medicine Today*, published monthly by Phillips Publishing Company, Inc., 7811 Montrose Rd., Potomac, MD 20854. 301-340-2100. $69/year.

Health Confidential, Board Room, Inc., 55 Railroad Ave., Greenwich, CT 06830. Published monthly. $49/year.

Health Hunter, a publication of the Center for the Improvement of Human Functioning Internatinal, Inc., 3100 N. Hillside Ave., Wichita, KS 67219. Published 10 times yearly. $25/year.

Health Naturally—Canada's Self-Help Care magazine, Box 159, Nobel, Ontario, Canada, P0G 1G0. $12.84 (Canada), $18.84 (U.S.), 6 issues per year. 705-342-1360.

Health News and Review, A Quarterly Health Newspaper. Published quarterly by Keats Publishing Company, 27 Pine St., P.O. Box 876, New Canaan, CT 06840–0876. $11.80/year.

Dr. Christiane Northrup's Health Wisdom for Women. Published monthly by Phillips Publishing, Inc., 7811 Montrose Rd., Potomac, MD 20854. 301-424-3700. $69.

Human Ecologist, published by Human Ecology Action League, Inc., P.O. Box 49126, Atlanta, GA 30359–1126. This 36-page journal is published quarterly. It is sent to HEAL members. Membership dues, $20/year. Contributions are tax deductible.

Latitudes, Exploring attention disorders, autism, hyperactivity, learning disabilities and Tourette syndrome, 1120 Royal Palm Beach Blvd., #283, Royal Palm Beach, FL 33411. $24/year, 6 issues. 407-798-0472.

Let's Live—America's foremost health and preventive magazine. 444 N. Larchmont Blvd., Los Angeles, CA. Published monthly. $19.95/year.

Lyme & Disease Update, publisher and editor, W. Charlene Glover, P.O. Box 15711–0711, Evansville, IN 47716. $19/year. Published monthly. 812-471-1990.

Mastering Food Allergies, Marjorie Hurt Jones, R.N., 2615 N. 4th St., #616, Couer d'Alene, ID 83814. (For information about her newsletter, send a long SASE.) $20/year, published six times a year.

Network News, National Women's Health Network, 514 Kent St., N.W., #400, Washington, DC 20004. Published bimonthly . All members receive a subscription to this newsletter. Membership $25.

NOHA News, published by Nutrition for Optimal Health (NOHA), P.O. Box 380, Winnetka, IL 60093. $8/year, published almost monthly.

Nutrition in Healing, a monthly newsletter by Jonathan B. Wright, M.D., and Alan R. Gaby, M.B., Publishers Management Corp., P.O. Box 84909, Phoenix, AZ 85071. 800-528-0559. $69.95/year.

Prevention, 33 E. Minor St., Emmaus, PA 18098–0099. 610-967-5171. Subscription rate: U.S., 1 year, $21.97. Published monthly.

Share, Care and Prayer Newsletter, 905 N. First Ave., Arcadia, CA 91006. Fax #818-446-2609. A donation of $20 or more.

Townsend Letters for Doctors, 911 Tyler St., Port Townsend, WA 98368–6541. 206-385-6021. $42/10 issues yearly.

The Well Mind Association of Greater Washington, Inc., 1141 Georgia Ave., Suite 326, Wheaton, MD 20902. 301-949-8282. $25/year—includes membership in association.

Wolf's Digest of Alternative Medicine, P.O. Box 2049, Sequim, WA 98382. $23.95/10 issues per year. 800-683-7014.

Women's Health Connection, P.O. Box 6338, Madison, WI 53716–0338, published 6 times a year, $12. 800-366-6632.

Books

Age Erasers for Women, Editors, *Prevention,* Rodale Press, 1994.

Ali, Majid, *The Canary and Chronic Fatigue,* Life Span Press, Denvill, NJ, 1993.

Appleton, N., *Secrets of Natural Healing with Food,* Rudra Press, 1993.

Appleton, N., *Healthy Bones,* Avery Press, Garden City, NY, 1995.

Ashford, N.A. and Miller, C.S., *Chemical Exposures: Low Levels and High Stakes,* Van Nostrand Reinhold, New York, NY, 1991.

Balch, P. and Balch, J., ℞ *Dietary Wellness,* PAB Publishing, Greenfield, IN, 1992.

Balch, J. and Balch, P., *Prescription for Nutritional Healing,* Avery Publishing Group, Garden City Park, NY, 1990.

Ballweg, M.L. and the Endometriosis Association, *Overcoming Endometriosis,* Contemporary Books, New York, NY, 1987.

Barnard, N.D., *Food for Life,* Harmony Books, New York, NY, 1993.

Barnes, B.O. and Galton, L., *Hypothyroidism, The Unsuspected Illness,* Harper and Row, New York, NY, 1976.

Baumslag, N. and Michels, D.L., *A Woman's Guide to Yeast Infections*, Pocket Books, New York, NY, 1992.

Beasley, J., *Betrayal of Health*, Times Books, New York, NY, 1992.

Becker, R. and Selden, G., *Body Electric—Electromagnetism and the Foundation of Life*, William Morrow, New York, NY, 1985.

Beebe, G., *Toxic Carpet*, published by Glen Beebe, P.O. Box 399086, Cincinnati, OH 45239, 1991.

Benson, H., *The Wellness Book*, Simon and Schuster, New York, NY, 1993.

Berthold-Bond, A., *Clean and Green—Complete Guide to Nontoxic and Environmentally Safe Housekeeping*, Ceres Press, Woodstock, NY, 1990.

Bland, J., *Bioflavonoids*, Keats Publishing Company, New Canaan, CT, 1984.

Bliznakov, E.G. and Hunt, G.L., *The Miracle Nutrient—CoEnzyme* Q_{10}, Bantam Books, New York, NY, 1987.

Borysenko, J., *Minding the Body, Mending the Mind*, Bantam Books, New York, NY, 1988.

The Boston Women's Health Book Collective, *The New Our Bodies, Ourselves*, Touchstone-Simon and Schuster, New York, NY, 1992.

Braley, J., *Dr. Braley's Food Allergy and Nutrition Revolution*, Keats Publishing, New Canaan, CT, 1992.

The Burton Goldberg Group, *Alternative Medicine—The Definitive Guide*, Future Medicine Publishing, Inc., Puyallup, WA, 1993.

Carper, J., *Food, Your Miracle Medicine*, HarperCollins, New York, NY, 1993.

Carper, J., *The Food Pharmacy to Good Eating*, Bantam Books, New York, NY, 1991.

Carter, J., *Racketeering in Medicine—The Suppression of Alternatives*, Hampton Roads Publishing Company, Norfolk, VA, 1992.

Castleman, M., *The Healing Herbs*, Rodale Press, Emmaus, PA, 1991.

Challem, J., *Getting the Most Out of Your Vitamins and Minerals*, Keats Publishing Company, New Canaan, CT, 1993.

Cheraskin, E., *The Vitamin Controversy—Questions and Answers*, Keats Publishing Company, New Canaan, CT, 1990.

Chopra, D., *Perfect Health—The Complete Mind/Body Guide*, Harmony Books, New York, NY, 1991.

Connolly, P., *Candida albicans Yeast-Free Cookbook*, Keats Publishing Company, New Canaan, CT, 1985.

Crook, W.G., *Chronic Fatigue Syndrome and the Yeast Connection*, Professional Books, Jackson, TN, 1992.

Crook, W.G., *Detecting Your Hidden Allergies*, Professional Books, Jackson, TN, 1988.

Crook, W.G., *Help for the Hyperactive Child—A Good Sense Guide for Parents*, Professional Books, Jackson, TN, 1991.

Crook, W.G., *Tracking Down Hidden Food Allergy*, Professional Books, Jackson, TN, 1978.

Crook, W.G. and Steven, L.J., *Solving the Puzzle of Your Hard-to Raise-Child*, Professional Books, Jackson, TN, 1987.

Crook, W.G., *The Yeast Connection*, Professional Books, Jackson, TN and Vintage Books, New York, NY, 1986.

Crook, W.G. and Jones, M.H., *The Yeast Connection Cookbook*, Professional Books, Jackson, TN, 1989.

Dadd, D.L., *Non-Toxic, Natural and Earth Wise: How to Protect Yourself and Your Family From Harmful Products and Live in Harmony With the Earth*, Jeremy P. Tarcher, Inc., Los Angeles, CA, 1990.

Dean, C., Dr., *Carolyn Dean's Complementary Natural Prescriptions for Common Ailments*, Keats Publishing Company, New Canaan, CT, 1994.

Dossey, L., *Meaning in Medicine—Doctor's Tales*, Bantam Books, New York, NY, 1991.

Dossey, L., *Healing Words: The power of prayer in the practice of medicine*, Harper, San Francisco, CA, 1993.

Dumke, N.M., *Allergy Cooking With Ease*, Starburst Publishers, P.O. Box 4123, Lancaster, PA, 17604, 1992.

Dumke, N.M., *The EPD Patient's Cooking and Lifestyle Guide*, Allergy Alert Co., Louisville, CO, 1994.

Erasmus, U., *Fats That Heal and Fats That Kill*, Alive Books, Burnaby, B.C., Canada, 1993.

Gaby, A.R., *Preventing and Reversing Osteoporosis*, Prima Publishing, Rocklin, CA, 1993.

Gaby, A.R., *Magnesium*, Keats Publishing Company, New Canaan, CT, 1994.

Gates, D. and Schatz, L., *The Body Ecology Diet*, BED Publications, Atlanta, GA, 1993.

Gerlach, E., *Autism Treatment Guide*, Four Leaf Press, 2020 Garfield St., Eugene, OR 97405–1545, 1993.

Gibbons, D., *Self-Help Way to Treat Colitis and Other IBS Conditions*, Keats Publishing Company, New Canaan, CT, 1992.

Gillespie, L., *You Don't Have to Live with Cystitis*, Avon Books, New York, NY, 1988.

Gittleman, A.L., *Guess What Came to Dinner—Parasites, and your health*, Avery, Garden City Park, New York, NY, 1993.

Gittleman, A.L., *Super Nutrition for Women*, Bantam Books, New York, NY, 1991.

Glassburn, V., *Who Killed Candida*, Teach Services, Inc., Brushton, NY, 1991.

Goldbeck, N. and D., *The Goldbeck's Guide to Good Food*, New American Library, New York, NY, 1987.

Goleman, D. and Gurin, J., *Mind/Body Medicine*, Consumer Reports Books, Yonkers, NY, 1993.

Goldstrich, J.D., *The Cardiologist's Painless Prescription for a Healthy Heart and a Longer Life*, 9-Heart-9 Publishing, 8215 West Chester Dr., Suite 307, Dallas, TX, 1994.

Golos, N. and Goldbitz, F., *If It's Tuesday, It Must Be Chicken*, Keats Publishing, New Canaan, CT, 1983.

Goodman, S., *Vitamin C—The Master Nutrient*, Keats Publishing Company, New Canaan, CT, 1991.

Greenberg, R. and Nori, A., *Freedom From Allergy Cookbook*, Third Edition, Blue Poppy Press, Vancouver, BC, 1991.

Greenwood, S., *Menopause Naturally*, Volcano Press, Volcano, CA, 1992.

Gursche, S., *Healing with Herbal Juices*, Alive Books, Burnaby, B.C., Canada.

Haas, E.M., *Staying Healthy with Nutrition*, Celestial Arts, Berkeley, CA, 1992.

Heimlich, J., *What Your Doctor Won't Tell You—Alternative Therapies*, HarperCollins, New York, NY, 1990.

Heinerman, J., *The Healing Benefits of Garlic*, Keats Publishing, New Canaan, CT, 1994.

Hoffman, R.L., *Lyme Disease*, Keats Publishing Company, New Canaan, CT, 1994.

Hoffman, R.L., *Tired All the Time*, Poseidon Press/Simon and Schuster, New York, NY, 1993.

Hoffman, R.L., *Seven Weeks to a Settled Stomach*, Simon and Schuster, New York, NY, 1992.

Hunter, B.T., *Gluten Intolerance*, Keats Publishing Company, New Canaan, CT, 1987.

Hunter, B.T., *Grain Power*, Keats Publishing Company, New Canaan, CT, 1994.

Hunter, B.T., *Brewer's Yeast, Wheat Germ, and Other High Powered Foods*, Keats Publishing Company, New Canaan, CT, 1982.

Jacobson, M.F. and Fritschner, S., *The Fast Food Guide*, Second Edition, Wertman, New York, NY, 1991.

Jacobson, M.F. and Maxwell, B., *What Are We Feeding Our Kids?* Workman Publishing Company, New York, NY, 1994.

Kamen, B., *Hormone Replacement Therapy, Yes or No?*, Nutrition Encounters, Inc., Novata, CA, 1993.

Krohn, J., Taylor S.A., and Larson, E.M., *Allergy Relief and Prevention*, Hartley and Marks, Point Roberts, WA, 1991.

Langer, S.E. and Scheer, J.F., *Solved: The Riddle of Illness*, Keats Publishing, New Canaan, CT, 1984.

Langer, S.E., *Solved: The Riddle of Weight-Loss*, Healing Arts Press, Rochester, VT, 1988.

Lark, S., *Premenstrual Syndrome Self-Help Book*, Celestial Arts, Berkeley, CA, 1984.

Larson, J.M., *Alcholism—The Biochemical Connection*, Villard Books, New York, NY, 1992.

Levin, A.S. and Zellerbach, M., *The Type I/Type II Allergy Relief Program*, Jeremy P. Tarcher, Inc., Los Angeles, CA, 1983.

Lewis, L., *52 Ways to Live a Long and Healthy Life*, The Summit Group, Ft. Worth, TX, 1993.

Lin, D.J., *Free Radicals and Disease Prevention*, Keats Publishing, New Canaan, CT, 1993.

Lonsdale, D., *Why I Left Orthodox Medicine*, Hampton Roads Publishing Company, Hampton Roads, VA, 1994.

Martorano, J., Morgan, M. and Fryer, W., *Unmasking PMS*, Evans and Company, New York, NY, 1993.

McDougall, J.A., *The McDougall Program—12 Days to Dynamic Health*, Plume Penguin, New York, NY, 1990.

McIlhaney, J.S., Jr., with Nethery, S., *1250 Health-Care Questions Women Ask*, Focus on the Family Publishing, Colorado Springs, CO 1992.

Mindell, E., *Earl Mindell's Herb Bible*, Simon and Schuster, New York, NY, 1992.

Mindell, E., *Garlic: The Miracle Nutrient*, Keats Publishing Company, New Canaan, CT, 1994.

Mowrey, D.B., *Herbal Tonic Therapies*, Keats Publishing Company, New Canaan, CT, 1993.

Moyers, B., *Healing and the Mind*, Doubleday, New York, NY, 1993.

Murray, G., *Gingko biloba*, Keats Publishing Company, New Canaan, CT, 1993.

Murray, M.T., *The Healing Power of Herbs*, Prima Publishing, Rocklin, CA, 1991.

Murray, M.T., *The Healing Power of Foods*, Prima Publishing, Rocklin, CA, 1993.

Murray, M. and Pizzorno, J., *Encyclopedia of Natural Medicine*, Prima Publishing Company, Rocklin, CA, 1991.

Nambudripad, D.S., *Good-bye to Illness*, Delta Publishing, Buena Park, CA, 1993.

Northrup, C., *Women's Bodies, Women's Wisdom*, Bantam Books, 1994.

Null, G., *Healing Your Body Naturally*, Four Walls, Eight Windows, London, NY, 1992.

Null, G. and Feldman, M., *Reverse the Aging Process Naturally*, Villard Books, New York, NY, 1993.

Ornish, D., *Dr. Dean Ornish's Program for Reversing Heart Disease*, Ballantine Books, New York, 1990.

Oski, F., *Don't Drink Your Milk—Facts about the world's most overrated nutrient—Ninth Edition*, Teach Services, Brushton, NY, 1992.

Ott, J.N., *Health and Light*, Pocket Books, New York, NY, 1983.

Passwater, R., *The Antioxidants*, Keats Publishing Company, New Canaan, CT, 1995.

Passwater, R., *Pycnogenol*, Keats Publishing Company, New Canaan, CT, 1994.

Perlmutter, D., *Life Guide—A Guide to a Longer and Healthier Life*, Life Guide Press, Naples, FL, 1994.

Podell, R.N., *When Your Doctor Doesn't Know Best*, Simon and Schuster, New York, NY, 1994.

Quillin, P., with Quillin, N., Beating Cancer with Nutrition, The Nutrition Times Press, Tulsa, OK, 1994.

Randolph, T.G. and Moss, R.W., *An Alternative Approach to Allergies: Revised Edition*, Harper and Row, New York, NY, 1989.

Rea, W. J., *Chemical Sensitivity* (Volumes I and II), CRC Press, Inc., 200 Corporate Blvd. N.W., Boca Raton, FL 33431, 1993. (Volume III, 1995).

Remington, D.W. and Higa, B., *Back to Health: Yeast Control*, Vitality House International, Provo, UT, 1986.

Robbins, J., *Diet for a New World*, Avon Books, 1992.

Rona, Z.P., *The Joy of Health, A Doctor's Guide to Nutrition and Alternative Medicine*, Llewellyn Publishers, St. Paul, MN and Hownslow Press, Willowdale, Ontario, Canada, 1992.

Rosenbaum, M. and Susser, M., *Solving the Puzzle of Chronic Fatigue Syndrome*, Life Sciences Press, Tacoma, WA, 1992.

Rosenvold, L., *Can a Gluten-Free Diet Help? How?*, Keats Publishing, New Canaan, CT, 1992.

Rousseau, D., Rea, W. and Enwright, G., *Your Home, Your Health and Well Being*, Hartley and Marks, Inc., Ten Speed Press, Point Roberts, WA, 1988.

Schmidt, M.A., Smith, L.H. and Sehnert, K.W., *Beyond Antibiotics*, North Atlantic Books, Berkeley, CA, 1993.

Schmidt, M.A., *Childhood Ear Infections—Home Care*, North Atlantic Books, Berkeley, CA, 1991.

Siegel, B.S., *Peace, Love and Healing*, Harper and Row, New York, NY, 1989.

Siguel, E.N., *Essential Fatty Acids in Health and Disease*, Nutrek Press, Brookline, MA, 1994.

Smith, L.M., *Feed Your Body Right*, M. Evans, New York, NY, 1994.

Soyka, F. and Edmonds, A., *The Ion Effect: How air electricity rules your life*, Bantam Books, Toronto, Canada, 1978.

Thrash, A. and Thrash, C.L., *Nutrition for Vegetarians*, New Lifestyle Books, Seale, AL, 1994.

Trowbridge, J. and Walker, M., *The Yeast Syndrome*, Bantam Books, New York, NY, 1986.

Truss, C.O., *The Missing Diagnosis*, Box 26508, Birmingham, AL 35226, 1983 and 1986.

Weil, A., *Health and Healing*, Houghton Mifflin, Boston, MA, 1988 (Revised, 1995).

Weil, A., *Natural Health, Natural Medicine*, Houghton Mifflin, Boston, MA, 1990 (Revised, 1995).

Weil, A.T., *Spontaneous Healing*, Knopf, New York, NY, 1995.

Weiner, M.A. and Goss, K., *Maximum Immunity*, Houghton Mifflin Company, Boston, MA, 1986.

Werbach, M.R., *Nutritional Influences on Illness*, Second Edition, Third Line Press, Tarzana, CA, 1993.

Werbach, M., *Healing Through Nutrition*, HarperCollins, New York, NY, 1993.

Wunderlich, R., *Candida albicans*, Keats Publishing Company, New Canaan, CT, 1986.

Index

About the Author

---◆---

William G. Crook, M.D., received his medical education and training at the University of Virginia, the Pennsylvania Hospital, Vanderbilt and Johns Hopkins. He is a fellow of the American Academy of Pediatrics, the American College of Allergy and Immunology and the American Academy of Environmental Medicine. He is a member of the American Medical Association, the American Academy of Allergy and Immunology, Alpha Omega Alpha and other medical organizations.

As a practicing physician, medical writer and lecturer, Dr. Crook is concerned about problems which affect millions of people all over the world. These include adults—especially women—who feel "sick all over," yet have been unable to find help. He is also concerned about children who are troubled by repeated ear infections, hyperactivity, attention deficits and other behavior and learning problems.

Dr. Crook is the author of eleven previous books and numerous reports in the medical and lay literature. For fifteen years he wrote a nationally syndicated health column, "Child Care" (*General Features* and the *Los Angeles Times* Syndicates).

Various of his publications have been translated into French, German, Japanese and Norwegian.

The Yeast Connection and the Woman is the fourth in his series of books which deal with the relationship of *Candida albicans* to many puzzling health disorders. The titles include *The Yeast Connection* (a bestseller with over one million copies in print), *The Yeast Connection Cookbook* and *Chronic Fatigue Syndrome and the Yeast Connection*.

Dr. Crook has been a popular guest on local, regional, national and international television and radio programs, including Oprah Winfrey, Sally Jessy Raphael, Regis Philbin, The 700 Club, Good

Morning Australia, TV Ontario and the British Broadcasting Company.

He has addressed professional and lay groups in 39 states, six Canadian provinces, Australia, England, Italy, Mexico, The Netherlands, New Zealand and Venezuela. And he has served as a visiting professor at Ohio State University, and the Universities of California (San Francisco) and Saskatchewan.

During the past decade Dr. Crook has presented his observations on the relationship of superficial yeast infections to chronic illness at the following medical schools: Georgetown, Johns Hopkins, Medical College of Georgia, Thomas Jefferson University, Louisiana State University, UCLA (Torrance), Vanderbilt and the Universities of California (San Francisco), Cincinnati, Minnesota, South Alabama, South Florida, Tennessee and Texas (San Antonio).

According to Douglas Sandberg, M.D., Professor of Pediatrics, University of Miami,

"Dr. William Crook brings to the reader years of experience as a practicing physician, forthright honesty, a dynamic informal writing style and intense desire to improve the health of people of all ages. In addition, Dr. Crook possesses the attribute relatively rare in a physician—an open mind."

Dr. Crook lives in Jackson, Tennessee, with his wife, Betsy. They have three daughters and four grandchildren. His interests include golf, oil painting and travel.

Other Books and Publications
by Dr. William G. Crook

You can get copies of *The Yeast Connection and the Woman*, as well as numerous other helpful books and publications by Dr. Crook, from most book stores, your health food store or pharmacy. You may also order directly from Wellness Health and Pharmaceuticals using the handy order form below.

ITEM	QTY.	PRICE	TOTAL
BOOKLETS:			
Yeasts		3.45	
Allergy		3.45	
Hypoglycemia		3.45	
Hyperactivity/ADD		3.45	
Chronic Fatigue Syndrome		3.45	
BOOKS:			
The Yeast Connection and the Woman		17.95	
The Yeast Connection		12.95	
Tracking Down Hidden Food Allergy		8.95	
The Yeast Connection Cookbook		14.95	
Help for the Hyperactive Child	✓	14.95	
Chronic Fatigue Syndrome and the Yeast Connection		15.95	
Solving The Puzzle of Your Hard-to-Raise Child		19.95	
Detecting Your Hidden Allergies		10.95	
Add $3.50 for single title orders/$5.00 for multiple titles.			
		GRAND TOTAL	

Prices subject to change without notice.

SHIP TO:

_____

Name   Phone

_____

Street address

_____

City   State   Zip

To order these publications, call 1-800-227-2627 or 1-205-879-6551. (Visa or Mastercard accepted.)

Or you can mail your check or money order along with this form to:

Wellness Health & Pharmaceuticals
2800 South 18th Street, Birmingham, AL 35209

If you order 5 or more copies of a single title, you will be given a 30% discount on that title.

REDUCE SUGAR OR SUGARFREE
  "   MILK PRODUCTS OR MILKFREE
  " "   YEAST PRODUCTS OR YEASTFREE
HIGH PROTEIN DIET
VITAMIN SUPPLEMENTS
ANTI YEAST MEDICATION — NYSTATIN
NUTRITIONAL SUPPLEMENTS
REMOVE ODOROUS CHEMICALS
MINERALS
PRIMROSE OILS
EXERCISE
REDUCE ANTIBIOTICS OR NONE AT ALL
  (TAKE NYSTATIN, DIFLUCAN, OR SPORANOX)
  WHEN TAKING ANTIBIOTICS.

R

ANTICANDIDA MEDICATION
ANTIFUNGAL   "
IMMUNOTHERAPY FOR ALLERGIES
AVOIDANCE OF ENVIRONMENTAL CHEMICALS
ORAL ANTIFUNGAL THERAPY

CANDIDA EXTRACTS
AMPHOTERACIN B
NYZORAL

ALLERGIC CYSTITIS

HIGH DOSES OF VIT. C
CALCIUM + MAGNESIUM.